Food for Diabetics

17th Edition

By Don Orwell

http://SuperfoodsToday.com

Copyright © 2017 by Don Orwell.

All legal rights reserved. You cannot offer this book for free or sell it. You do not have reselling legal rights to this book. This eBook may not be recreated in any file format or physical format without having the expressed written approval of Don Orwell. All Violators will be sued.

While efforts have been made to assess that the information contained in this book is valid, neither the author nor the publisher assumes any accountability for errors, interpretations, omissions or usage of the subject matters herein.

Disclaimer:

The Information presented in this book is created to provide useful information on the subject areas discussed. The publisher and author are not accountable for any particular health or allergic reaction needs that may involve medical supervision and are not liable for any damage or damaging outcomes from any treatment, application or preparation, action, to any person reading or adhering to the information in this book. References are presented for informational reasons only and do not represent an endorsement of any web sites or other sources. Audience should be informed that the websites mentioned in this book may change.

This publication includes opinions and ideas of its author and is meant for informational purposes only. The author and publisher shall in no event be held liable for any damage or loss sustained from the usage of this publication.

Your Free Gift

As a way of saying thanks for your purchase, I'm offering you my FREE eBook that is exclusive to my book and blog readers.

Superfoods Cookbook - Book Two has over 70 Superfoods recipes and complements Superfoods Cookbook Book One and it contains Superfoods Salads, Superfoods Smoothies and Superfoods Deserts with ultra-healthy non-refined ingredients. All ingredients are 100% Superfoods.

It also contains Superfoods Reference book which is organized by Superfoods (more than 60 of them, with the list of their benefits), Superfoods spices, all vitamins, minerals and antioxidants. Superfoods Reference Book lists Superfoods that can help with 12 diseases and 9 types of cancer.

http://www.SuperfoodsToday.com/FREE

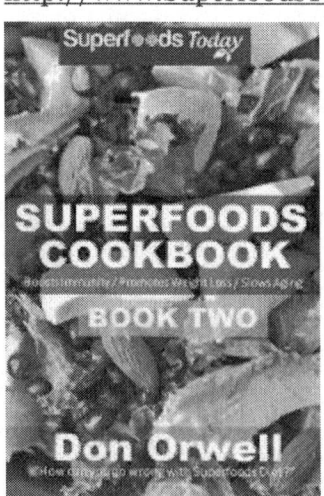

Table of Contents

Food for Diabetics 1
    Introduction 20
Superfoods Recipes for Diabetics 21
Condiments 21
    Basil Pesto 21
    Cilantro Pesto 22
    Sundried Tomato Pesto 24
Broths 25
    Vegetable broth 25
    Chicken Broth 27
    Beef Broth 28
Pastes 30
    Curry Paste 30
    Tomato paste 32
    Precooked beans 35
Breakfast - Oatmeal 36
    Superfoods Oatmeal Breakfast 36
    Oatmeal Yogurt Breakfast 39
    Cocoa Oatmeal 41
    Flax and Blueberry Vanilla Overnight Oats 43
    Apple Oatmeal 44
    Almond Butter Banana Oats 45
    Coconut Pomegranate Oatmeal 47

    Blue Milk Oatmeal 48

    Yogurt, Sesame Seeds and Blueberry Oatmeal 49

Chia Pudding Recipes 50

    Cacao & Raspberry Chia Pudding 50

    Blueberry Chia Pudding 51

Savory Breakfasts 52

    Regular egg recipes 52

    Omelet with Leeks 53

    Egg pizza crust 54

    Omelet with Superfoods veggies 55

    Egg Muffins 57

    Steak and Eggs 60

        Egg Bake 62

    Frittata 64

    Superfoods Naan / Pancakes / Crepes 66

    Zucchini Pancakes 67

    Cottage Cheese Sesame Balls 69

    Frittata with Carrots, Green Peas and Asparagus 71

    Frittata with Asparagus and Tomato 73

    Leeks, Spinach, Eggs & Yogurt 74

    Broccoli Frittata 75

Superfoods Smoothies 77

    Fruits and Veggies preparation 79

GREEN SMOOTHIES 80

- Kale Kiwi Smoothie 80
- Zucchini Apples Smoothie 81
- Dandelion Smoothie 82
- Fennel Honeydew Smoothie 83
- Broccoli Apple Smoothie 85
- Salad Smoothie 86
- Avocado Kale Smoothie 87
- Watercress Smoothie 88
- Beet Greens Smoothie 89
- Broccoli Leeks Cucumber smoothie 90
- Cacao Spinach Smoothie 91
- Flax Almond Butter Smoothie 92
- Apple Kale Smoothie 93

Rainbow Smoothie 94
- 3 Colors Rainbow Smoothie 94

Salad Dressings 95
- Italian Dressing 95
- Yogurt Dressing 95

Salads 96
- Large Fiber Loaded Salad with Italian Dressing 96
- Large Fiber Loaded Salad with Yogurt Dressing 98
- Large Fiber Loaded Salad as a meal on its own – only 258 calories per serving 100
- Greek Salad 102
- Cucumber, Cilantro, Quinoa Tabbouleh 104

Almond, Quinoa, Red Peppers & Arugula Salad 105

Asparagus, Quinoa & Red Peppers Salad 106

Chickpeas, Quinoa, Cucumber & Tomato Salad 108

Strawberry Spinach Salad 109

Tuna Bean Salad 111

Quinoa Salad 113

Cauliflower & Eggs Salad 115

Quinoa & almond Superfoods Tabbouleh 116

Greek Cucumber Salad 118

Mediterranean Salad 120

Pomegranate Avocado salad 122

Superfoods Salad 123

Roasted Beet Salad 125

Carrot, Quinoa, Tomato & Spinach Salad in a Jar 126

Tomato, Cucumber, Corn & Lettuce Salad in a Jar 127

Chickpeas, Onion, Tomato & Parsley Salad in a Jar 128

Arugula, Carrot, Corn & Spinach Salad in a Jar 129

Shrimp, Cucumber & Arugula Salad in a Jar 130

Tomato, Cucumber, Pumpkin & Dandelion Jar Salad 131

Carrot, Peppers, Cucumber & Cabbage Salad in a Jar 132

Tomato, Cucumber, Carrot & Parsley Salad in a Jar 133

Apple Coleslaw 134

Chicken, Roasted Veggies & Arugula Salad 136

Broccoli, Quinoa, Shrimps & Scallops Salad 137

Tuna, Tomato, Arugula & Eggs Salad 138

Avocado, Tomato, Arugula Salad 140

Chicken, Tomato, Spinach & Cucumber Salad 142

Apple, Spinach & Eggs Salad 143

Artichoke, Arugula & Lamb Salad 144

Tuna, Tomato, Eggs & Lettuce Salad 145

Soups 146

Cream of Broccoli Soup 146

Lentil Soup 148

Cold Cucumber Avocado Soup 150

Bouillabaisse 151

Gaspacho 153

Italian Beef Soup 154

Creamy roasted mushroom 156

Black Bean Soup 158

Squash soup 160

Kale White Bean Pork Soup 162

Avgolemono – Greek lemon chicken soup 164

Egg-Drop Soup 166

Creamy Tomato Basil Soup 168

Minestrone 169

Grilled Meats & Salad 171

Chicken and Large Fiber Loaded Salad with Italian Dressing 171

Salmon with Large Fiber Loaded Salad with Italian Dressing 173

- Herb Crusted Salmon 174
- Ground Beef Patty with Large Fiber Loaded Salad with Yogurt Dressing 176
- Lean Pork with Fiber Loaded Salad with Yogurt Dressing 178
- Caribbean Chicken salad 180
- Tuna with Large Fiber Loaded Salad with Italian Dressing 182

Stews, Chilies and Curries 184
- Stuffed Peppers with beans 184
- Vegetarian Chili 186
- Lentil Stew 188
- Braised Green Peas with Beef 190
- White Chicken Chili 193
- Kale Pork 195
- 30-Minute Squash Cauliflower and Green Peppers Coconut Curry . 197
- Crockpot Red Curry Lamb 199
- Easy Lentil Dhal 200
- Gumbo 202
- Chickpea Curry 205
- Red Curry Chicken 206
- Braised Green Beans with Pork 207
- Ratatouille 210
- Barbecued Beef 212
- Beef Tenderloin with Roasted Shallots 214
- Chili 216
- Glazed Meatloaf 218

Eggplant Lasagna 220

Stuffed Eggplant 222

Stuffed Red Peppers with Beef 223

Superfoods Goulash 225

Frijoles Charros 226

Chicken Cacciatore 228

Cabbage Stewed with Meat 230

Beef Stew with Peas and Carrots 232

Green Chicken Stew 234

Irish Stew 236

Hungarian Pea Stew 238

Chicken Tikka Masala 240

Greek Beef Stew (Stifado) 242

Beef, Parsnip, Celery Stew 244

Chicken Mushrooms & Olives Stew 246

Chicken Pasanda Curry 248

Osso Bucco & Garlic Stew 249

Beef Meatballs with White Beans 250

Duck Stew 252

Pork, Celery and Basil Stew 254

Meat Stew with Red Beans 256

Vegetarian Garbanzo Chili 258

Red Peppers Pork Curry 260

Beef Ratatouille 261

Chicken, Green Peas and Red Peppers Stew 262

Crock Pot Turkey Roast Mediterranean style 263

Slow Cooker Pot Roast 264

Crock Pot Whole Chicken 265

Beef, Leeks & Mushrooms Stew 266

Chicken, Garlic & Tomato Stew 267

Minced Pork, Tomato & Red Peppers Stew 268

Beef, Eggplant, Celery & Peppers Stew 269

Chicken & Onion Stew 270

Leeks, Mushrooms & Pork Neck Meat 271

Broccoli, Pork & Peppers 274

Haitian Chicken Broccoli 275

Leeks, Cauliflower, Chicken & Carrot 276

Okra & Pork Stew 277

Chicken, Black Beans and Cauliflower 278

Celery, Carrots & Cauliflower Pork 279

Slow Cooked Carnitas 280

Beef & Apple 281

Bigos - Polish Pork, Venison & Cabbage Stew 282

Cumin Lamb 283

Mexican Lamb Chili 284

Moroccan Lamb, Tomato Sauce & Green Peppers Stew 286

Pork, Mushrooms & Herbs Stew 287

Chicken Green Curry 288

Two Beans Chili 289

Chicken & Artichoke Hearts 291

Green Peppers, Chicken and Green Onions 292

Black Bean Chicken Chili 293

Haitian Spinach Shrimp Stew 295

Duck Curry 296

Eggplant Red Pepper Stew 297

Irish Lamb Stew 298

Shrimp, Onion & Cilantro Stew 299

Venison Green Beans Onion Stew 300

Pork Cauliflower Stew 301

Sweet Potato Veal Stew 302

Pork Broccoli Carrot Stew 302

Moroccan Lamb & Mushrooms Stew 304

Shrimp Peppers Stew 305

Afghan Stew 306

Hunter's Green Beans Chicken Stew 309

Kale Chicken Jambalaya 310

Minced Pork and Veal Stew 311

Olives & Chicken Stew 312

Pulled Pork 313

Chicken, Olives, Capers & Eggplant Stew 314

Turkish Chicken Stew 315

Veal & Red Peppers Stew 316

Chinese Eggplant, Chicken & Green Onions Stew 317
Pumpkin, Chicken, & Chinese Celery Stew 317
Spicy Shrimp & Eggplant Stew 318
Veal, Tomato, Garlic, Corn & Zucchini Stew 319
Chicken, Chickpeas, Tomato, Peppers & Eggplant Stew 320
Pork, Chinese Celery & Mushrooms Stew 321
Shrimp, Yellow Peas & Green Onions Stew 322
Pork & Bok Choy Stew 323
Shrimp & Red Peppers Stew 324
Pork, Mushrooms, Red Peppers & Zucchini Stew 325
Beef, Leeks & Mushrooms Stew 326
Chicken & Butternut Squash Stew 328
Chicken, Garlic & Tomato Stew 329
Minced Pork, Tomato & Red Peppers Stew 330
Beef, Eggplant, Celery & Peppers Stew 331
Chicken & Onion Stew 332
Pork & Black Eyed Peas Stew 333
Zucchini Rolls 334
Beef Pot Roast with Broccoli 335
Mixed Seafood, Saffron & Sundried Tomatoes 336
Chicken and Sweet Potato 337
Black Bean Cuban Stew 338
Chicken and Garbanzo Stew 339
Spicy Beef Stew – Yukgaejang (Korean Recipe) 340

Kale, Quinoa and Beans Stew 341

Veal & Sweet Potato Stew 342

Teriyaki Chicken & Carrots 343

Spicy Garbanzo and Spinach Stew 344

Cacciucco - Shrimp, Mussels, Fish & Scallops Stew 345

Lamb and Peppers Stew 346

Plantain Chili 347

BBQ Pork 348

Penang Chicken Curry 349

Chicken Fennel Stew 350

Garbanzo Kale Curry 351

Mexican Veal 352

Okra Pork Spinach Stew 353

Red Curry 354

Shrimp & Green Peas 355

Shrimp & Peppers 356

BBQ Pork Ribs 357

Pork Shoulder Stew 358

Fish, Onion & Fennel Stew 359

Kale & Shiitake Stew 360

Kale & Chicken Stew 361

Mackerel & Bamboo Shoots Stew 362

Korean Spicy Fish Soup – Mae Un Tang 363

Mushrooms & Pork Ribs Stew 364

- Olives Jambalaya 365
- Pork & Cauliflower Stew 366
- Shui Zhu Yu - Sichuan Fish Stew 367
- Haleem – Beef & Lentils Stew 368
- Hong Shao Rou Pork Stew 369
- Pork Jambalaya 370
- Khoresht – Green Peas Stew 371
- Kimchee Jjiagae – Kimchee Stew 372
- Locro Argentine Stew 373
- Mixed Fish Stew 374
- Onion, Leeks & Chicken Breast Stew 375
- Pork & Onion Stew 376
- Shrimp Gumbo Stew 377
- Cholent – Jewish Brisket & Beans Stew 378
- Beef Daube Stew 379
- Dinuguan – Filipino Stew... 380
- Fabada Asturiana – Spanish Pork Belly & Beans Stew 381
- Ghormeh Sabzi – Persian Stew 382
- Goulash – Spicy Beef Stew 383
- Letscho Chicken 384
- Narial Murgh Shorba Stew 385

Stir Fries 386
- Pork and Bok Choy / Celery Stir Fry 386
- Lemon Chicken Stir Fry... 388

Pan seared Brussels sprouts 390

Beef and Broccoli Stir Fry 391

Garbanzo Stir Fry 393

Thai Basil Chicken 396

Shrimp with Snow Peas 398

Pork and Green Beans Stir Fry 400

Cashew chicken 402

Chinese Celery, Mushrooms & Fish Stir Fry 404

Pork, Green Pepper and Tomato Stir Fry 405

Pork, Red & Green Peppers, Onion & Carrots Stir Fry 406

Chicken, Carrots & Snow Peas Stir Fry 407

Beef, Green beans, Broccoli & Carrot Stir Fry 408

Pork, Onion & Bok Choy Stir Fry 409

Chicken, Red Peppers & Bok Choy Stir Fry 410

Cauliflower & Shiitake Stir Fry 411

Pork, Cabbage & Bok Choy Stir Fry 412

Chicken & Chinese Celery Stir Fry 413

Meats 414

Baked Chicken Breast with Fresh Basil 414

Roast Chicken with Rosemary 416

Carne Asada 417

Meatballs 418

Baked Beef Meatballs 418

Middle Eastern Meatballs 420

Casseroles 422

    Broccoli Chicken Casserole 422

    Beef Meatballs Broccoli Casserole 424

    Beef Meatballs Cauliflower Casserole 426

    Cabbage Roll Casserole 428

    Pork Chop Casserole 430

    Chicken & Mushrooms Casserole 431

    Pork & Red Peppers Casserole 432

    Chicken, Carrot and Cherry Tomatoes Casserole 433

    Chicken, Carrot and Onions Italian Casserole 434

    Red Peppers, Zucchini and Eggplant Casserole 436

    Chia, Flax & Broccoli Casserole 438

    Osso Bucco Casserole 439

    Chicken, Olives & Garlic Casserole 440

    Pork, Sweet Potatoes & Tomato Casserole 442

    Eggplant, Zucchini and Tomato Casserole 444

    Zucchini & Chicken Casserole 446

    Shrimp, Tomato Paste and Red Peppers Casserole 447

    Mushrooms Casserole 448

    Chicken Eggplant Casserole 451

    Beef Meatballs Green Beans Casserole 453

    Chicken, Tomato Paste and Olives Casserole 455

    Chicken, Carrot and Mushrooms Casserole 457

    Pork Liver Casserole 458

- Salmon Broccoli Casserole 459
- Salmon, Tomato Paste and Mushrooms Casserole 461
- Zucchini Noodles & Slivered Almonds Casserole................................ 462
- Lamb and Red Kidney Beans Casserole.. 463
- Beet & Beef Casserole.. 464
- "Breaded" "fried" food 466
  - Breaded Tilapia.. 466
  - Breaded Chicken... 468
  - Lemon Pork with Asparagus 470
- Pizza 472
- Side dishes.. 474
  - Roasted curried cauliflower 474
  - Roasted cauliflower with Tahini sauce 476
  - Baked Sweet Potatoes 477
  - Asparagus with mushrooms and hazelnuts 478
  - Chard and Cashew Sauté.. 480
  - Cauliflower rice side dish 481
- Crockpot.. 482
  - Slow Cooker Pepper Steak 482
  - Pork Tenderloin with peppers and onions 484
  - Beef Bourguinon 486
  - Italian Chicken 488
  - Ropa Vieja 490
  - Lemon Roast Chicken... 492

- Fall Lamb and Vegetable Stew...494
- Slow cooker pork loin...496
- Sauerbraten..498

Fish..500
- Cioppino..500
- Flounder with Orange Coconut Oil 502
- Grilled Salmon 503
- Crab Cakes...505

Sweets...507
- Superfoods Dark Chocolate...507
- Fruits dipped in Superfoods chocolate 508
- Superfoods No-Bake Cookies 510
- Raw Brownies 512
- Superfoods Ice cream 513
- Apple Spice Cookies..514
- Superfoods Macaroons 515
- Superfoods Stuffed Apples..516
- Whipped Coconut cream 517
- Granola Mix...519
- Upside down Apple Cake 521
- Raw Vegan Reese's Cups..523
- Raw Vegan Coffee Cashew Cream Cake 525
- Raw Vegan Chocolate Cashew Truffles...527
- Raw Vegan Double Almond Raw Chocolate Tart.................................529

Raw Vegan Bounty Bars 531
Raw Vegan Tartlets with Coconut Cream 533
Raw Vegan "Peanut" Butter Truffles 535
Raw Vegan Chocolate Pie... 537
Raw Vegan Chocolate Walnut Truffles 539
Other Books from this Author.. 541

Introduction

Hello,

My name is Don Orwell and my blog SuperfoodsToday.com is dedicated to Superfoods lifestyle. This book is suitable for diabetics with **diabetes type 2**. You can read everything about Superfoods Diet, the way I lost weight and Superfoods lifestyle in my free book on Amazon:

http://superfoodstoday.com/AmazonFree

Superfoods Recipes for Diabetics

Allergy labels: SF – Soy Free, GF – Gluten Free, DF – Dairy Free, EF – Egg Free, V - Vegan, NF – Nut Free

Condiments

Basil Pesto
- 1 cup basil
- 1/3 cup cashews
- 2 garlic cloves, chopped
- 1/2 cup olive oil

Process basil, cashews and garlic until smooth. Add oil in a slow stream. Process to combine. Transfer to a bowl. Season with salt and pepper. Stir to combine. Allergies: SF, GF, DF, EF, V

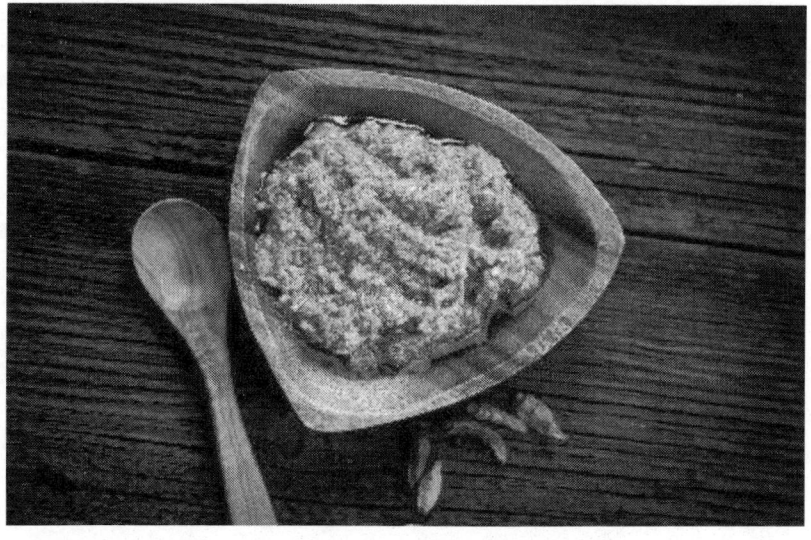

Cilantro Pesto

- 1 cup cilantro
- 1/3 cup cashews
- 2 garlic cloves, chopped
- 1/2 cup olive oil or avocado oil

Process cilantro, cashews and garlic. Add oil in a slow stream. Process to combine. Transfer to a bowl. Season with salt and pepper. Stir to combine. Allergies: SF, GF, DF, EF, V

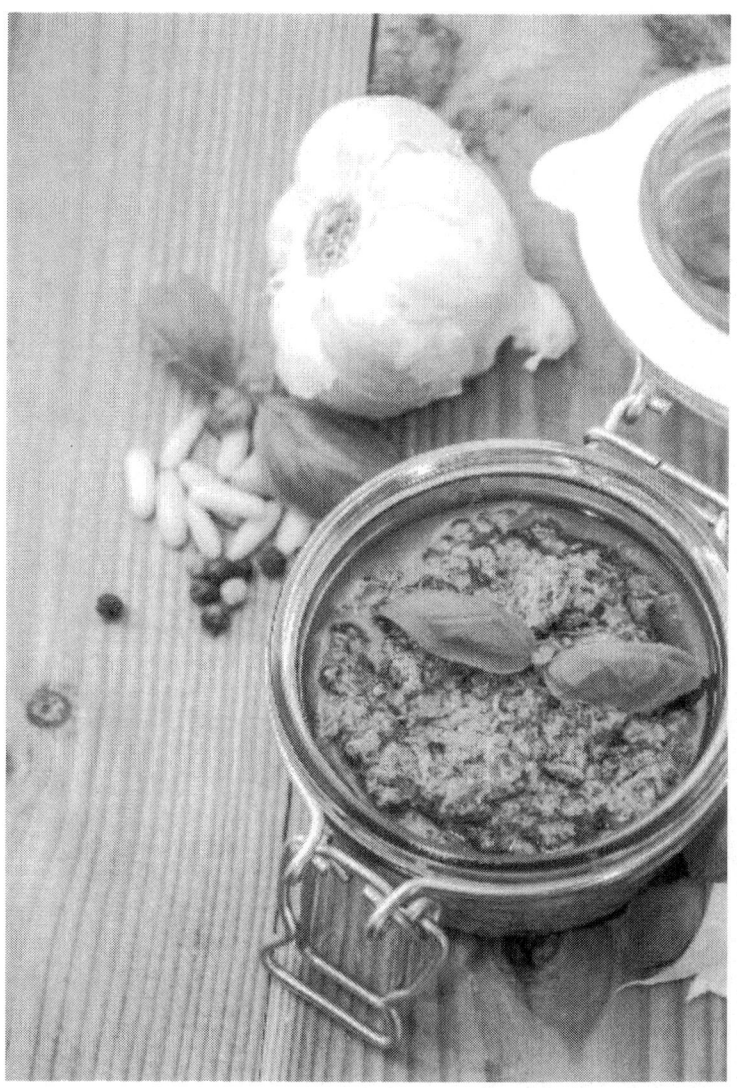

Sundried Tomato Pesto

- 3/4 cup sundried tomatoes
- 1/3 cup cashews
- 2 garlic cloves, chopped
- 1/2 cup olive oil or avocado oil

Process tomato, cashews and garlic. Add oil in a slow stream. Process to combine. Transfer to a bowl. Season with salt and pepper. Stir to combine. Allergies: SF, GF, DF, EF, V

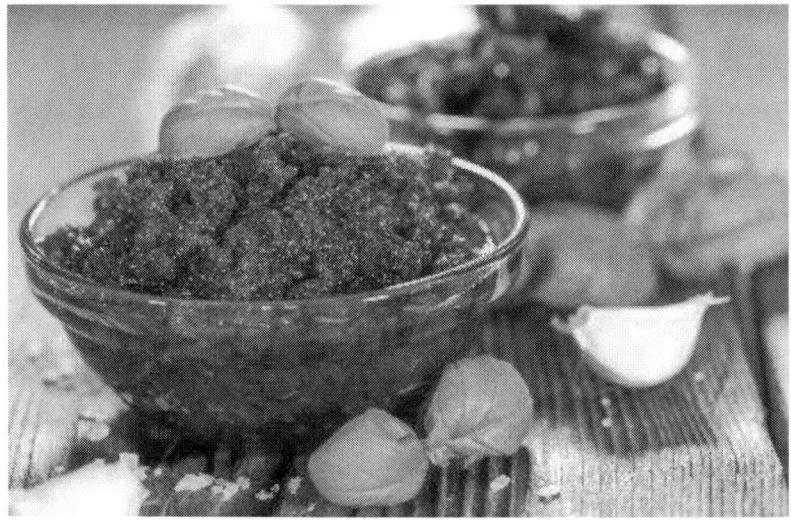

Broths

Some recipes require a cup or more of various broths, vegetable, beef or chicken broth. I usually cook the whole pot and freeze it.

Vegetable broth

Servings: 6 cups

Ingredients

- 1 tbsp. coconut oil
- 1 large onion
- 2 stalks celery, including some leaves
- 2 large carrots
- 1 bunch green onions, chopped
- 8 cloves garlic, minced
- 8 sprigs fresh parsley
- 6 sprigs fresh thyme
- 2 bay leaves
- 1 tsp. salt
- 2 quarts water

Instructions - Allergies: SF, GF, DF, EF, V, NF

Chop veggies into small chunks. Heat oil in a soup pot & add onion, scallions, celery, carrots, garlic, parsley, thyme, and bay leaves. Cook over high heat for 5 to 7 minutes, stirring occasionally.

Bring to a boil and add salt. Lower heat and simmer, uncovered, for 30 minutes. Strain. Other ingredients to consider: broccoli stalk, celery root

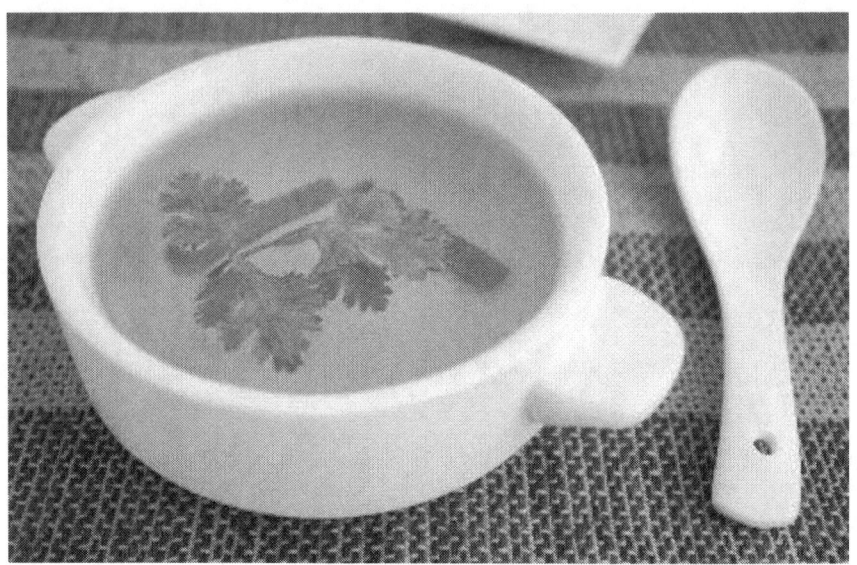

Chicken Broth

Ingredients

- 4 lbs. fresh chicken (wings, necks, backs, legs, bones)
- 2 peeled onions or 1 cup chopped leeks
- 2 celery stalks
- 1 carrot
- 8 black peppercorns
- 2 sprigs fresh thyme
- 2 sprigs fresh parsley
- 1 tsp. salt

Instructions - Allergies: SF, GF, DF, EF, NF

Put cold water in a stock pot and add chicken. Bring just to a boil. Skim any foam from the surface. Add other ingredients, return just to a boil, and reduce heat to a slow simmer. Simmer for 2 hours. Let cool to warm room temperature and strain. Keep chilled and use or freeze broth within a few days. Before using, defrost and boil.

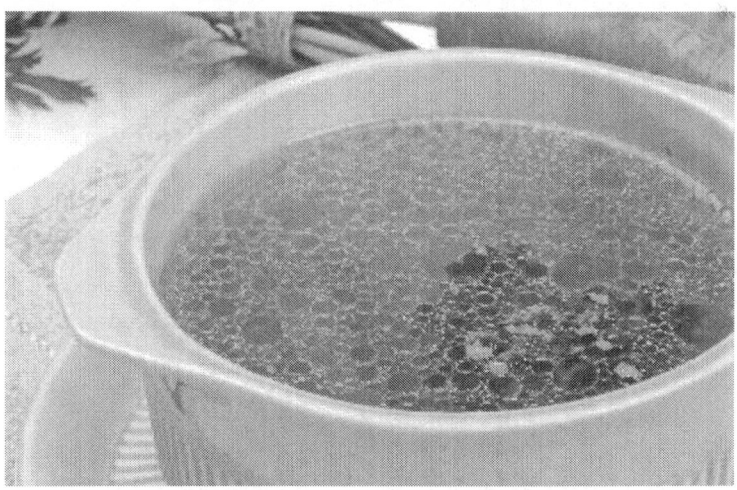

Beef Broth

Ingredients

- 4-5 pounds beef bones and few veal bones
- 1 pound of stew meat (chuck or flank steak) cut into 2-inch chunks
- olive oil or avocado oil
- 1-2 medium onions, peeled and quartered
- 1-2 large carrots, cut into 1-2 inch segments
- 1 celery rib, cut into 1 inch segments
- 2-3 cloves of garlic, unpeeled
- Handful of parsley, stems and leaves
- 1-2 bay leaves
- 10 peppercorns

Instructions - Allergies: SF, GF, DF, EF, NF

Heat oven to 375°F. Rub olive oil over the stew meat pieces, carrots, and onions. Place stew meat or beef scraps, stock bones, carrots and onions in a large roasting pan. Roast in oven for about 45 minutes, turning everything half-way through the cooking.

Place everything from the oven in a large stock pot. Pour some boiling water in the oven pan and scrape up all of the browned bits and pour all in the stock pot.

Add parsley, celery, garlic, bay leaves, and peppercorns to the pot. Fill the pot with cold water, to 1 inch over the top of the bones. Bring the stock pot to a regular simmer and then reduce the heat to low, so it just barely simmers. Cover the pot loosely and let simmer low and slow for 3-4 hours.

Scoop away the fat and any scum that rises to the surface once in a while.

After cooking, remove the bones and vegetables from the pot. Strain the broth. Let cool to room temperature and then put in the refrigerator.

The fat will solidify once the broth has chilled. Discard the fat (or reuse it) and pour the broth into a jar and freeze it.

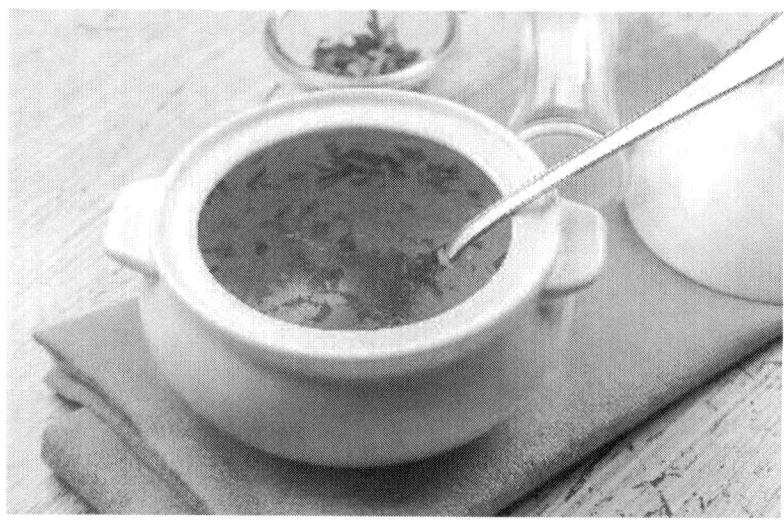

Pastes

Curry Paste

This should not be prepared in advance, but there are several curry recipes that are using curry paste and I decided to take the curry paste recipe out and have it separately. So, when you see that the recipe is using curry paste, please go to this part of the book and prepare it from scratch. Don't use processed curry pastes or curry powder; make it every time from scratch. Keep the spices in original form (seeds, pods), ground them just before making the curry paste. You can dry heat in the skillet cloves, cardamom, cumin and coriander and then crush them coarsely with mortar and pestle.

Ingredients

- 2 onions, minced
- 2 cloves garlic, minced
- 2 teaspoons fresh ginger root, finely chopped
- 6 whole cloves
- 2 cardamom pods
- 2 (2 inch) pieces cinnamon sticks, crushed
- 1 tsp. ground cumin
- 1 tsp. ground coriander
- 1 tsp. salt
- 1 tsp. ground cayenne pepper
- 1 tsp. ground turmeric

Instructions - Allergies: SF, GF, DF, EF, V, NF

Heat oil in a frying pan over medium/high heat and fry onions until transparent. Stir in garlic, cumin, ginger, cloves, cinnamon, coriander, salt, cayenne, and turmeric. Cook for around 1 minute over medium heat, stirring constantly. At this point other curry ingredients should be added.

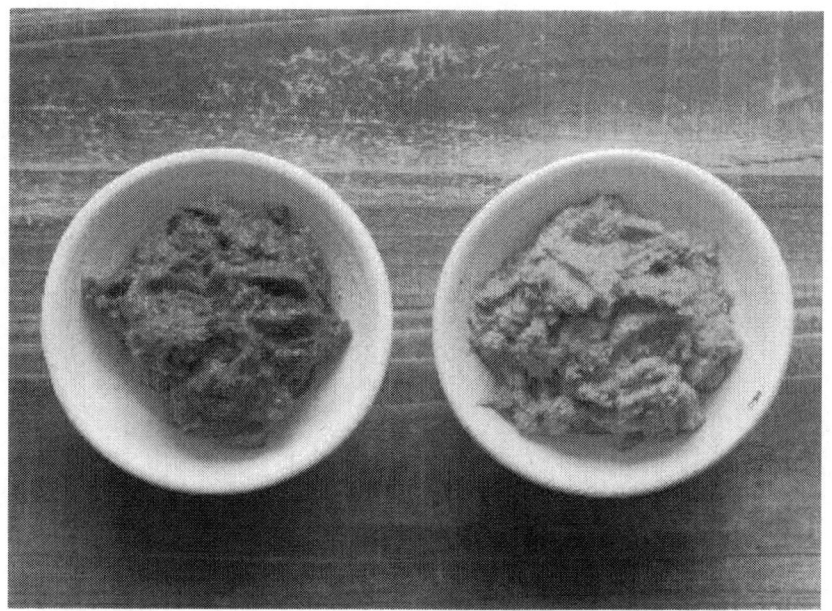

Tomato paste

Some recipes (chili) require tomato paste. I usually prepare 20 or so liters at once (when tomato is in season, which is usually September) and freeze it.

Ingredients

- 5 lbs. chopped plum tomatoes
- 1/4 cup extra-virgin olive oil or avocado oil plus 2 tbsp.
- salt, to taste

Instructions - Allergies: SF, GF, DF, EF, V, NF

Heat 1/4 cup of the oil in a skillet over medium heat. Add tomatoes. Season with salt. Bring to a boil. Cook, stirring, until very soft, about 8 minutes.

Pass the tomatoes through the finest plate of a food mill. Push as much of the pulp through the sieve as possible and leave the seeds behind.

Bring it to boil, lower it and then boil uncovered, so the liquid will thicken (approx. 30-40 minutes). That will give you homemade tomato juice. You get tomato paste if you boil for 60 minutes, it gets thick like store bought ketchup.

Store sealed in an airtight container in the refrigerator for up to one month, or freeze, for up to 6 months.

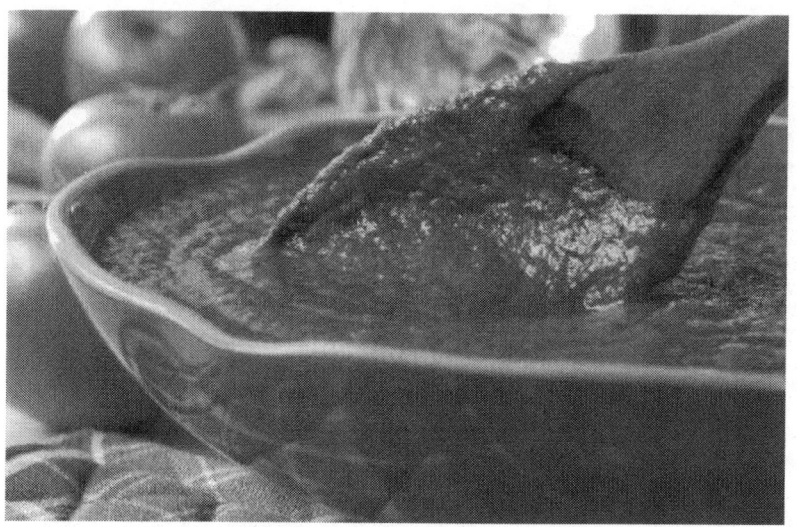

Healthy Superfoods Casserole Sauce

- 2 beaten eggs
- Salt, pepper
- 1 cup of low-fat Greek yogurt
- 1 Tbsp. olive oil
- 1/2 cup of low fat parmesan or shredded cheddar cheese

Optional:
- 1 tsp of flax seeds meal
- 1/2 tsp. oregano or thyme or any other herbs

Precooked beans

Again, some recipes require that you cook some beans (butter beans, red kidney, garbanzo) in advance. Cooking beans takes around 3 hours and it can be done in advance or every few weeks and the rest get frozen. Soak beans for 24 hours before cooking them. After the first boil, throw the water, add new water and continue cooking. Some beans or lentils can be sprouted for few days before cooking and that helps people with stomach problems.

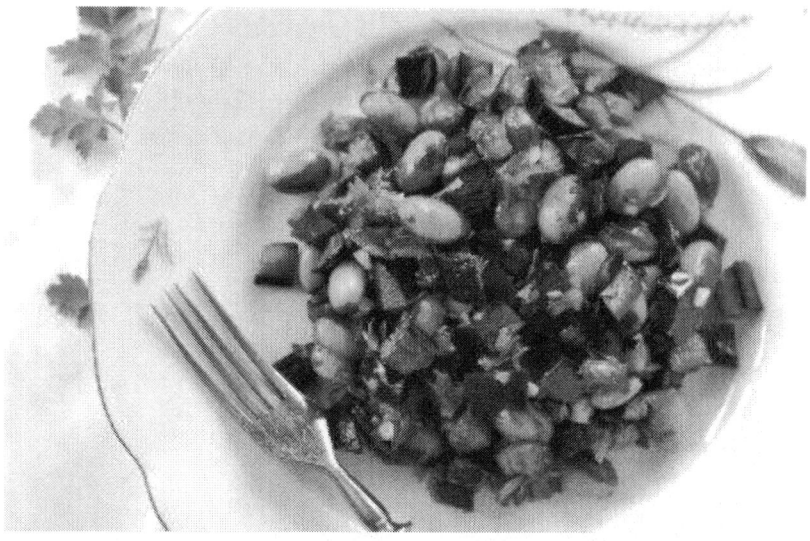

Breakfast - Oatmeal

Superfoods Oatmeal Breakfast
Serves 1 - Allergies: SF, GF, DF, EF, V, NF

- 1 cup cooked oatmeal
- 1 tsp. of ground flax seeds
- 1 tsp. of sunflower seeds
- A dash of cinnamon
- Half of the tsp. of cocoa

Cook oatmeal with hot water and after that mix all ingredients. Sweeten if you have to with a teaspoon of lucuma powder. Optional: You can replace sunflower seeds with pumpkin seed or chia seed. You can add a handful of blueberries or any berries instead of cocoa.

Nutrition Facts

Serving Size 52 g

Amount Per Serving

Calories 207 — Calories from Fat 58

	% Daily Value*
Total Fat 6.4g	10%
Saturated Fat 0.9g	4%
Cholesterol 0mg	0%
Sodium 5mg	0%
Potassium 246mg	7%
Total Carbohydrates 28.8g	10%
Dietary Fiber 7.3g	29%
Sugars 0.5g	
Protein 8.2g	

Vitamin A 0% • Vitamin C 0%
Calcium 4% • Iron 13%

Nutrition Grade A-

* Based on a 2000 calorie diet

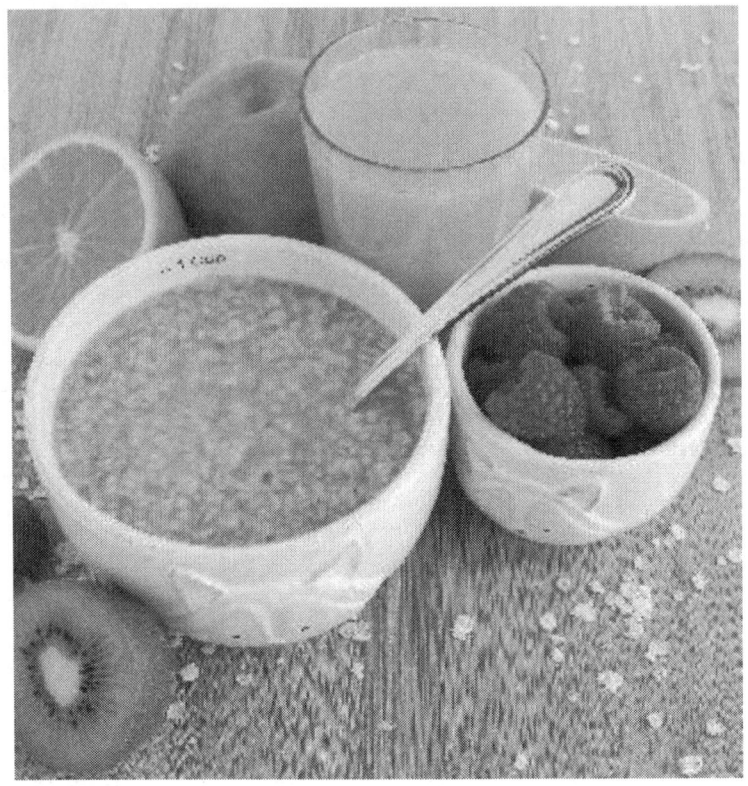

Oatmeal Yogurt Breakfast

Serves 1 - Allergies: SF, GF, EF, NF

- 1/2 cup dry oatmeal
- Handful of blueberries (optional)
- 1 cup of low-fat yogurt

Mix all ingredients and wait 20 minutes or leave overnight in the fridge if using steel cut oats.

Nutrition Facts

Serving Size 247 g

Amount Per Serving

Calories 255 — Calories from Fat 37

	% Daily Value*
Total Fat 4.2g	6%
Saturated Fat 2.1g	11%
Cholesterol 11mg	4%
Sodium 131mg	5%
Potassium 557mg	16%
Total Carbohydrates 36.6g	12%
Dietary Fiber 3.6g	15%
Sugars 16.8g	
Protein 14.3g	

Vitamin A 2%	Vitamin C 12%
Calcium 35%	Iron 10%

Nutrition Grade A

* Based on a 2000 calorie diet

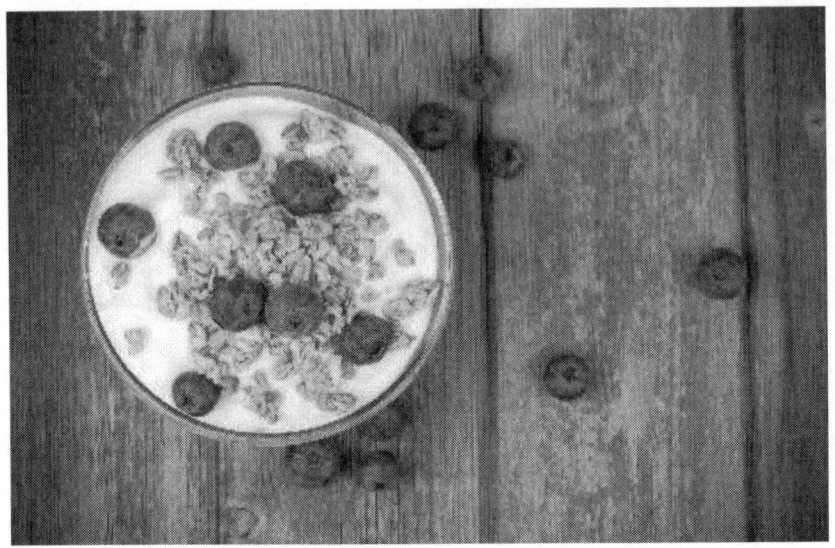

Cocoa Oatmeal

Serves 1

Ingredients - Allergies: SF, GF, DF, NF

- 1/2 cup oats
- 2 cups water
- A pinch tsp. salt
- 1/2 tsp. ground vanilla bean
- 2 tbsp. cocoa powder
- 1 tbsp. lucuma powder
- 2 tbsp. ground flax seeds meal
- a dash of cinnamon
- 2 egg whites

Instructions

In a saucepan over high heat, place the oats and salt. Cover with 2 cups water. Bring to a boil and cook for 3-5 minutes, stirring occasionally. Keep adding 1/2 cup water if necessary as the mixture thickens.

In a separate bowl, whisk 4 tbsp. water into the 4 tbsp. cocoa powder to form a smooth sauce. Add the vanilla to the pan and stir.

Turn the heat down to low. Add the egg whites and whisk immediately. Add the flax meal, and cinnamon. Stir to combine. Remove from heat, add lucuma powder and serve immediately.

Topping suggestions: sliced strawberries, blueberries or few almonds.

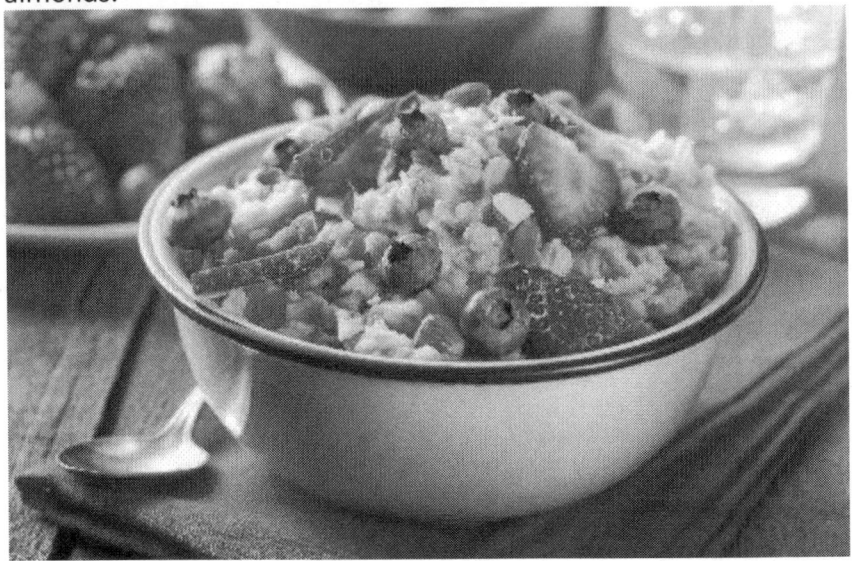

Flax and Blueberry Vanilla Overnight Oats
Serves 1

Ingredients - Allergies: SF, GF, EF, V, NF

- 1/2 cup oats
- 1/3 cup water
- 1/4 cup low-fat yogurt
- 1/2 tsp. ground vanilla bean
- 1 tbsp. flax seeds meal
- A pinch of salt
- Blueberries, almonds, blackberries, lucuma powder for topping

Instructions

Add the ingredients (except for toppings) to the bowl in the evening. Refrigerate overnight.

In the morning, stir up the mixture. It should be thick. Add the toppings of your choice.

Apple Oatmeal

Serves 1

Ingredients - Allergies: SF, GF, DF, EF, V, NF

- 1 grated apple
- 1/2 cup oats
- 1 cup water
- Dash of cinnamon
- 2 tsp. lucuma powder

Instructions

Cook the oats with the water for 3-5 minutes.

Add grated apple and cinnamon. Stir in the lucuma powder.

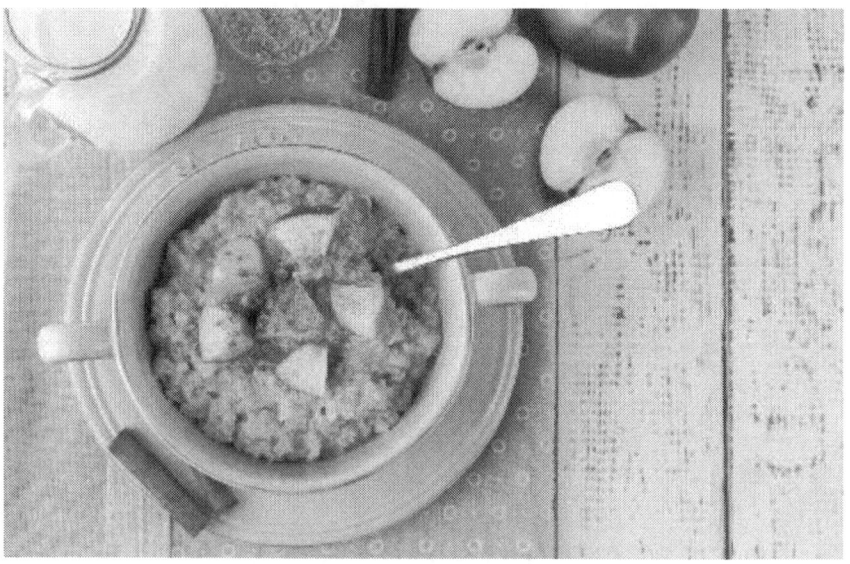

Almond Butter Banana Oats

Serves 1

Ingredients - Allergies: SF, GF

- 1/2 cup oats
- 3/4 cup water
- 1 egg white
- 1 banana
- 1 tbs. flax seeds meal
- 1 tsp lucuma powder
- pinch cinnamon
- 1/2 tbs. almond butter

Instructions

Combine oats and water in a bowl. Beat the egg white, then whisk it in with the uncooked oats. Boil on stovetop. Check consistency and continue to heat as necessary until the oats are fluffy and thick. Mash banana and add to oats. Heat olive oil in a skillet over medium/high for around 1 minute

Stir in flax, lucuma powder, and cinnamon. Top with almond butter!

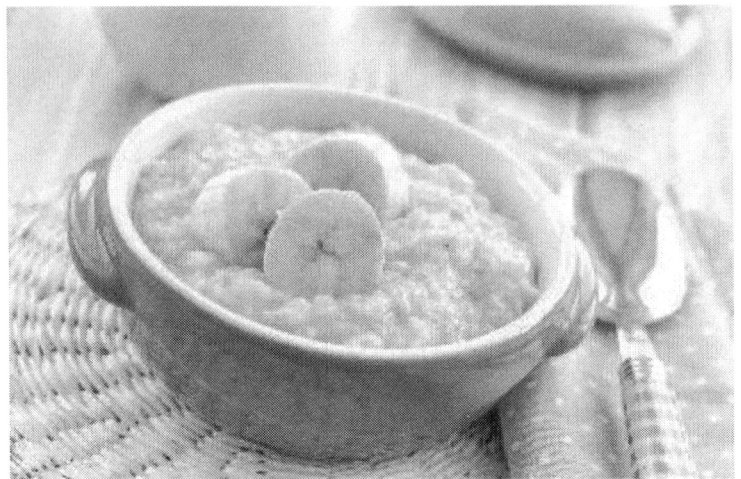

Coconut Pomegranate Oatmeal

Serves 1

Ingredients - Allergies: SF, GF, DF, EF, V, NF

- 1/2 cup oats
- 1/3 cup coconut milk
- 1 cup water
- 2 tbs. shredded unsweetened coconut
- 1-2 tbs. flax seeds meal
- 1 tbs. lucuma powder
- 3 tbs. pomegranate seeds

Instructions

Cook oats with the coconut milk, water, and salt.

Stir in the coconut, lucuma powder and flaxseed meal. Sprinkle with extra coconut and pomegranate seeds.

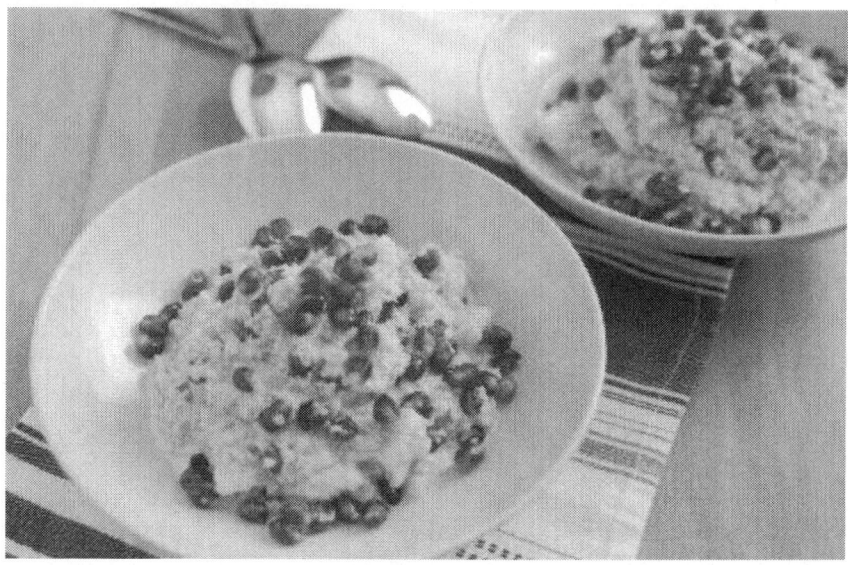

Blue Milk Oatmeal

Serves 1

Ingredients - Allergies: SF, GF, EF, V, NF

- 1/2 cup oats
- 3/4 cup almond milk
- 1/4 cup fresh chopped cranberries
- ½ cup blueberries
- 1 banana, chopped

Instructions

Cook the oats with the almond milk for 3-5 minutes and add blueberries. Mix in cranberries and banana. After some time, blueberries will turn milk blue ☺.

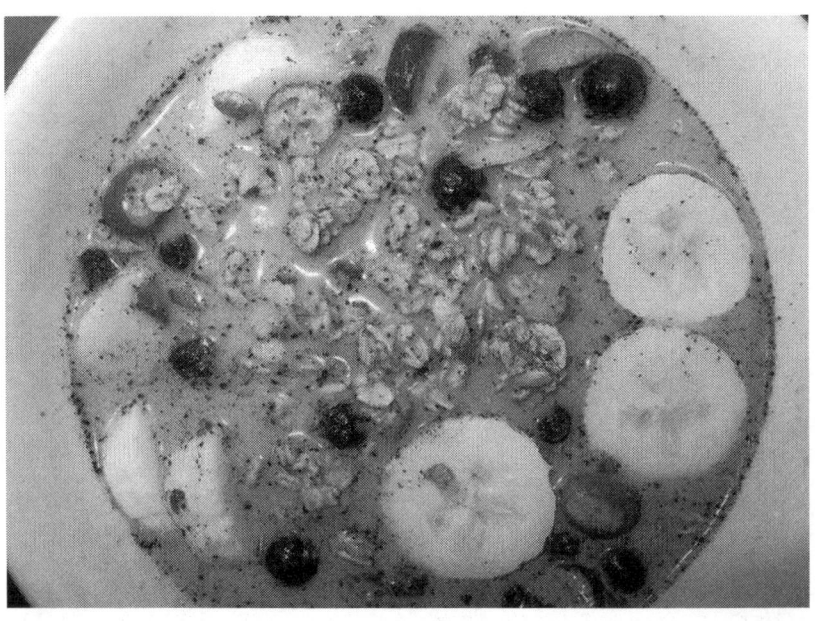

Yogurt, Sesame Seeds and Blueberry Oatmeal
Serves 1

Ingredients - *Allergies: SF, GF, EF, V, NF*

- 1/2 cup oats
- 3/4 cup yogurt
- 1/4 cup sesame seeds
- 1/2 tsp. cinnamon
- 4 almonds
- 1/2 cup blueberies, chopped

Instructions

Mix yogurt, sesame seeds and oats and let them soak for 15 minutes. Add cinnamon, almonds and blueberries.

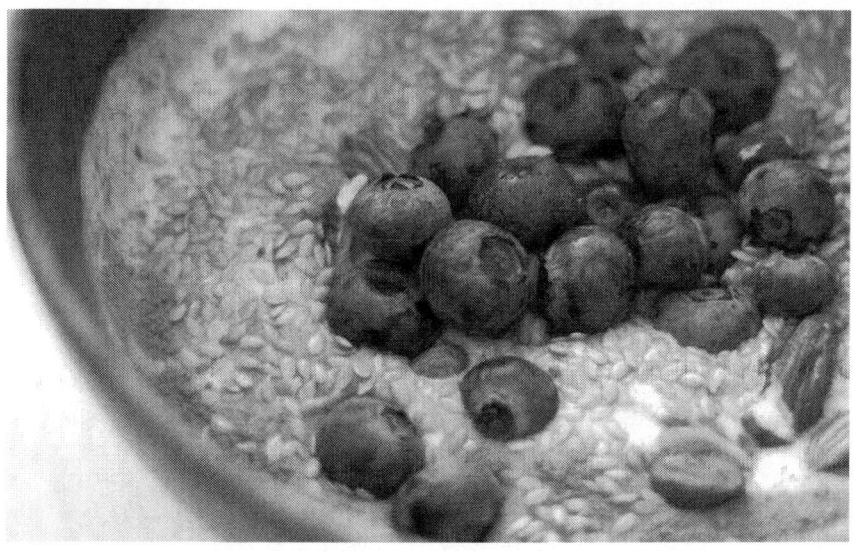

Chia Pudding Recipes

Cacao & Raspberry Chia Pudding
Serves 2

Ingredients

- 1/4 cup Chia seeds
- 1 cup coconut milk
- 1 tablespoon Raw honey
- 1 Tsp. cacao powder
- 1/2 cup yogurt
- 1/2 cup raspberries

Instructions

Mix coconut milk, honey, cacao and chia seeds and leave overnight in the fridge. Divide into 2 glasses, top each with 1/4 cup yogurt and 1/4 cup raspberries.

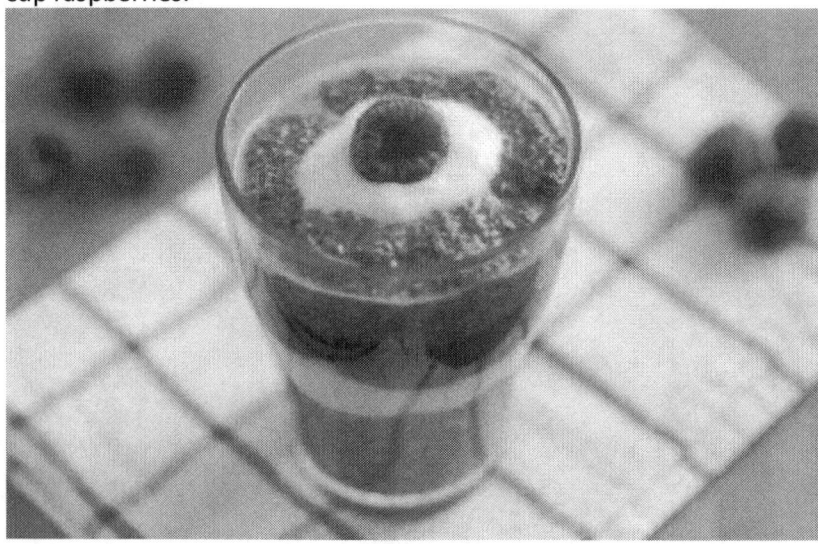

Blueberry Chia Pudding
Serves 2

Ingredients

- 1/4 cup Chia seeds
- 1 cup coconut milk
- 1 tablespoon Raw honey
- 1/2 cup blueberry smoothie
- 1/4 cup chopped almonds

Instructions

Mix coconut milk, honey, blueberry smoothie and chia seeds and leave overnight in the fridge. Divide into 2 glasses and top each almonds.

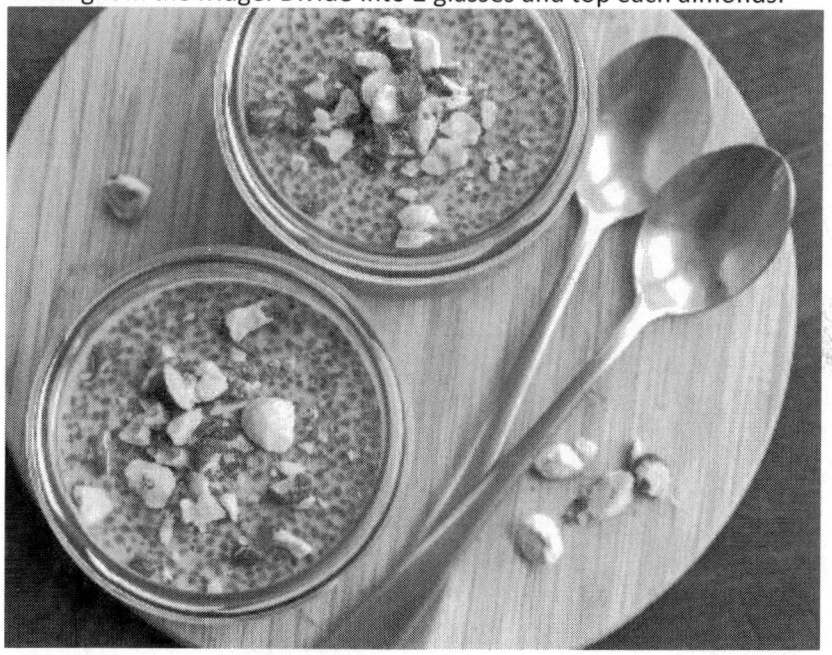

Savory Breakfasts
Serves 1

Regular egg recipes
Allergies: SF, GF, DF, NF

Eggs are great way to start a day and you can enjoy them hard boiled, scrambled, poached or in the omelet with veggies. Eat some breakfast veggies with eggs.

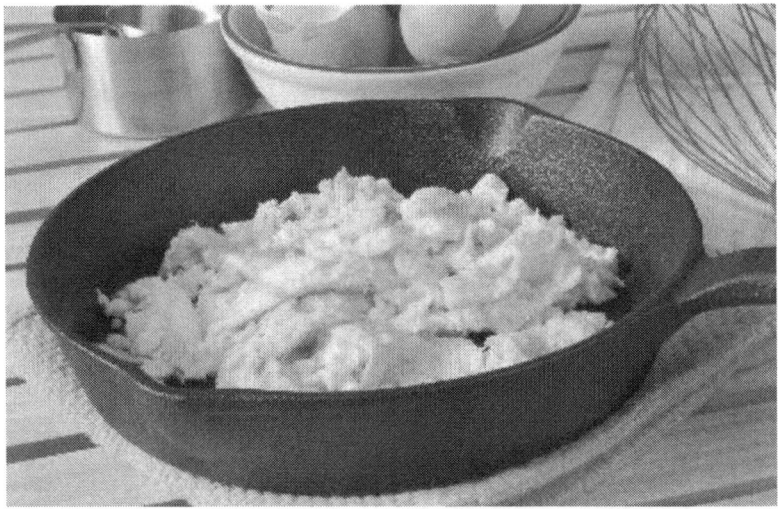

Omelet with Leeks

Serves 1 - Allergies: SF, GF, DF, NF

Cook leeks in little coconut oil until they get soft and then mix the beaten eggs in.

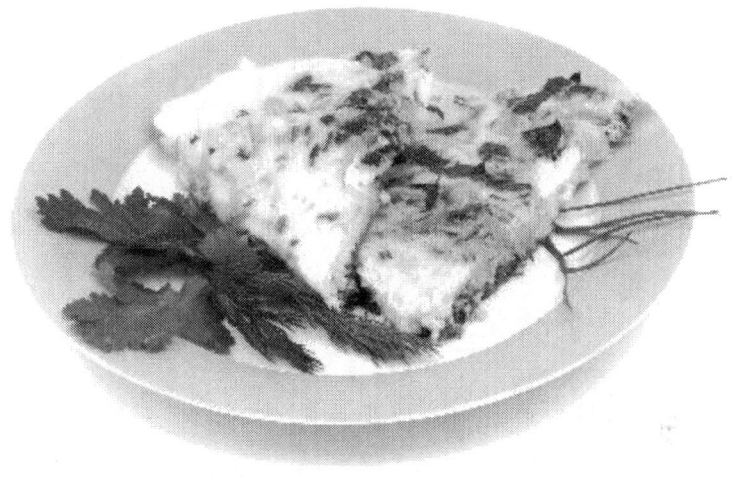

Egg pizza crust

Ingredients - Allergies: SF, GF, DF, NF

- 3 eggs
- 1/2 cup of coconut flour
- 1 cup of coconut milk
- 1 crushed garlic clove

Mix and make an omelet.

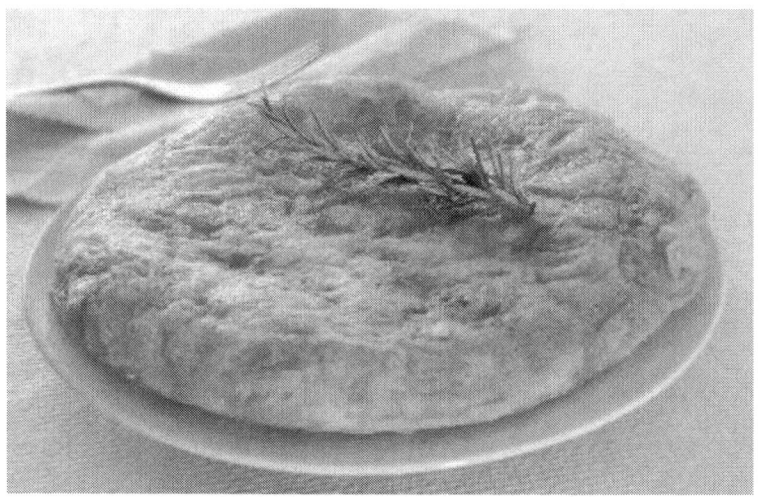

Omelet with Superfoods veggies

Serves 1

Ingredients - Allergies: SF, GF, DF, NF

- 2 large eggs
- Salt
- Ground black pepper
- 1 tsp. olive oil or cumin oil
- 1 cup spinach, cherry tomatoes and 1 spoon of yogurt cheese
- Crushed red pepper flakes and a pinch of dill (optional)

Instructions

Whisk 2 large eggs in a small bowl. Season with salt and ground black pepper and set aside. Heat 1 tsp. olive oil in a skillet over medium/high heat. Add baby spinach, tomatoes, cheese and cook, tossing, until wilted (Approx. 1 minute). Add eggs; cook, stirring occasionally, until just set, about 1 minute. Stir in cheese. Sprinkle with crushed red pepper flakes and dill.

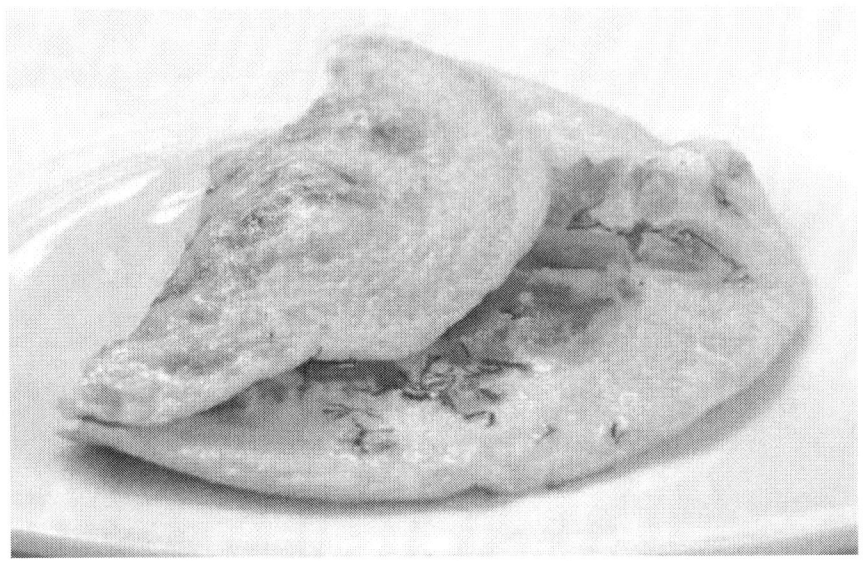

Egg Muffins

Ingredients - Allergies: SF, GF, DF, NF

Serving: 8 muffins

- 8 eggs
- 1 cup diced green bell pepper
- 1 cup diced onion
- 1 cup spinach
- 1/4 tsp. salt
- 1/8 tsp. ground black pepper
- 2 tbsp. water

Instructions

Heat the oven to 350 degrees F. Oil 8 muffin cups. Beat eggs together. Mix in bell pepper, spinach, onion, salt, black pepper, and water. Pour that mixture in the muffin cups. Bake in the oven until muffins are done in the middle.

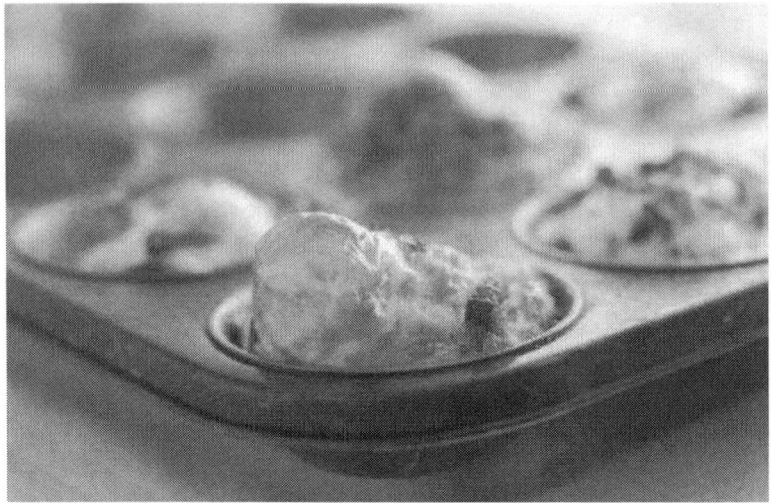

Smoked Salmon Scrambled Eggs

Ingredients, serves 2 - Allergies: SF, GF, DF, NF

- 1 tsp <u>coconut</u> oil
- 4 eggs
- 1 Tbs water
- 4 oz smoked salmon, sliced
- 1/2 avocado
- ground black pepper, to taste
- 4 chives, minced (or use 1 green onion, thinly sliced)

Instructions

Heat a skillet over medium heat. Add oil to a pan when hot. Meanwhile, scramble eggs. Add scrambled eggs to the hot skillet, along with smoked salmon. Stirring continuously, cook scrambled eggs until soft & fluffy.

Remove from heat. Top with avocado, black pepper, and chives to serve.

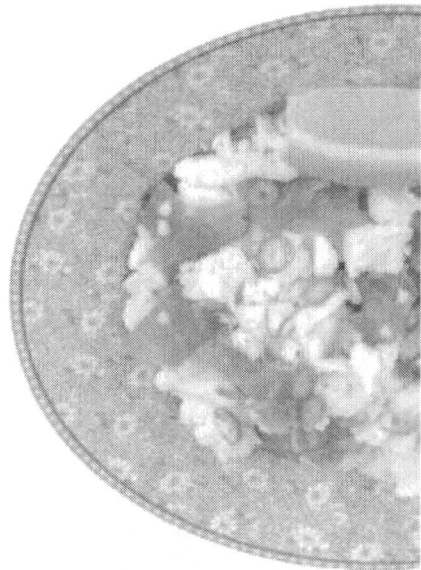

Steak and Eggs

Serves 2

Ingredients - Allergies: SF, GF, DF, NF

- 1/2 lb boneless beef steak or pork tenderloin
- 1/4 tsp ground black pepper
- 1/4 tsp sea salt (optional)
- 2 tsp coconut oil
- 1/4 onion, diced
- 1 red bell pepper, diced
- 1 handful spinach or arugula
- 2 eggs

Instructions

Season sliced steak or pork tenderloin with sea salt & black pepper. Heat a sauté pan over high heat. Add 1 tsp coconut oil, onions, and meat when pan is hot, and sauté until steak is slightly cooked. Add spinach and red bell pepper, and cook until steak is done to your liking. Meanwhile, heat a small fry pan over medium/high heat. Add remaining coconut oil, and fry two eggs. Top each steak with a fried egg to serve.

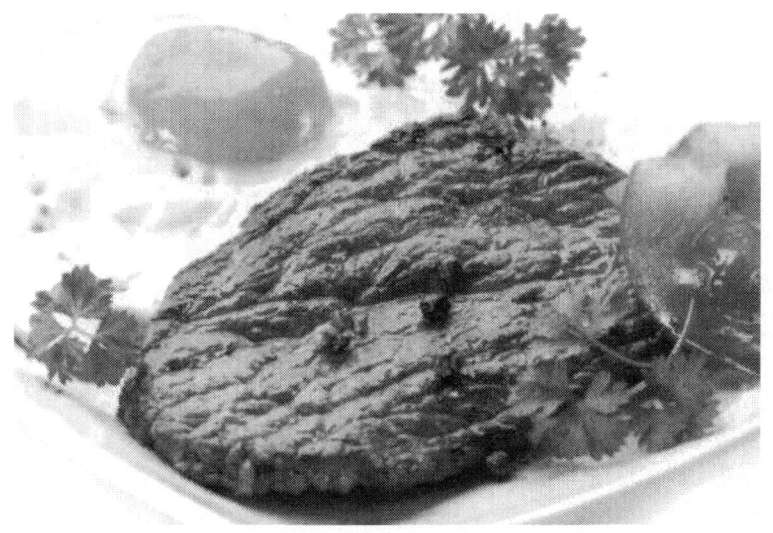

Egg Bake

Ingredients - Allergies: SF, GF, DF, NF

Serves 6

- 2 cups chopped red peppers or spinach
- 1 cup zucchini
- 2 tbsp. coconut oil
- 1 cup sliced mushrooms
- 1/2 cup sliced green onions
- 8 eggs
- 1 cup coconut milk
- 1/2 cup almond flour
- 2 tbsp. minced fresh parsley
- 1/2 tsp. dried basil
- 1/2 tsp. salt
- 1/4 tsp. ground black pepper

Instructions

Preheat oven to 350 degrees F. Put coconut oil in a skillet. Heat it to medium heat. Add mushrooms, onions, zucchini and red pepper (or spinach) until vegetables are tender, about 5 minutes. Drain veggies and spread them over the baking dish.

Beat eggs in a bowl with milk, flour, parsley, basil, salt, and pepper. Pour egg mixture into baking dish.

Bake in preheated oven until the center is set (approx. 35 to 40 minutes).

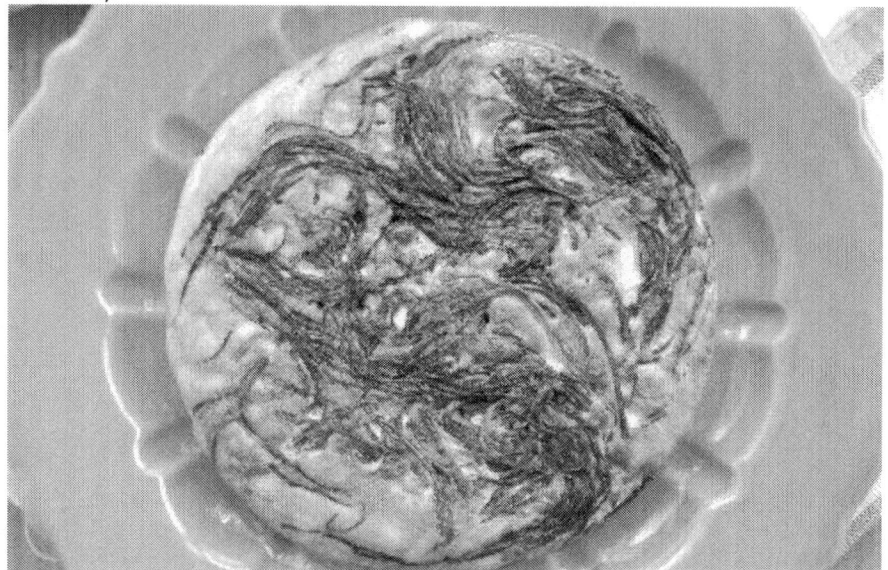

Frittata

6 servings

Ingredients - Allergies: SF, GF, DF, NF

- 2 tbsp. olive oil or avocado oil
- 1 Zucchini, sliced
- 1 cup torn fresh spinach
- 2 tbsp. sliced green onions
- 1 tsp. crushed garlic, salt and pepper to taste
- 1/3 cup coconut milk
- 6 eggs

Instructions

Heat olive oil in a skillet over medium heat. Add zucchini and cook until tender. Mix in spinach, green onions, and garlic. Season with salt and pepper. Continue cooking until spinach is wilted.

In a separate bowl, beat together eggs and coconut milk. Pour into the skillet over the vegetables. Reduce heat to low, cover, and cook until eggs are firm (5 to 7 minutes).

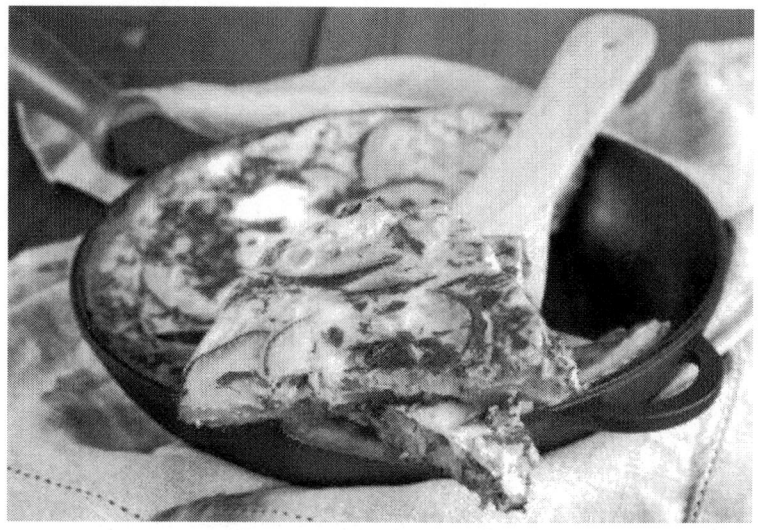

Superfoods Naan / Pancakes / Crepes

Ingredients - Allergies: SF, GF, DF, EF, V

- 1/2 cup <u>almond</u> flour
- 1/2 cup Tapioca Flour
- 1 cup Coconut Milk
- Salt
- <u>coconut</u> oil

Instructions

Mix all the ingredients together.

Heat a pan over medium/high heat and pour batter to desired thickness. Once the batter looks firm, flip it over to cook the other side.

If you want this to be a dessert crepe or pancake, then omit the salt. You can add minced garlic or ginger in the batter if you want, or some spices.

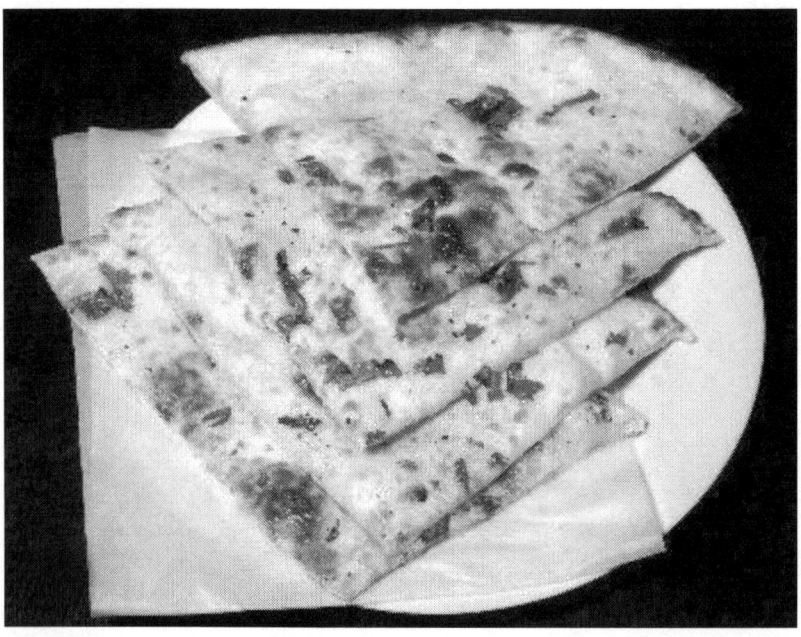

Zucchini Pancakes

Serves 3

Ingredients - Allergies: SF, GF, DF

- 2 medium zucchini
- 2 tbsp. chopped onion
- 3 beaten eggs
- 6 to 8 tbsp. almond flour
- 1 tsp. salt
- 1/2 tsp. ground black pepper
- coconut oil

Instructions

Heat the oven to 300 degrees F.

Grate the zucchini into a bowl and stir in the onion and eggs. Stir in 6 tbsp. of the flour, salt, and pepper.

Heat a large pan over medium/high heat & add coconut oil in the pan. When the oil is hot, lower the heat to medium-low and add batter into the pan. Cook the pancakes about 2 minutes on each side, until browned. Place the pancakes in the oven.

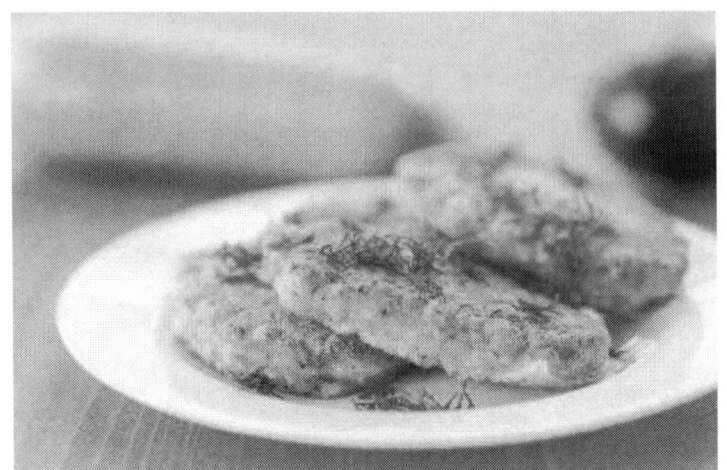

Cottage Cheese Sesame Balls

Ingredients - Allergies: SF, GF, EF

- 16 ounce farmers cheese or cottage cheese
- 1 cup finely chopped almonds
- 1and 1/2 cups oatmeal

In a large bowl, combine blended cottage cheese, almonds and oatmeal. Make balls and roll in sesame seeds mix.

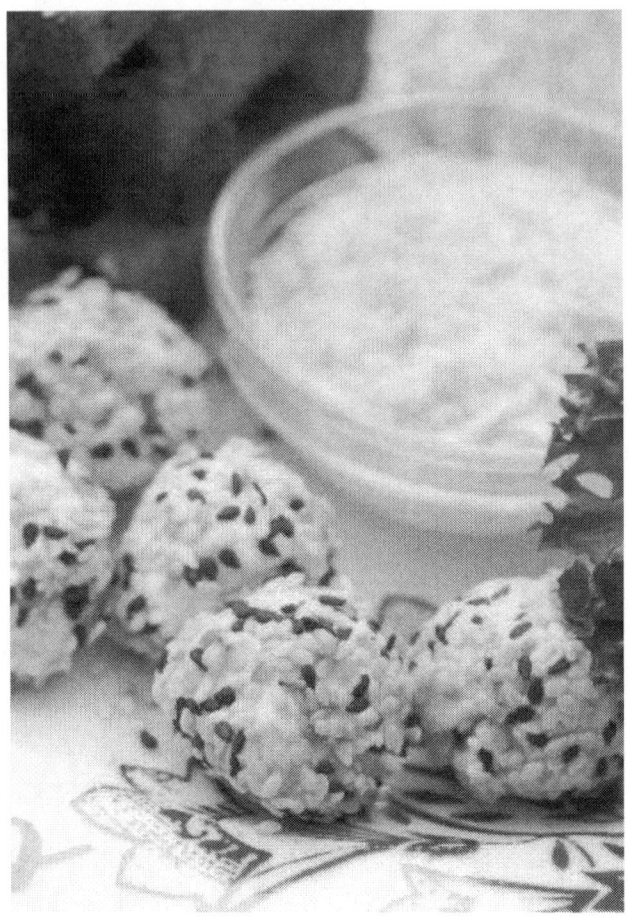

Frittata with Carrots, Green Peas and Asparagus
Serves 1

Ingredients - Allergies: SF, GF, DF, NF

- 2 large eggs
- Salt
- Ground black pepper
- 1 tsp. olive oil or avocado oil
- 1/2 cup cooked green peas
- 1/2 cup chopped carrot
- 1/2 cup asparagus
- 1 tbsp. fresh dill

Instructions

Whisk 2 large eggs in a small bowl. Season with salt and ground black pepper and set aside. Heat 1 tsp. oil in a skillet over medium/high heat. Add carrots and asparagus and cook, tossing, approx. 5 minutes. Add cooked and drained green peas. Add eggs; cook, stirring occasionally, until just set, about 1 minute. Sprinkle with dill.

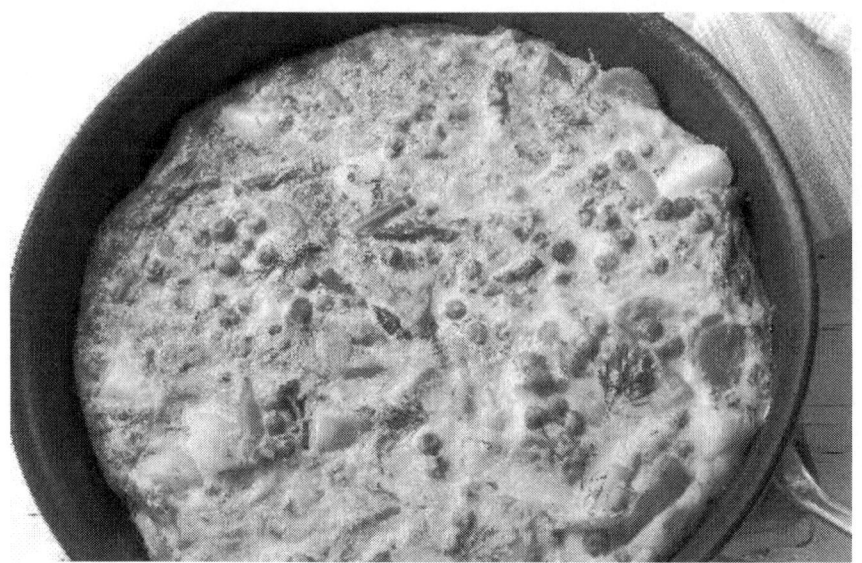

Frittata with Asparagus and Tomato
Serves 1

Ingredients - Allergies: SF, GF, DF, NF

- 2 large eggs
- Salt
- Ground black pepper
- 1 tsp. olive oil or avocado oil
- 1 cup asparagus
- 1/2 cup sliced tomatoes

Instructions

Whisk 2 large eggs in a small bowl. Season with salt and ground black pepper and set aside. Heat 1 tsp. oil in a skillet over medium/high heat. Add asparagus and cook, tossing approx. 4-5 minutes. Add tomatoes and eggs and cook, stirring occasionally, until just set, about 1 minute. Sprinkle with dill (optional).

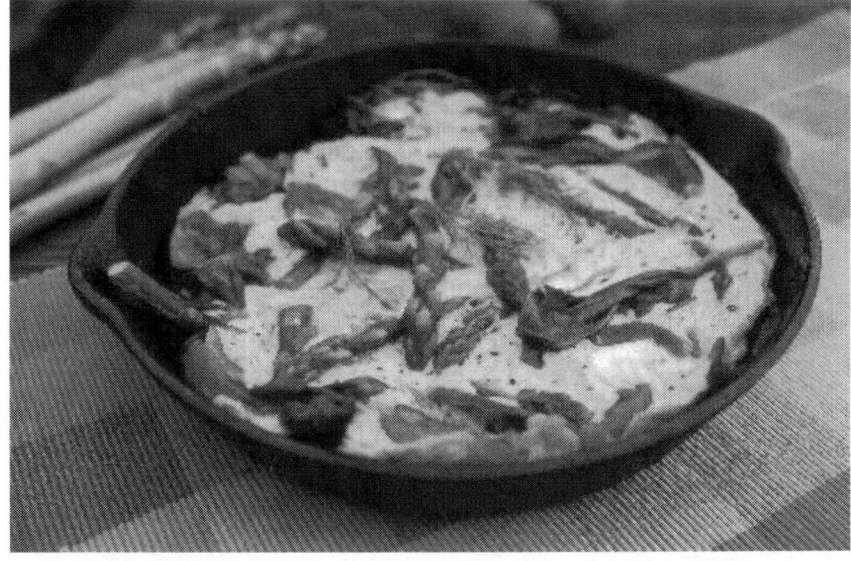

Leeks, Spinach, Eggs & Yogurt

Serves 1

Ingredients - Allergies: SF, GF, DF, NF

- 2 large eggs
- Salt
- Ground black pepper
- 1 tsp. olive oil or avocado oil
- 1/2 cup sliced leeks
- 1/3 cup spinach
- 1/3 cup thick Greek yogurt

Instructions

Heat 1 tsp. olive oil in a skillet over medium/high heat. Add leeks and coook for 5 minutes. Add spinach, salt and pepper and cook, tossing, until wilted (Approx. 1 minute). Break eggs on top and fry until done. Top with yogurt.

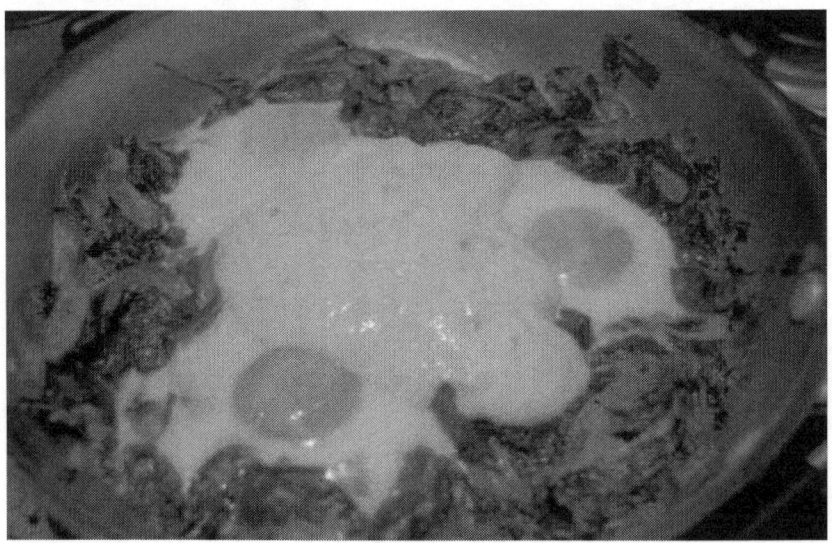

Broccoli Frittata

Serves 1

Ingredients - Allergies: SF, GF, DF, NF

- 2 large eggs
- Salt
- Ground black pepper
- 1 tsp. olive oil or avocado oil
- 1 cup Broccoli

Instructions

Whisk 2 large eggs in a small bowl. Season with salt and ground black pepper and set aside. Heat 1 tsp. olive oil in a skillet over medium/high heat. Add broccoli and cook, tossing, approx. 4-5 minutes. Add eggs; cook, stirring occasionally, until just set.

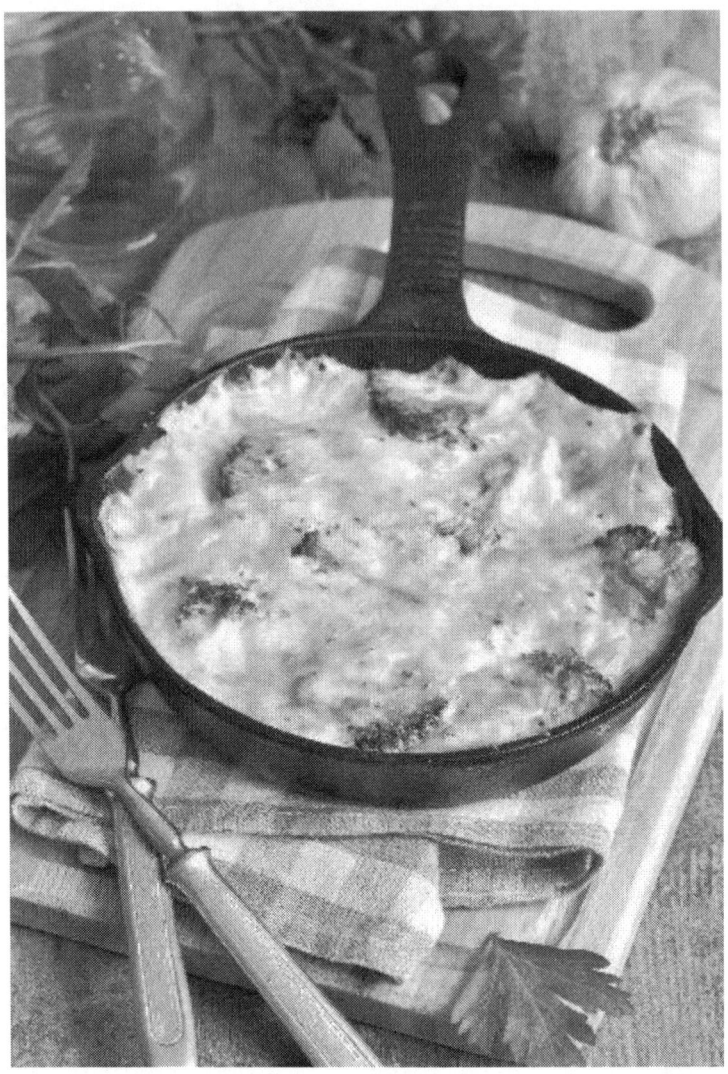

Superfoods Smoothies

Put the liquid in first. Surrounded by tea or yogurt, the blender blades can move freely. Next, add chunks of fruits or vegetables. Leafy greens are going into the pitcher last. Preferred liquid is green tea, but you can use almond or coconut milk or herbal tea.

Start slow. If your blender has speeds, start it on low to break up big pieces of fruit. Continue blending until you get a puree. If your blender can pulse, pulse a few times before switching to a puree mode. Once you have your liquid and fruit pureed, start adding greens, very slowly. Wait until previous batch of greens has been completely blended. I use blenders because they're sturdy and offer 7 year warranty. That was definitely the best investment in my health.

Thicken? Added too much tea or coconut milk? Thicken your smoothie by adding ice cubes, flax meal, chia seeds or oatmeal. Once you get used to various tastes of smoothies, add any seaweed, spirulina, chlorella powder or ginger for additional kick. Experiment with any Superfoods in powder form at this point. Think of adding any nut butter or sesame paste too or some Superfoods oils.

Rotate! Rotate your greens; don't always drink the same smoothie! At the beginning try 2 different greens every week and later introduce third and fourth one weekly. And keep rotating them. Don't use spinach and kale all the time. Try beets greens, they have a pinch of pink in them and that add great color to your smoothie. Here is the list of leafy green for you to try: spinach, kale, dandelion, chards, beet leaves, arugula, lettuce, collard greens, bok choy, cabbage, cilantro, parsley.

Flavor! Flavor smoothies with ground vanilla bean, cinnamon, ½ tsp. of lucuma powder, nutmeg, cloves, almond butter, cayenne pepper, ginger or just about any seeds or chopped nuts combination.

Not only are green smoothies high in nutrients, vitamins and fiber, they can also make any vegetable you probably don't like (be it kale, spinach or broccoli) taste great. The secret behind blending the perfect smoothie is using sweet fruits or nuts or seeds to give your drink a unique taste.

There's a reason kale and spinach seem to be the main ingredients in almost every green smoothie. Not only do they give smoothies their verdant color, they are also packed with calcium, protein and iron.

Although blending alone increases the accessibility of carotenoids, since the presence of fats is known to increase carotenoid absorption from leafy greens, it is possible that coconut oil, nuts and seeds in a smoothie could increase absorption further.

Fruits and Veggies preparation

- Wash fruits and veggies
- Pluck leaves and stems from berries
- Core apples (optional)
- Peel orange, lemon, lime, grapefruit, kiwi, beet, pomegranate, ginger, dragon fruit and banana
- Peel and take the seeds out of papaya
- Remove seeds from peppers, apricots, peaches, cherries, plums and prunes
- Mangos, melons and avocados should be peeled, and inner seed taken out
- Watermelons should have their outer rind removed.
- Scoop out the flesh from passion fruit
- Cut fruits and veggies in 2-inch slices

If you can't find some ingredient, replace it with the closest one.

All details about each ingredient (vitamins, minerals, antioxidants etc.) can be found in my free Superfoods Reference book:
http://superfoodstoday.com/Free

GREEN SMOOTHIES

Kale Kiwi Smoothie

- 1 cup Kale, chopped

- 2 Apples

- 3 Kiwis

- 1 tablespoon <u>flax</u> seeds

- 1 tablespoon royal jelly

- 1 cup crushed ice

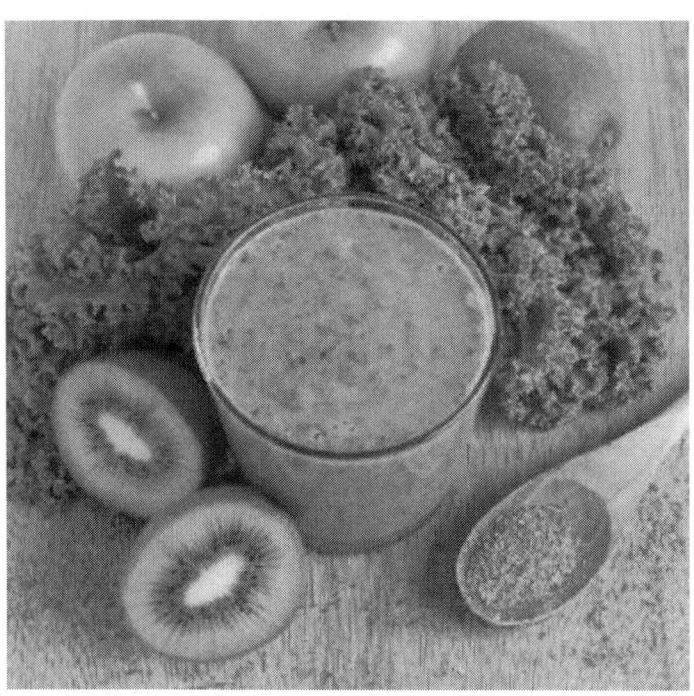

Zucchini Apples Smoothie

- 1/2 cup zucchini
- 2 Apples
- 3/4 avocado
- 1 stalk Celery
- 1 Lemon
- 1 tbsp. Spirulina
- 1 1/2 cups crushed ice

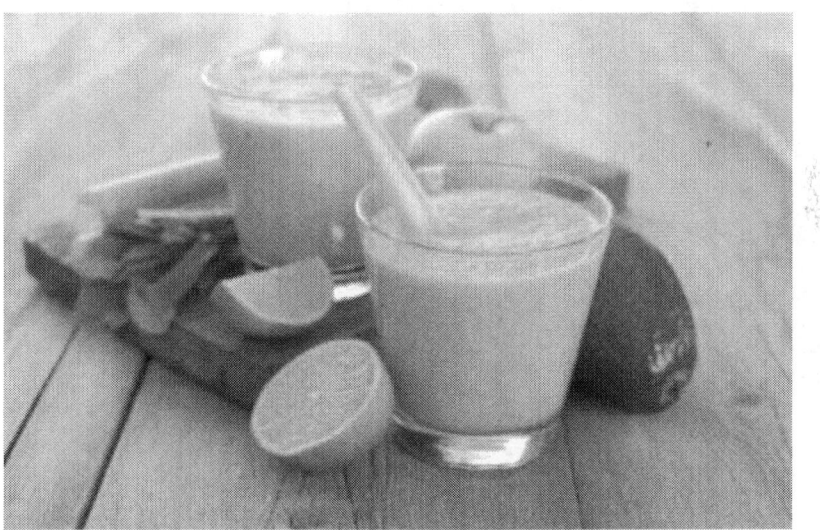

Dandelion Smoothie

- 1 cup Dandelion greens
- 1 cup Spinach
- ½ cup tahini
- 1 Red Radish
- 1 tbsp. chia seeds
- 1 cup lavender tea

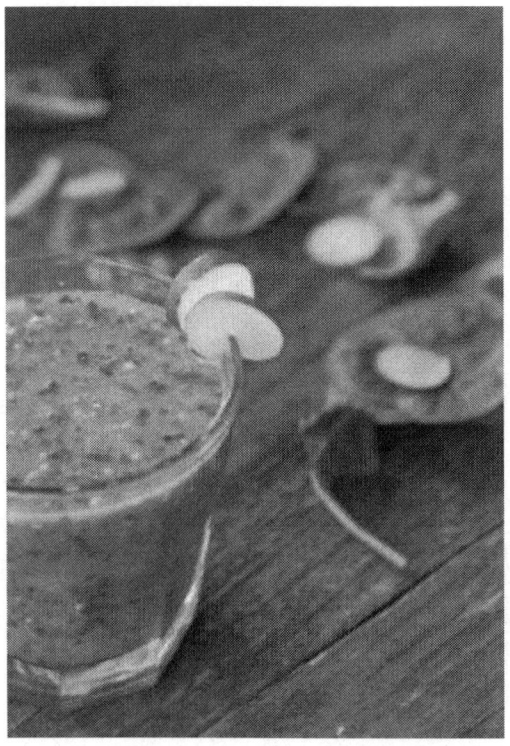

Fennel Honeydew Smoothie

- ½ cup fennel

- 1 cup Broccoli

- 1 tbsp. Cilantro

- 1 cup Honeydew

- 1 cup crushed ice

- 1 tbsp. Chlorella

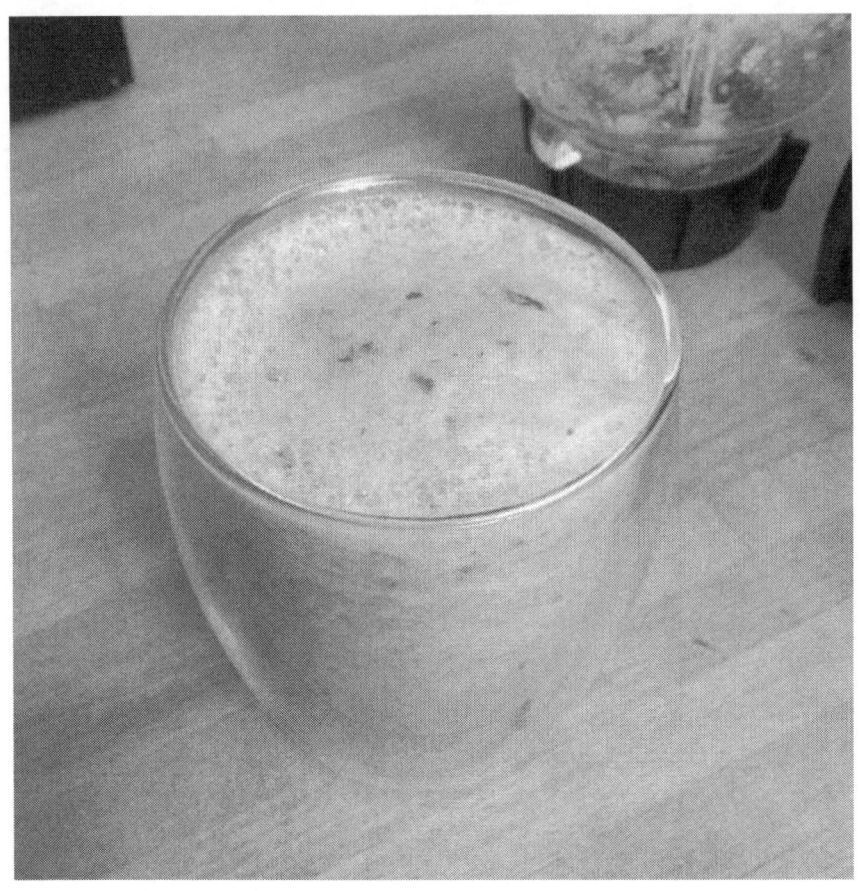

Broccoli Apple Smoothie

- 1 Apple
- 1 cup Broccoli
- 1 tbsp. Cilantro
- 1 Celery stalk
- 1 cup crushed ice
- 1 tbsp. crushed Seaweed

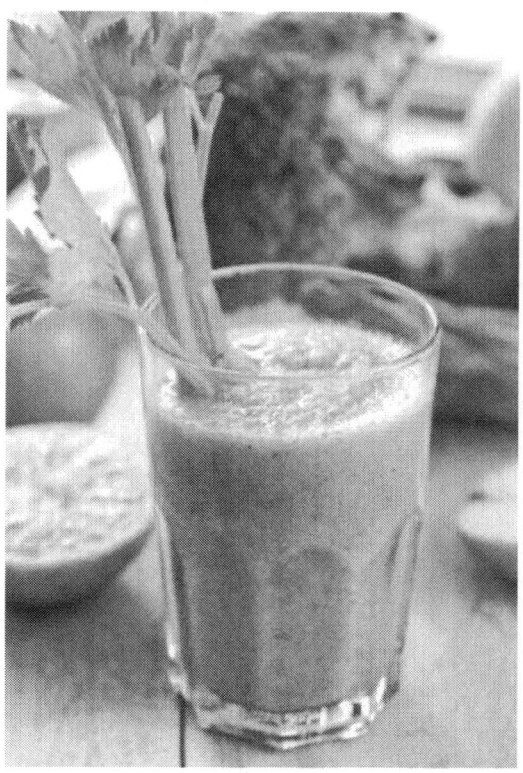

Salad Smoothie

- 1 cup spinach
- ½ cucumber
- 1/2 small onion
- 2 tablespoons Parsley
- 2 tablespoons lemon juice
- 1 cup crushed ice
- 1 tbsp. olive oil or cumin oil
- ¼ cup Wheatgrass

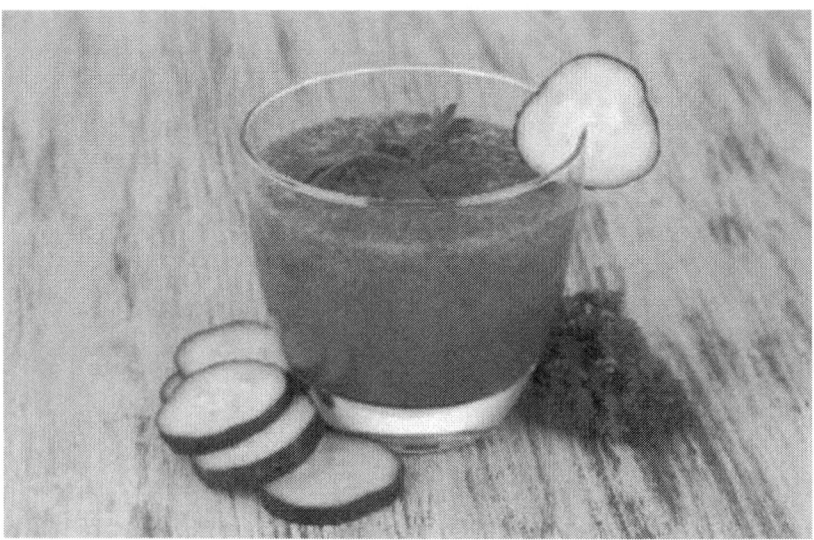

Avocado Kale Smoothie

- 1 cup Kale
- ½ Avocado
- 1 cup Cucumber
- 1 Celery Stalk
- 1 tbsp. chia seeds
- 1 cup chamomile tea
- 1 tbsp. Spirulina

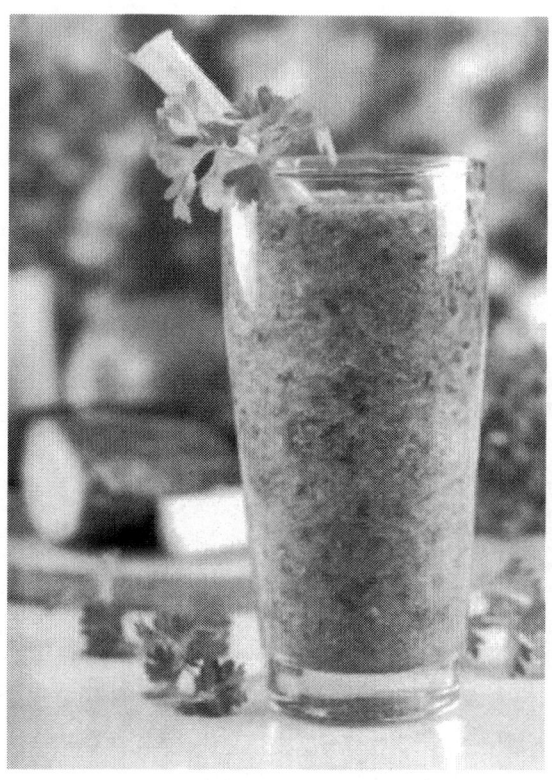

Watercress Smoothie

- 1 cup Watercress
- ½ cup almond butter
- 2 small cucumbers
- 1 cup coconut milk
- 1 tbsp. Chlorella
- 1 tbsp. Black cumin seeds – sprinkle on top and garnish with parsley

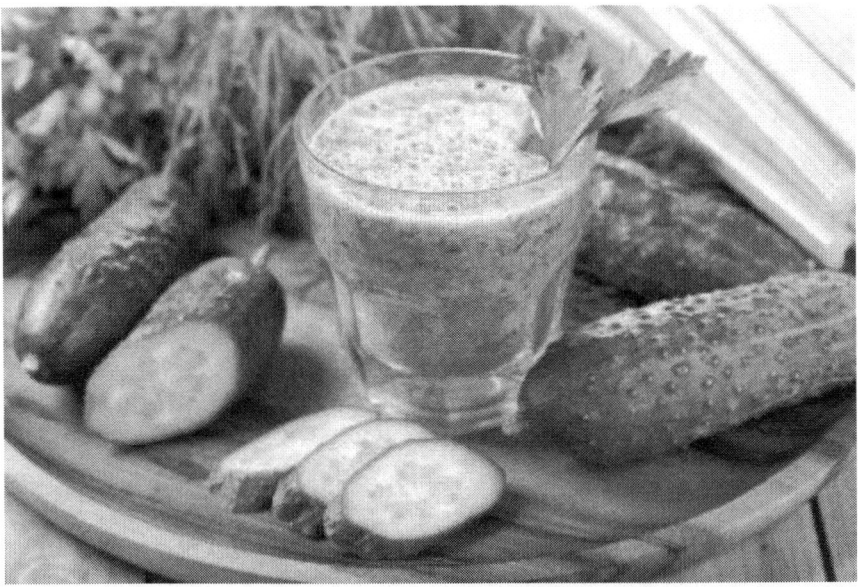

Beet Greens Smoothie

- 1 cup Beet Greens

- 2 tbsp. Pumpkin seeds butter

- 1 cup Strawberry

- 1 tbsp. Sesame seeds

- 1 tbsp. hemp seeds

- 1 cup chamomile tea

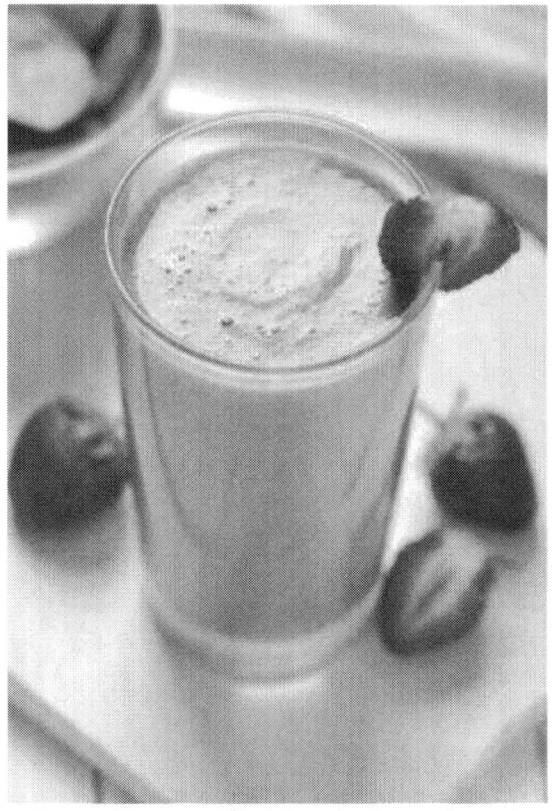

Broccoli Leeks Cucumber smoothie

- 1 cup Broccoli
- 2 tbsp. Cashew butter
- 2 Leeks
- 2 Cucumbers
- 1 Lime
- ½ cup Lettuce
- ½ cup Leaf Lettuce
- 1 tbsp. Matcha
- 1 cup crushed ice

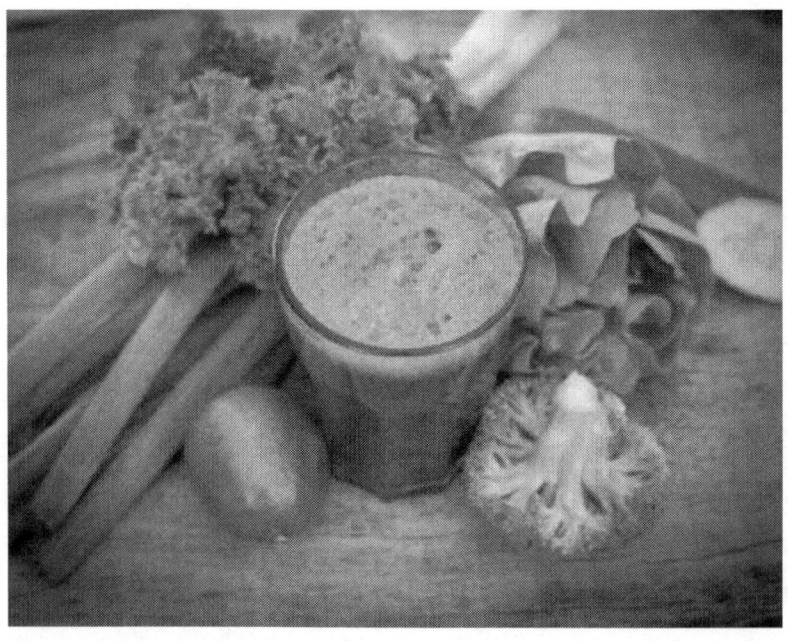

Cacao Spinach Smoothie

- 2 cups spinach
- 1 cup blueberries, frozen
- 1 tablespoons dark cocoa powder
- ½ cup unsweetened almond milk
- 1/2 cup crushed ice
- 1 tsp lucuma powder
- 1 tbsp. Matcha powder

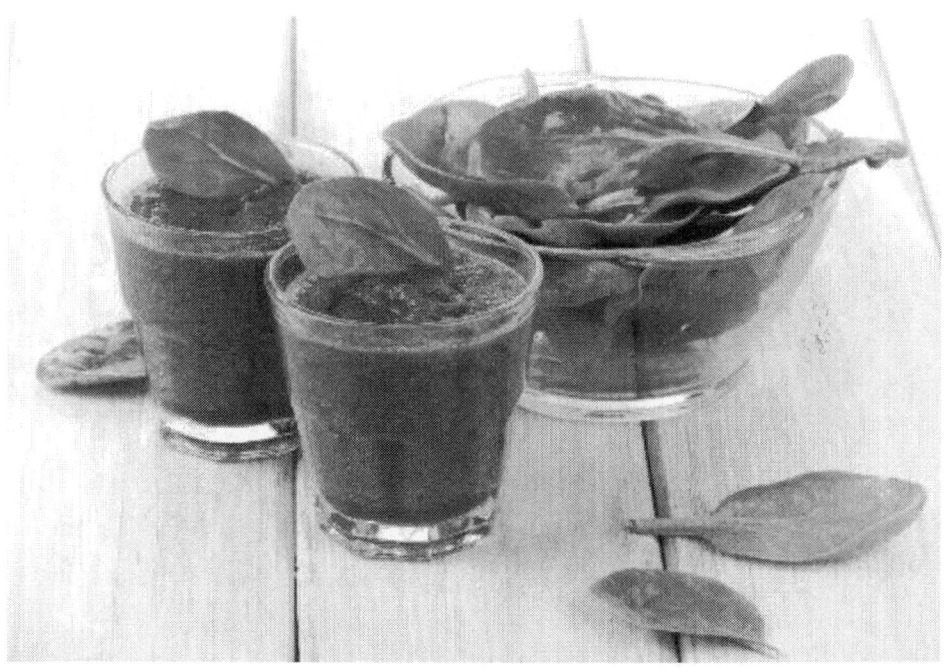

Flax Almond Butter Smoothie

- ½ cup plain yogurt
- 2 tablespoons almond butter
- 2 cups spinach
- 1 banana, frozen
- 3 strawberries
- 1/2 cup crushed ice
- 1 teaspoon flax seeds

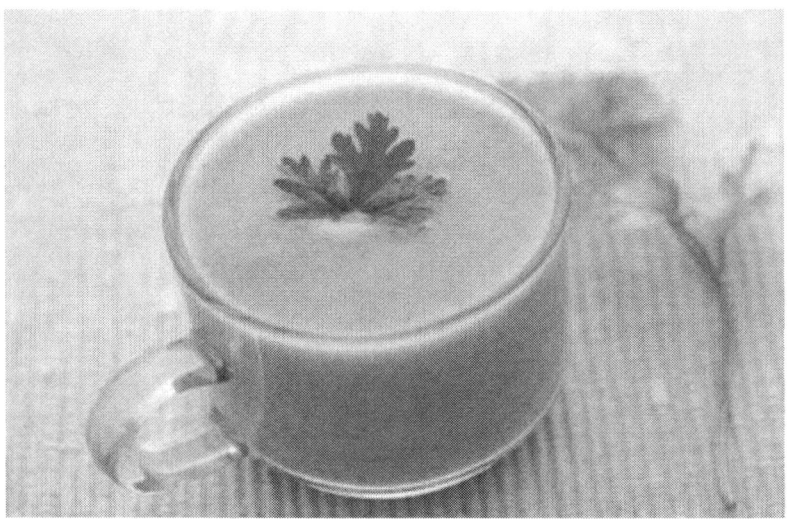

Apple Kale Smoothie

- 1 cup kale
- ½ cup coconut milk
- 1 tbsp. Maca
- 1 banana, frozen
- ¼ teaspoon cinnamon
- 1 Apple
- Pinch of nutmeg
- 1 clove
- 3 ice cubes

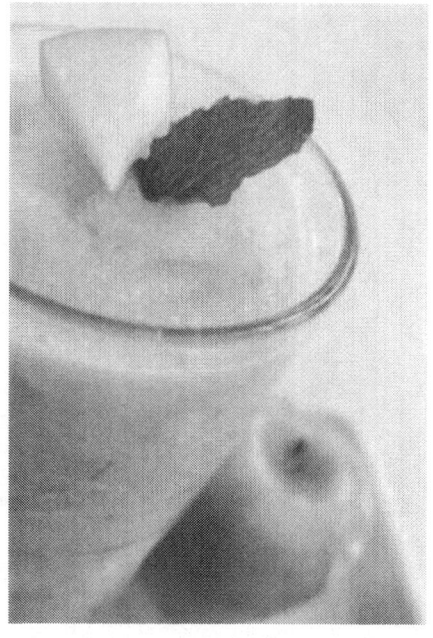

Rainbow Smoothie

3 Colors Rainbow Smoothie
- Blend 1 Large beet with some crushed ice

- Blend 3 carrots with some crashed ice

- Blend 1 cucumber, 1 cup of leaf lettuce and ½ cup Wheatgrass

- Serve them separate to preserve the distinct color

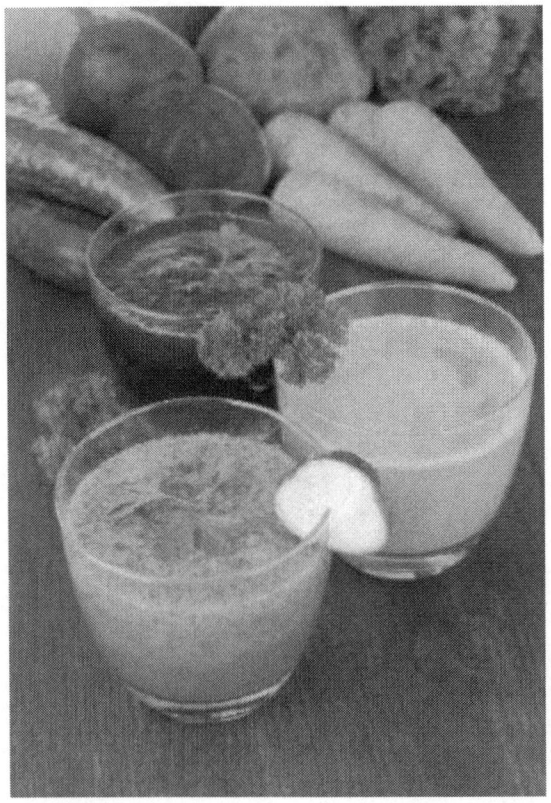

Salad Dressings

Italian Dressing

Serves 1 - Allergies: SF, GF, DF, EF, V, NF

- 1 tsp. olive oil or cumin oil
- lemon
- minced garlic
- salt
- 1 Tbsp. of Spirulina, Chlorella, Maca or Matcha (optional)

Yogurt Dressing

Serves 1 - Allergies: SF, GF, DF, EF, V, NF

- half a cup of plain low-fat Greek yogurt or low-fat buttermilk
- olive oil or avocado oil
- minced garlic
- salt
- lemon

Occasionally I would add a tsp. of mustard or some herbs like basil, oregano, marjoram, chives, thyme, parsley, dill or mint. If you like spicy hot food, add some cayenne in the dressing. It will speed up your metabolism and have interesting hot spicy effect in cold yogurt or buttermilk.

Salads

Large Fiber Loaded Salad with Italian Dressing

Serves 1 - Allergies: SF, GF, EF, NF

- 1 cup of spinach
- 1 cup of shredded cabbage, sauerkraut or lettuce. Cabbage has more substance.
- Italian or Yogurt dressing
- Cayenne pepper (optional)
- Few sprigs of cilantro (optional)
- 2 spring (green) onions (optional)

Nutrition Facts

Serving Size 105 g

Amount Per Serving

Calories 64	Calories from Fat 44
	% Daily Value*
Total Fat 4.9g	**7%**
Saturated Fat 0.7g	**4%**
Cholesterol 0mg	**0%**
Sodium 36mg	**2%**
Potassium 286mg	**8%**
Total Carbohydrates 5.1g	**2%**
Dietary Fiber 2.4g	**10%**
Sugars 2.4g	
Protein 1.8g	
Vitamin A 58%	Vitamin C 57%
Calcium 6%	Iron 6%

Nutrition Grade A

* Based on a 2000 calorie diet

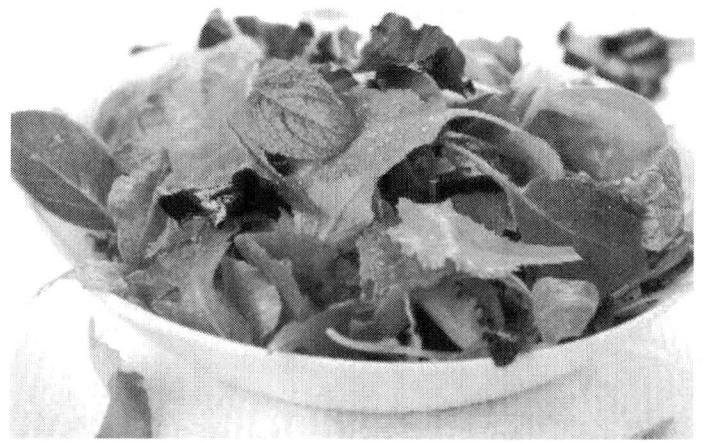

Large Fiber Loaded Salad with Yogurt Dressing

Serves 1 - Allergies: SF, GF, EF, NF

- 1 cup of spinach
- 1 cup of shredded cabbage or lettuce. Cabbage has more substance.
- Italian or Yogurt dressing
- Cayenne pepper (optional)
- Few sprigs of cilantro (optional)
- 2 spring (green) onions (optional)

Nutrition Facts

Serving Size 226 g

Amount Per Serving

Calories 136	Calories from Fat 40
	% Daily Value*
Total Fat 4.5g	7%
Saturated Fat 1.7g	8%
Cholesterol 7mg	2%
Sodium 122mg	5%
Potassium 573mg	16%
Total Carbohydrates 13.8g	5%
Dietary Fiber 2.4g	10%
Sugars 11.0g	
Protein 8.7g	
Vitamin A 59%	Vitamin C 58%
Calcium 28%	Iron 7%

Nutrition Grade A

* Based on a 2000 calorie diet

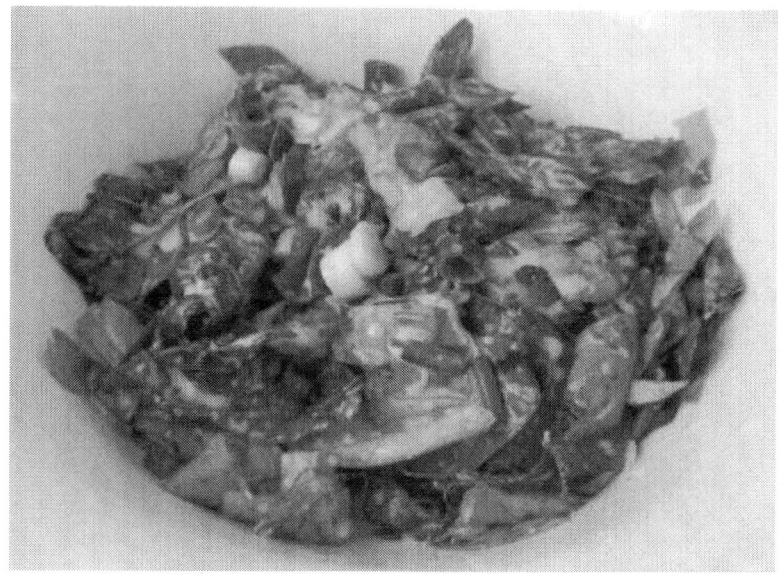

Large Fiber Loaded Salad as a meal on its own – only 258 calories per serving

Serves 1 - Allergies: SF, GF, EF, NF

This is what I eat every second evening and I can't get enough of it!!! This is the real secret to lose weight while having full stomach with grade A ingredients!!

- 1 cup of spinach
- 1 cup of shredded cabbage
- Yogurt dressing
- Cayenne pepper (optional)
- Few sprigs of cilantro (optional)
- 2 spring (green) onions
- 5 oz. low-fat farmers cheese

Pour yogurt dressing into the salad bowl. Add farmers' cheese and mix thoroughly. Cut spring onions in small pieces and add to the cheese mixture and mix. Add spinach and cabbage and mix thoroughly. Add spices (optional).

FOOD FOR DIABETICS

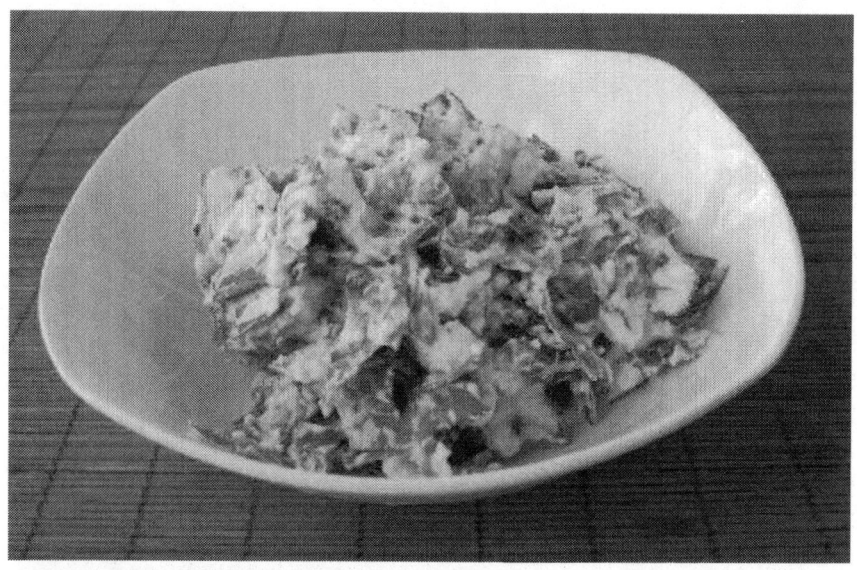

Nutrition Facts

Serving Size 401 g

Amount Per Serving

Calories 258	Calories from Fat 62
	% Daily Value*
Total Fat 6.8g	**11%**
Saturated Fat 2.0g	**10%**
Cholesterol 7mg	**2%**
Sodium 708mg	**30%**
Potassium 656mg	**19%**
Total Carbohydrates 21.5g	**7%**
Dietary Fiber 3.2g	**13%**
Sugars 15.9g	
Protein 26.6g	
Vitamin A 65% •	Vitamin C 68%
Calcium 30% •	Iron 9%

Nutrition Grade A-

* Based on a 2000 calorie diet

Greek Salad

Serves 4 - Allergies: SF, GF, EF, NF

- 1 head iceberg lettuce
- 1 head romaine lettuce
- 1 lb. plump tomatoes
- 6 oz. Greek or black olives, sliced
- 4 oz. sliced radishes
- 4 oz. low-fat feta or goat cheese
- 2 oz. anchovies (optional)

Dressing:
- 3 oz. olive oil or avocado oil
- 3 oz. fresh lemon juice
- 1 tsp. dried oregano
- 1 tsp. black pepper
- 1 tsp. salt
- 4 cloves garlic, minced

Wash and cut lettuce into pieces. Slice tomatoes in quarters. Combine olives, lettuce, tomatoes, and radishes in large bowl. Mix dressing ingredients together and toss with vegetables. Pour out into a shallow serving bowl. Crumble feta/goat cheese over all, and arrange anchovy fillets on top (if desired).

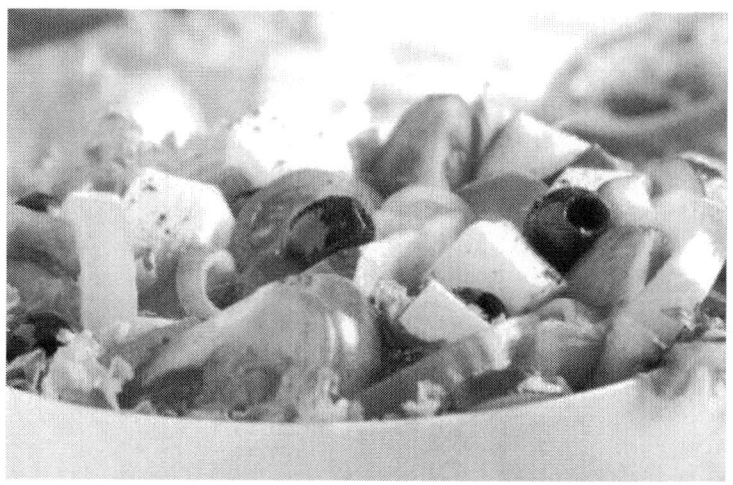

Cucumber, Cilantro, Quinoa Tabbouleh

Serves 2

Ingredients - Allergies: SF, GF, DF, EF, NF, V

- 1 cup cooked quinoa mixed with 1 tbsp. sesame seeds
- 1/2 cup chopped tomato and green pepper
- 1 cup chopped cucumber
- 1/2 cup chopped cilantro

Dressing:
- 1 tbsp. olive oil or cumin oil
- 1 tbsp. fresh lemon juice
- pinch of black pepper
- pinch of sea salt

Instructions: Mix all ingredients.

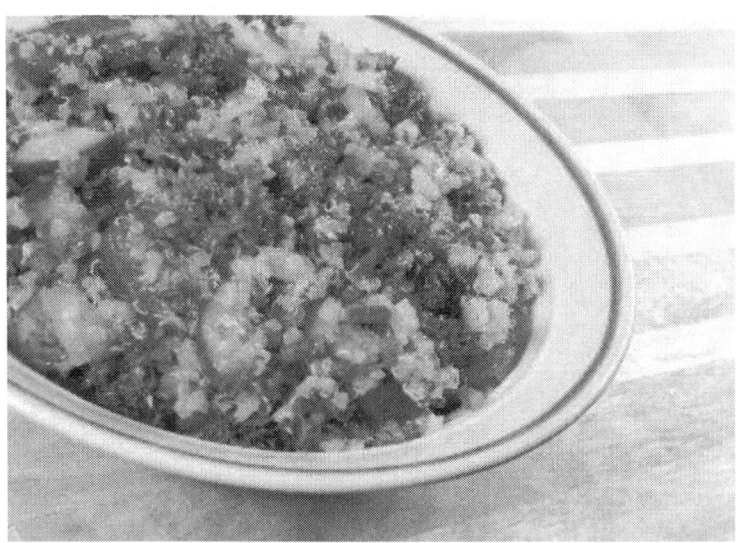

Almond, Quinoa, Red Peppers & Arugula Salad

Serves 2

Ingredients - Allergies: SF, GF, DF, EF, NF, V

- 1 cup cooked quinoa mixed with 1 tbsp. pumpkin seeds
- 1/2 cup chopped almonds
- 1 cup chopped arugula
- 1/2 cup sliced red peppers

Dressing:
- 1 tbsp. olive oil or cumin oil
- 1 tbsp. fresh lemon juice
- pinch of black pepper
- pinch of sea salt

Instructions: Mix all ingredients.

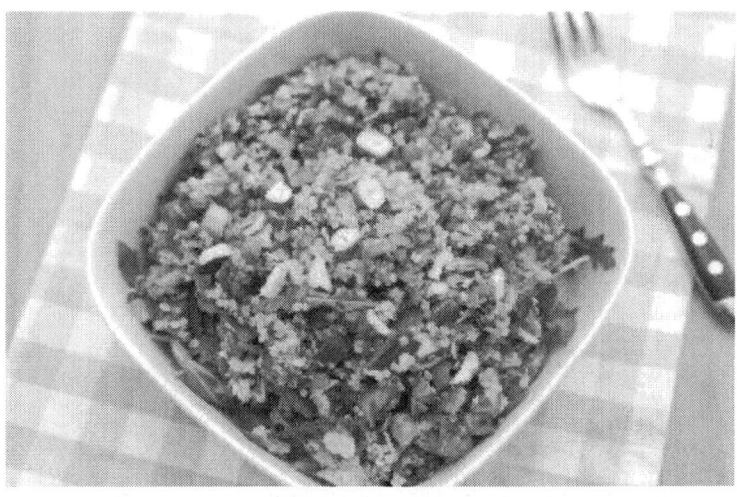

Asparagus, Quinoa & Red Peppers Salad

Serves 2

Ingredients - Allergies: SF, GF, DF, EF, NF, V

- 1 cup cooked quinoa mixed with 1 tbsp. sunflower seeds
- 1 cup sliced red peppers
- 1 cup grilled asparagus
- Garnish with lime and parsley

Dressing:
- 1 tbsp. olive oil or avocado oil
- 1 tbsp. fresh lemon juice
- pinch of black pepper
- pinch of sea salt

Instructions: Mix all ingredients.

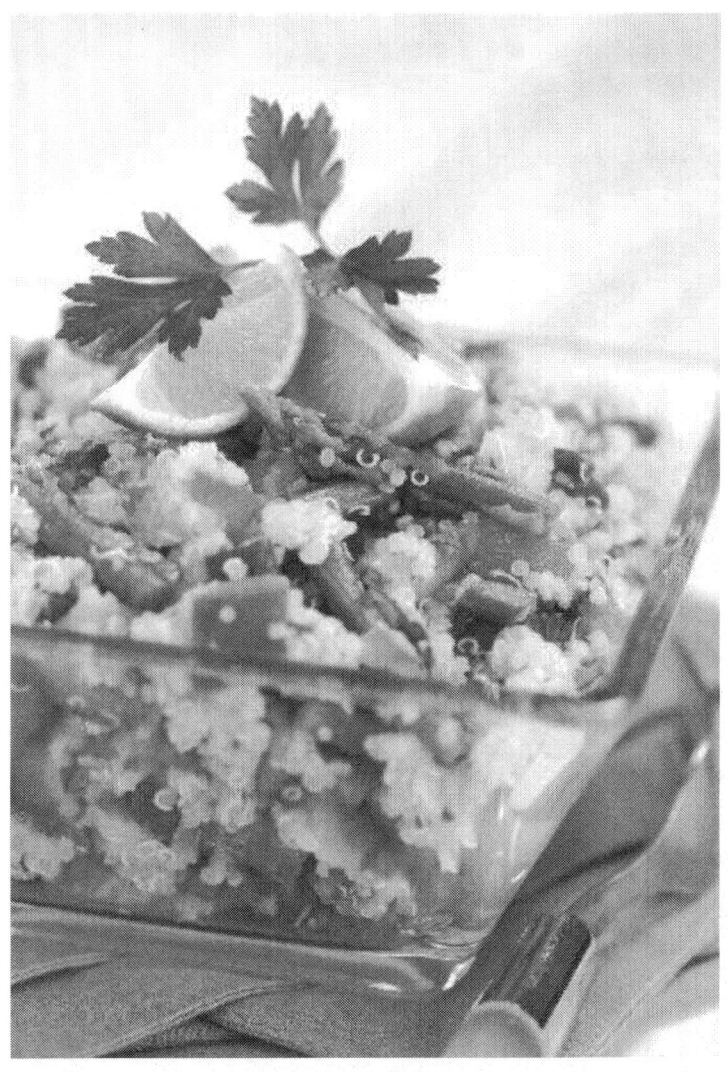

Chickpeas, Quinoa, Cucumber & Tomato Salad

Serves 2

Ingredients - Allergies: SF, GF, DF, EF, NF, V

- 1 cup cooked quinoa mixed with 1 tbsp. sesame seeds
- 1 cup cooked chickpeas
- 1 cup chopped cucumber and green onions
- 1/2 cup chopped tomato

Dressing:
- 1 tbsp. olive oil or avocado oil
- 1 tbsp. fresh lemon juice
- pinch of black pepper
- pinch of sea salt

Instructions: Mix all ingredients.

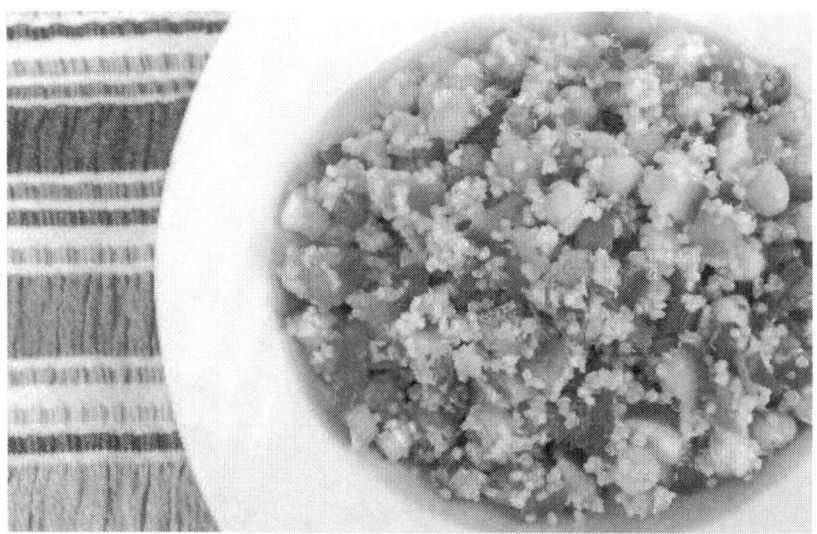

Strawberry Spinach Salad
Serves 4-6

Ingredients - Allergies: SF, GF, DF, EF, V

- 2 tbsp. black sesame seeds
- 1 tbsp. poppy seeds
- 1/2 cup olive oil or avocado oil
- 1/4 cup lemon juice
- 1/4 tsp. paprika
- 1 bag fresh spinach - chopped, washed and dried
- 1 quart strawberries, sliced
- 1/4 cup toasted slivered almonds

Instructions

Whisk together the sesame seeds, olive oil, poppy seeds, paprika, lemon juice and onion. Refrigerate.
In a large bowl, combine the spinach, strawberries and almonds. Pour dressing over salad. Toss and refrigerate 15 minutes before serving.

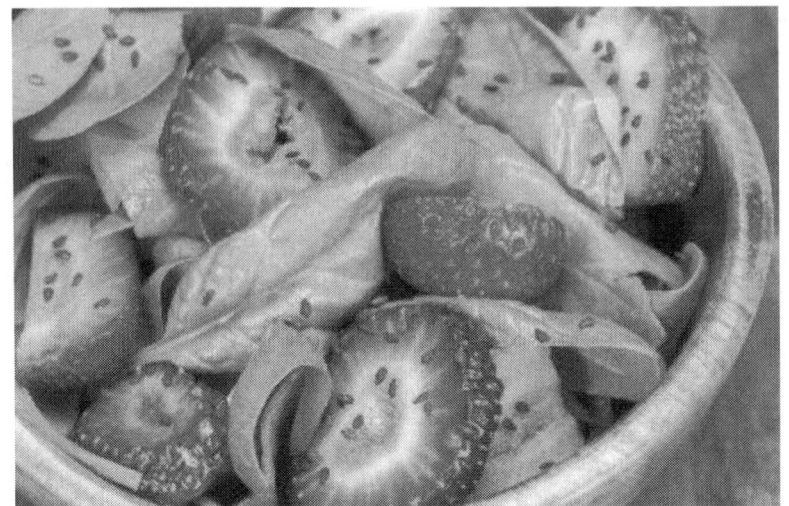

Tuna Bean Salad

Serves 1 - Allergies: SF, GF, DF, EF, NF

Ingredients

- 1 can tuna in water, drained
- 1/3 cup four bean mix (or just white or red beans), drained, rinsed
- 1 tomato, deseeded, chopped
- 1 large celery stick, trimmed, finely chopped
- 1/2 small onion, halved, thinly sliced
- 1/2 cup flat-leaf parsley leaves, chopped
- 1/2 lemon, rind finely grated, juiced
- 1 garlic clove, crushed & 1 tbsp. extra-virgin olive oil

Mix all ingredients and serve.

Nutrition Facts

Serving Size 335 g

Amount Per Serving

Calories 345	Calories from Fat 114
	% Daily Value*
Total Fat 12.6g	**19%**
Saturated Fat 2.3g	**11%**
Trans Fat 0.0g	
Cholesterol 28mg	**9%**
Sodium 115mg	**5%**
Potassium 1191mg	**34%**
Total Carbohydrates 27.1g	**9%**
Dietary Fiber 7.8g	**31%**
Sugars 6.1g	
Protein 31.5g	

Vitamin A 68%	•	Vitamin C 107%
Calcium 9%	•	Iron 29%

Nutrition Grade A

* Based on a 2000 calorie diet

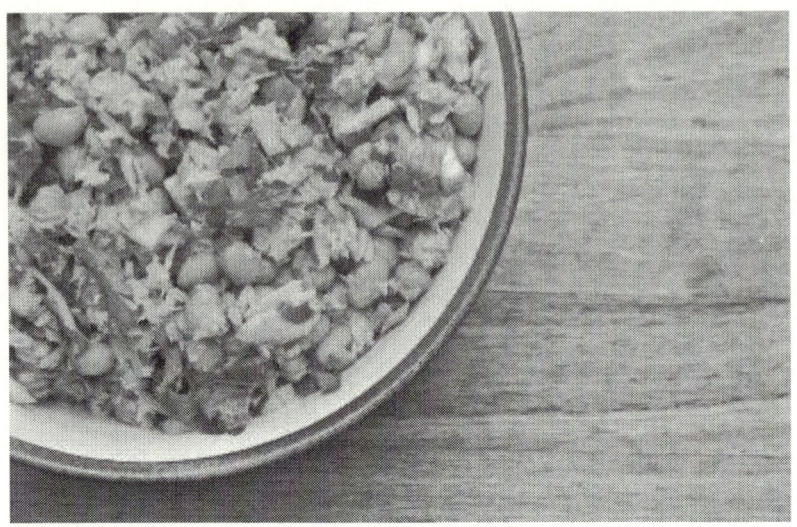

Quinoa Salad

Serves: 6

Ingredients - Allergies: SF, GF, EF

For the salad
- 2 cups cooked quinoa
- 2-3 cups frozen green peas
- 1/2 cup low-fat feta cheese
- 6oz.pork, cubed
- 1/2 cup freshly chopped basil and cilantro
- 1/2 cup almonds, pulsed in a food processor until crushed

For the dressing
- 1/3 cup lemon juice (1-2 large juicy lemons)
- 1/3 cup olive oil or avocado oil
- 1/4 tsp. salt (more to taste)
- a few teaspoons lucuma powder , to taste

Instructions

Bring a pot of water to boil and then lower the heat. Add the peas and cook covered until bright green. In the meantime, brown pork in a skillet. Toss the quinoa with the pork, peas, feta, herbs, and almonds.

Puree all the dressing ingredients in the food processor. Toss the dressing with the salad ingredients. Season generously with salt and pepper. Serve with baby spinach.

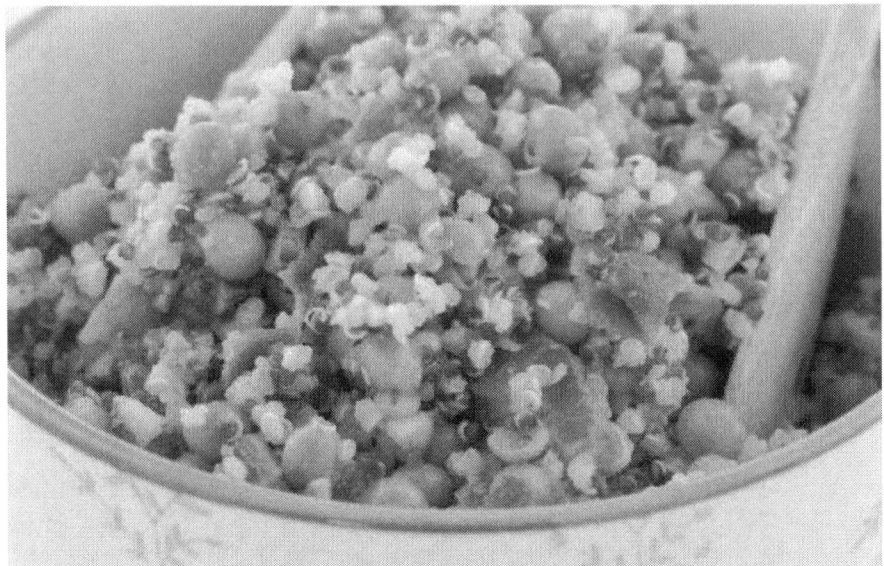

Cauliflower & Eggs Salad

Serves 1

Ingredients - Allergies: SF, GF, NF

- 1 cup chopped Cauliflower
- 2 hardboiled eggs - chopped,
- 2 oz. shredded cheddar cheese, low-fat
- 1 red onion, celery,
- 1 dill pickles,
- 1 tbsp. yellow mustard.

Mix all ingredients.

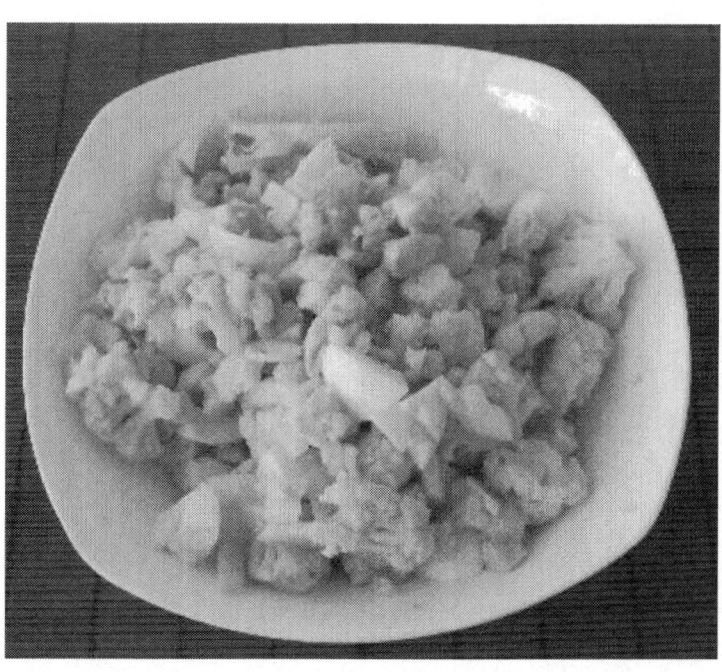

Quinoa & almond Superfoods Tabbouleh

Serves 2-3

Ingredients - Allergies: SF, GF, EF

- 2 cups cooked quinoa
- 1 bunch mint, leaves picked & 1 bunch flat leaf parsley
- 1/2 small red onion, finely chopped
- 1/4 Cup lemon juice& 1/4 Cup extra virgin olive oil or avocado oil
- 1/2 Cup whole almonds & 1/2 cup chia or sunflower seeds
- 1 Cup cherry tomatoes & 1 Avocado optional
- 1 Cup chopped Kale or Dandelion
- Low fat yogurt, to serve, optional

Instructions

Cook quinoa and let it cool. Chop off and discard half of the parsley stalks. Finely chop the remaining parsley bunch, mint and greens. Stir herbs in a salad bowl and add onion to drained quinoa. Combine lemon juice and olive oil and season well. Add other ingredients, mix and dress salad.

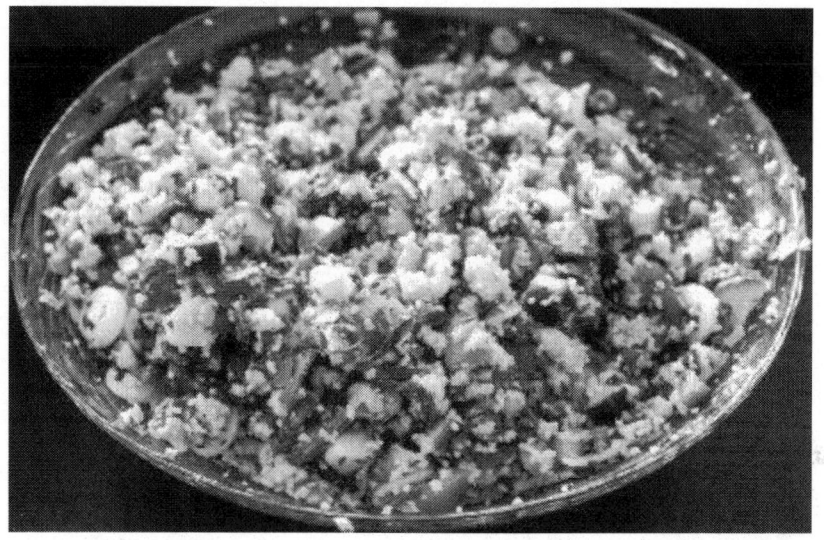

Greek Cucumber Salad

Serves 2-3

Ingredients - Allergies: SF, GF, EF, NF

- 2-3 cucumbers, sliced
- 2 teaspoons salt
- 3 tbsp. lemon juice
- 1/4 tsp. paprika
- 1/4 tsp. white pepper
- 1/2 clove garlic, minced
- 4 fresh green onions, diced
- 1 cup thick Greek Yogurt
- 1/4 tsp. paprika

Instructions

Slice cucumbers thinly, sprinkle with salt and mix. Set aside for one hour. Mix lemon juice, water, garlic, paprika and white pepper, and set aside. Squeeze liquid from cucumber slices a few at a time, and place slices in the bowl. Discard liquid. Add lemon juice mixture, green onions, and yogurt. Mix and sprinkle additional paprika or dill over top. Chill for 1-2 hours.

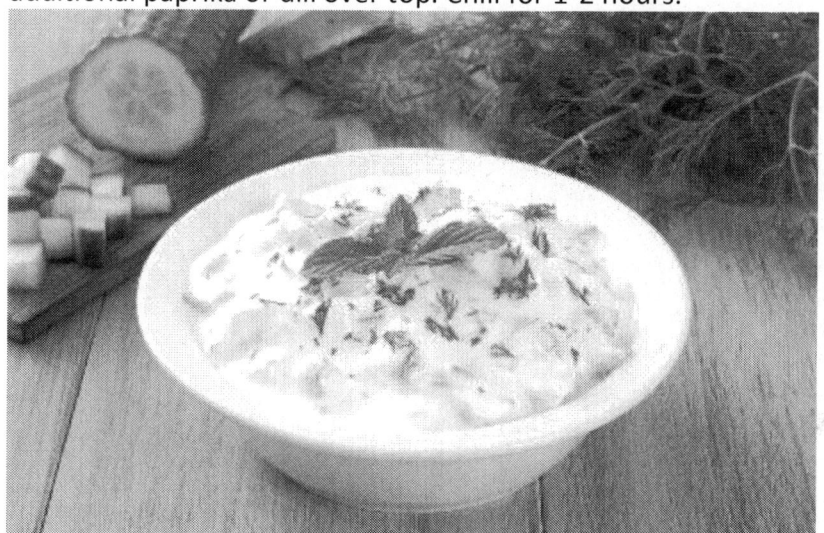

Mediterranean Salad

Serves 3-4

Ingredients - Allergies: SF, GF, DF, EF, V, NF

- 1 medium head romaine lettuce, torn
- 3 small tomatoes, diced
- 1 medium cucumber, sliced
- 1 small green bell pepper, sliced
- 1 small onion, cut into rings
- 6 radishes, thinly sliced
- 1/2 cup flat leaf parsley, chopped
- 1/3 cup olive oil or avocado oil
- 3 tbsp. lemon juice
- 1 garlic clove, minced
- Salt & pepper
- 1 tsp. fresh mint, minced

Instructions

Combine lettuce, tomatoes, cucumber, pepper, onion, radishes & parsley in a salad bowl. Whisk together olive oil, lemon juice, garlic, salt, pepper & mint. Pour over salad & toss to coat.

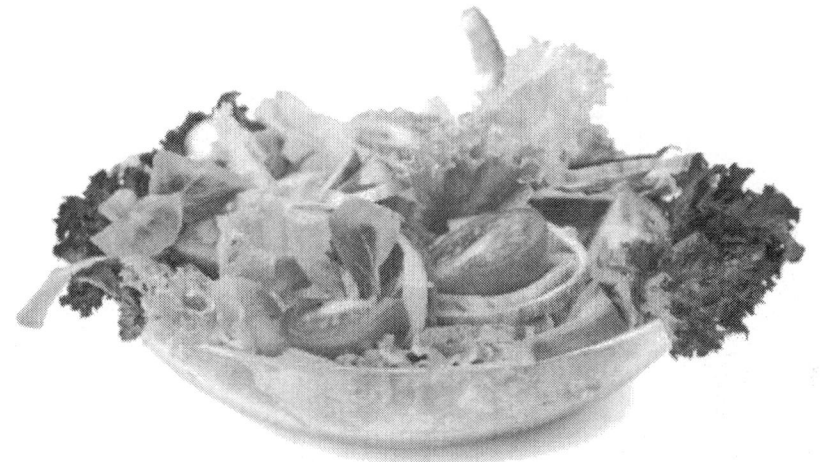

Pomegranate Avocado salad

Serves 1

Ingredients - Allergies: SF, GF, DF, EF, V

- 1 cup mixed greens, spinach, arugula, red leaf lettuce
- 1 ripe avocado, cut into 1/2-inch pieces
- 1/2 cup pomegranate seeds
- 1/4 cup pecan
- 1/4 cup blackberries
- 1/4 cup cherry tomatoes
- <u>olive</u> oil or <u>avocado</u> oil, salt, lemon juice

Instructions

Combine greens, pecan, cut avocado, tomatoes, pomegranates and blackberries in a salad bowl. Whisk together salt, olive oil and lemon juice and pour over salad.

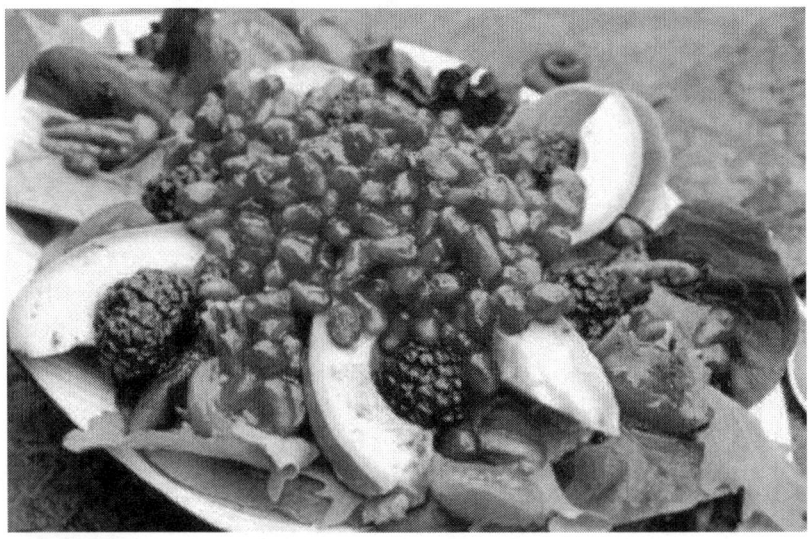

Superfoods Salad

Allergies: SF, GF

Typical superfoods salad should have:

1 part leafy greens - kale, spinach, dandelion and optional cilantro

1 part veggies -carrots, tomato, peppers, beets, broccoli, celery, and some pungent veggies - shallots, ginger or garlic

1 part fruits - pomegranates, avocado, blackberries, blueberries, sliced apple, grapefruit, raspberries

1/2 part of nuts & seeds - almond, walnuts, chia, flax meal, sunflower seeds, pumpkin seeds

1 part protein - low-fat feta, yogurt, 2 boiled eggs or tuna

1 part cooked quinoa (optional)

Make your own mix and use different ingredient every time

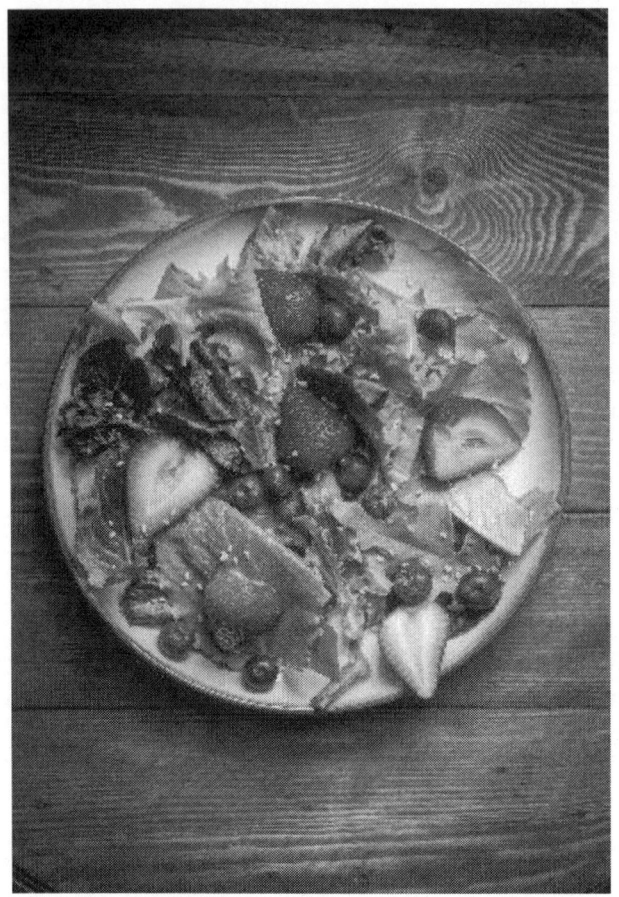

Roasted Beet Salad

Serves 3-4

Instructions - Allergies: SF, GF, DF, EF, V, NF

Toss 4 beets cut in half in a baking dish with olive oil, salt and pepper. Cover and roast at 425 degrees F until tender; let cool, then rub off the skins. Toss with any juices from the baking dish, capers, chopped pickles, a dash each of hot sauce, and chopped parsley or dill.

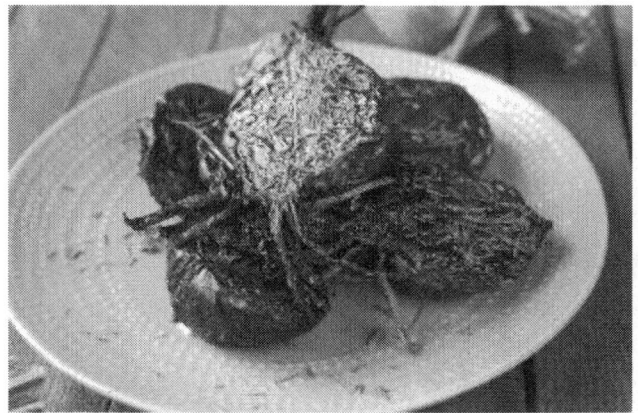

Carrot, Quinoa, Tomato & Spinach Salad in a Jar
Serves 2

Ingredients - Allergies: SF, GF, EF, NF

- 1/2 cup sunflower seeds and 1/2 cup carrots
- 1/2 cup of shredded cabbage and 1/2 cup of tomatoes
- 1 cup cooked quinoa mixed with 1 tbsp. chia seeds
- 1 cup spinach

Dressing:
- 1 tbsp. olive oil
- 1 tbsp. fresh lemon juice and pinch of sea salt

Instructions: Put ingredients in this order: dressing, sunflower seeds, carrots, cabbage, tomatoes and spinach.

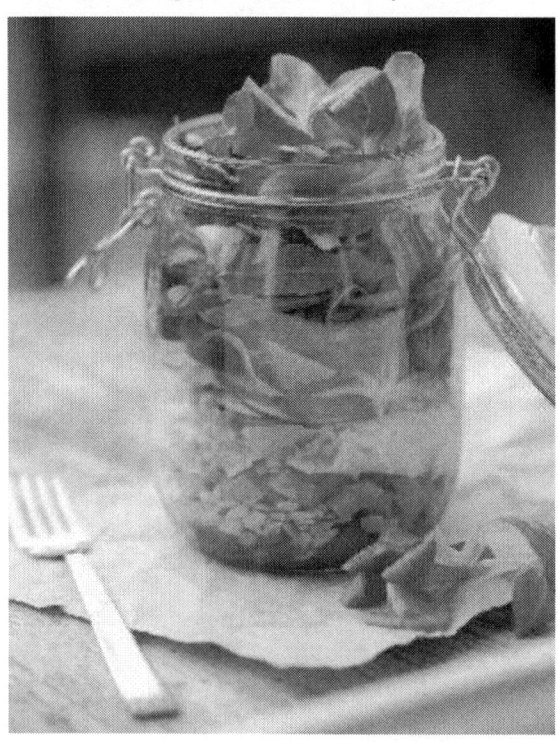

Tomato, Cucumber, Corn & Lettuce Salad in a Jar
Serves 2

Ingredients - Allergies: SF, GF, EF, NF

- 1/2 cup corn
- 1/2 cup tomatoes
- 1/2 cup of sliced cucumber
- 1 cup lettuce

Dressing:
- 1 tbsp. olive oil and 2 Tbsp. Greek Yogurt
- 1 tbsp. fresh lemon juice and pinch of sea salt

Instructions: Put ingredients in this order: dressing, sunflower seeds, carrots, cabbage, tomatoes and spinach.

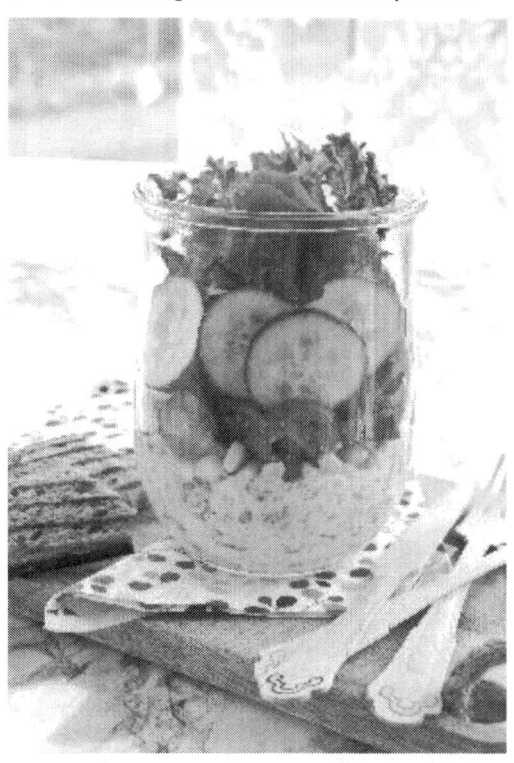

Chickpeas, Onion, Tomato & Parsley Salad in a Jar
Serves 2

Ingredients - Allergies: SF, GF, EF, NF
- 1 cup cooked chickpeas
- 1/2 cup chopped tomatoes
- 1/2 of a small onion, chopped
- 1 tbsp. chia seeds
- 1 Tbsp. chopped parsley

Dressing:
- 1 tbsp. olive oil and 1 tbsp. of Chlorella.
- 1 tbsp. fresh lemon juice and pinch of sea salt

Instructions: Put ingredients in this order: dressing, tomatoes, chickpeas, onions and parsley.

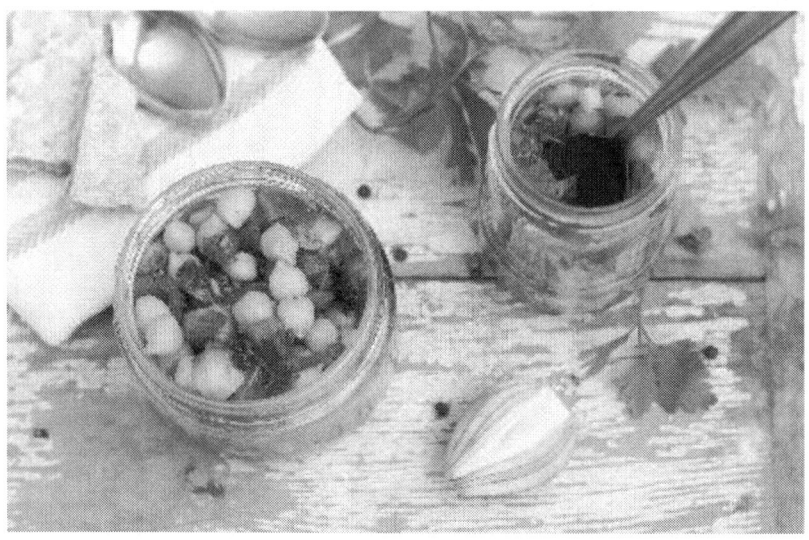

Arugula, Carrot, Corn & Spinach Salad in a Jar
Serves 2

Ingredients - Allergies: SF, GF, EF, NF

- 1 cup corn
- 1 cup tomatoes
- 1/2 cup of julienned carrot
- 1/2 cup spinach

Dressing:
- 1 tbsp. olive oil and 2 Tbsp. Greek Yogurt
- 1 tbsp. fresh lemon juice and pinch of sea salt

Instructions: Put ingredients in this order: dressing, tomatoes, corn, carrots, and arugula.

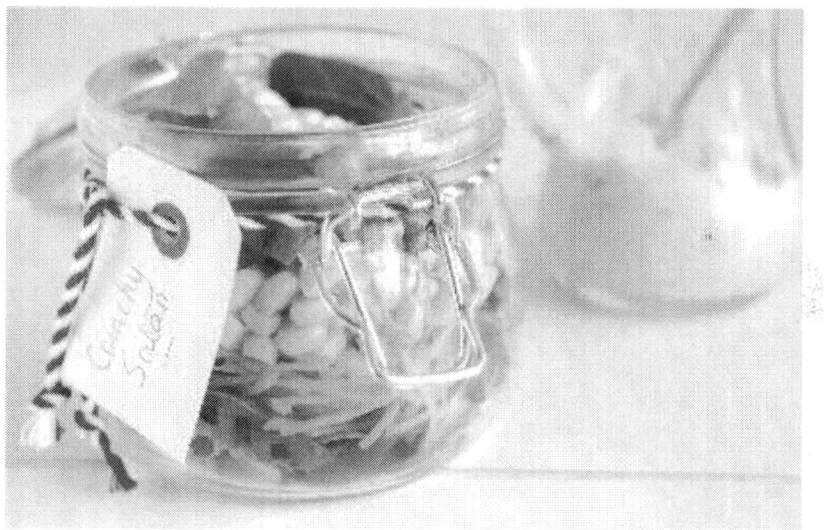

Shrimp, Cucumber & Arugula Salad in a Jar
Serves 2

Ingredients - Allergies: SF, GF, EF, NF

- 1 cup cooked shrimp
- 1/2 cup of cucumber
- 1 cup of arugula

Dressing:
- 1 tbsp. olive oil
- 1 tbsp. fresh lemon juice and pinch of sea salt

Instructions: Put ingredients in this order: dressing, cucumber, shrimp and arugula.

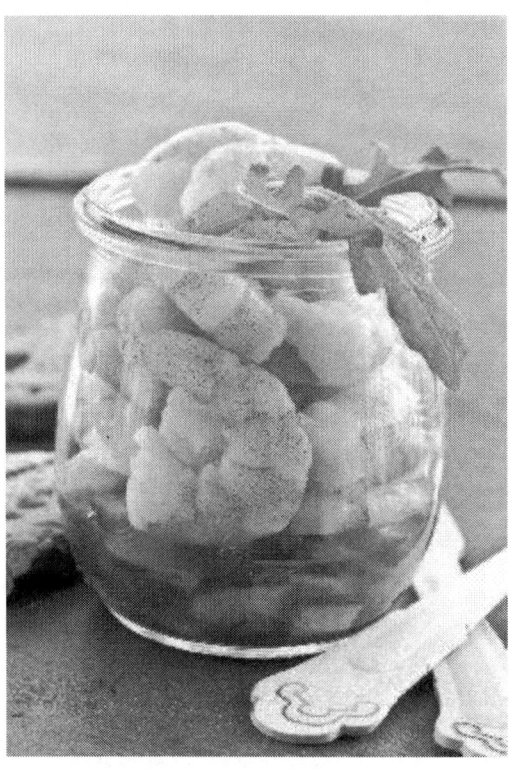

Tomato, Cucumber, Pumpkin & Dandelion Jar Salad
Serves 2

Ingredients - Allergies: SF, GF, EF, NF

- 1/2 cup cooked, cubed pumpkin
- 1/2 cup tomatoes
- 1/2 cup of sliced cucumber
- 1/2 cup Dandelion leaves

Dressing:
- 1 tbsp. olive oil and 1 tbsp. of Chlorella
- 1 tbsp. fresh lemon juice and pinch of sea salt

Instructions: Put ingredients in this order: dressing, tomatoes, cucumbers, pumpkin and dandelion leaves.

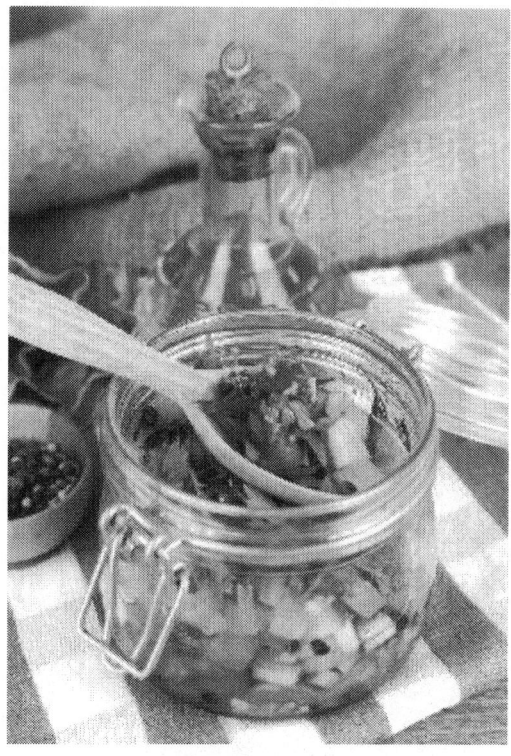

Carrot, Peppers, Cucumber & Cabbage Salad in a Jar
Serves 2

Ingredients - Allergies: SF, GF, EF, NF

- 1/2 cup chopped cucumber and 1/2 cup chopped carrots
- 1/2 cup of shredded red cabbage and 1/2 cup of red peppers
- 1 cup lettuce

Dressing:
- 1 tbsp. olive oil
- 1 tbsp. fresh lemon juice and pinch of sea salt

Instructions: Put ingredients in this order: dressing, cucumbers, peppers, cabbage, carrots and lettuce.

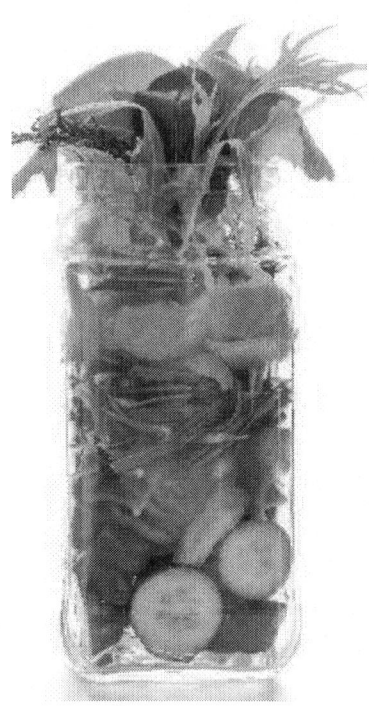

Tomato, Cucumber, Carrot & Parsley Salad in a Jar
Serves 2

Ingredients - Allergies: SF, GF, EF, NF

- 1/2 cup red tomatoes
- 1/2 cup yellow tomatoes
- 1/2 cup of sliced carrot
- 1 Tbsp. of chopped parsley

Dressing:
- 1 tbsp. olive oil and 2 Tbsp. Greek Yogurt
- 1 tbsp. fresh lemon juice and pinch of sea salt

Instructions: Put ingredients in this order: dressing, cucumbers, yellow tomato, carrots, red tomato and parsley.

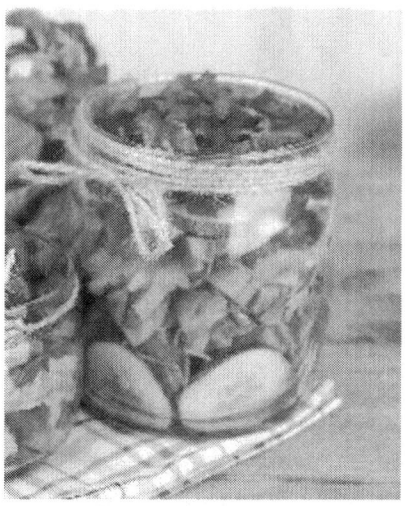

Apple Coleslaw

Serves 1-2

Ingredients - Allergies: SF, GF, DF, EF, V, NF

- 1 cup chopped cabbage (various color)
- 1 tart apple chopped
- 1 celery, chopped
- 1 red pepper chopped
- 5 tsp. olive oil or avocado oil
- juice of 1 lemon
- 2 Tbs lucuma powder (optional)
- dash sea salt

Instructions

Toss the cabbage, apple, celery, and pepper together in a large bowl. In a smaller bowl, whisk remaining ingredients. Drizzle over coleslaw and toss to coat.

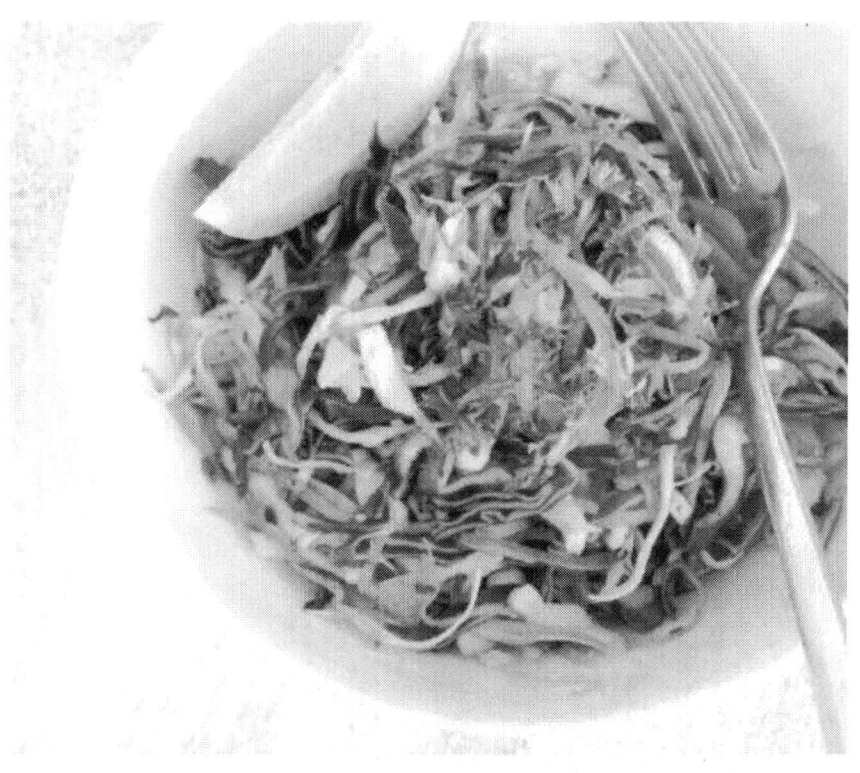

Chicken, Roasted Veggies & Arugula Salad

Serves 2

Ingredients - Allergies: SF, GF, DF, EF, NF

- 1 cup sliced grilled chicken
- 1/2 cup tomato
- 1/2 cup grilled veggies
- 1 cup arugula
- 1/2 cup chopped red peppers

Dressing:
- 1 tbsp. olive oil or avocado oil
- 1 tbsp. fresh lemon juice
- pinch of black pepper
- pinch of sea salt

Instructions: Mix all ingredients.

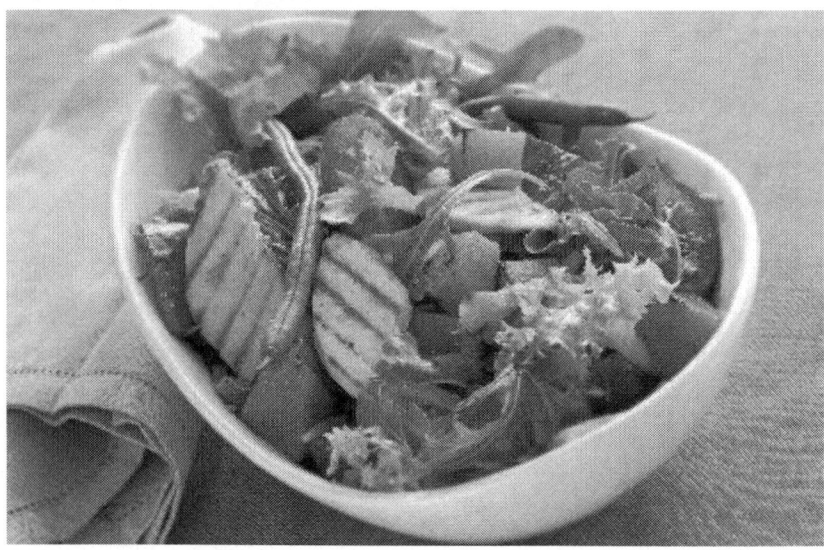

Broccoli, Quinoa, Shrimps & Scallops Salad

Serves 2

Ingredients - Allergies: SF, GF, DF, EF, NF

- 1 cup cooked quinoa mixed with 1 tbsp. ground flax seeds
- 1 cup stir fried broccoli
- 1/2 cup green peas
- 1 cup stir fried shrimp and scallops

Dressing:
- 1 tbsp. olive oil
- 1 tbsp. fresh lemon juice
- pinch of black pepper
- pinch of sea salt

Instructions: Mix all ingredients.

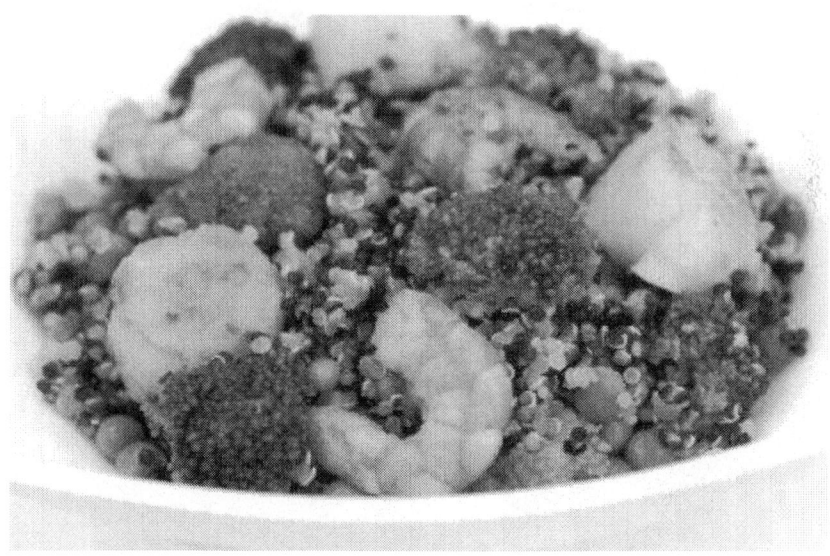

Tuna, Tomato, Arugula & Eggs Salad

Serves 2

Ingredients - Allergies: SF, GF, DF, NF

- 1 cup tuna chunks
- 1/2 cup chopped tomato
- 2 halved eggs
- 1 cup Arugula
- 1/2 cup sliced yellow peppers

Dressing:
- 1 tbsp. olive oil
- 1 tbsp. fresh lemon juice
- pinch of black pepper
- pinch of sea salt

Instructions: Mix all ingredients.

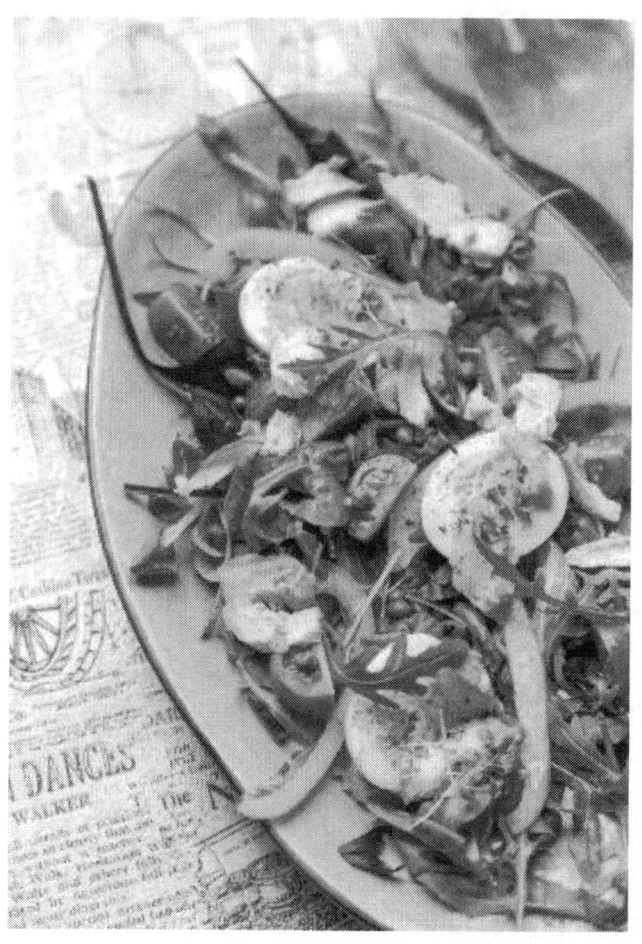

Avocado, Tomato, Arugula Salad

Serves 2

Ingredients - Allergies: SF, GF, DF, EF, NF, V

- 1 cup Orange tomatoes
- 1/2 cup chopped avocado
- 1/2 cup arugula radish
- 1 cup Red Tomatoes

Dressing:
- 1 tbsp. olive oil
- 1 tbsp. fresh lemon juice
- pinch of black pepper
- pinch of sea salt

Instructions: Mix all ingredients.

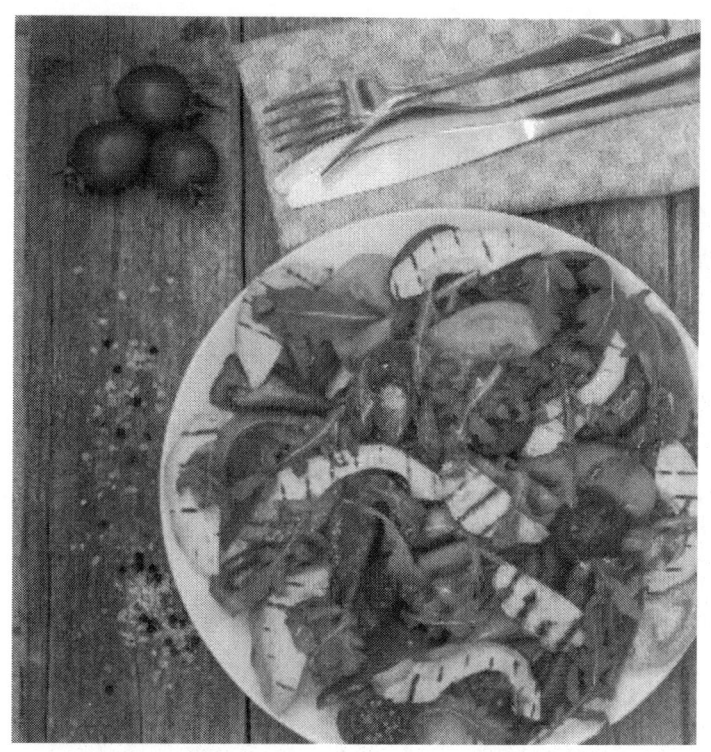

Chicken, Tomato, Spinach & Cucumber Salad

Serves 2

Ingredients - Allergies: SF, GF, DF, EF, NF, V

- 1 cup grilled chicken
- 1/2 cup chopped cucumber
- 1/2 cup chopped tomato
- 1 cup cooked spinach

Dressing:
- 1 tbsp. olive oil or avocado oil
- 1 tbsp. fresh lemon juice
- pinch of black pepper
- pinch of sea salt

Instructions: Mix all ingredients.

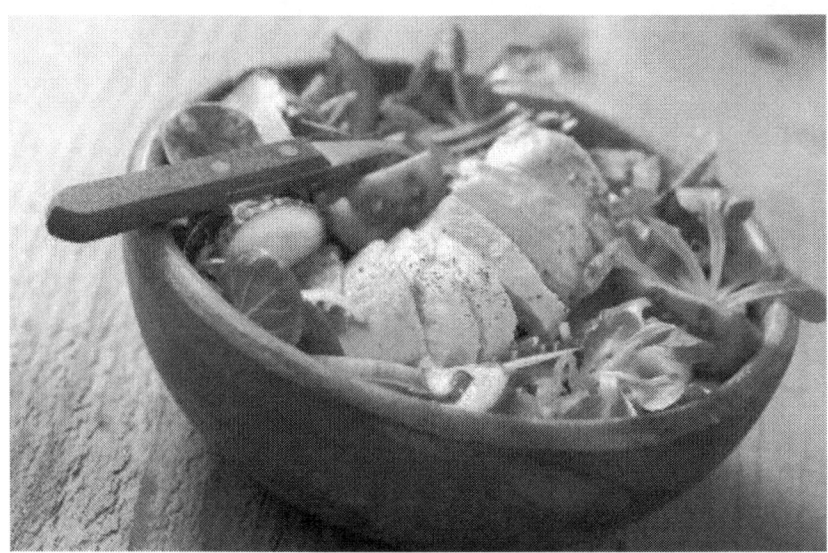

Apple, Spinach & Eggs Salad

Serves 2

Ingredients - Allergies: SF, GF, DF, NF, V

- 4 quartered hard boiled eggs
- 2 granny Smith apples, chopped
- 2 cups spinach
- 1/2 cup ground hazelnuts

Dressing:
- 1 tbsp. olive oil or avocado oil
- 1 tbsp. fresh lemon juice
- pinch of black pepper
- pinch of sea salt

Instructions: Mix all ingredients, top with ground hazelnuts.

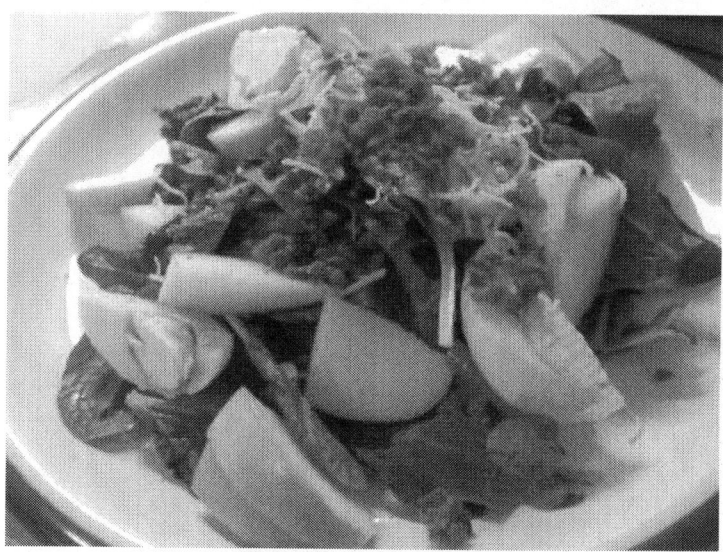

Artichoke, Arugula & Lamb Salad

Serves 2

Ingredients - Allergies: SF, GF, DF, EF, NF

- 1 cup sliced roasted lamb
- 1 cup roasted quartered artichoke hearts.
- 1/2 cup chopped red onion
- 1 cup Arugula

Dressing:
- 1 tbsp. olive oil or avocado oil
- 1 tbsp. fresh lemon juice
- pinch of black pepper
- pinch of sea salt

Instructions: Roast artichoke hearts for 20 minutes in the oven. Mix all ingredients.

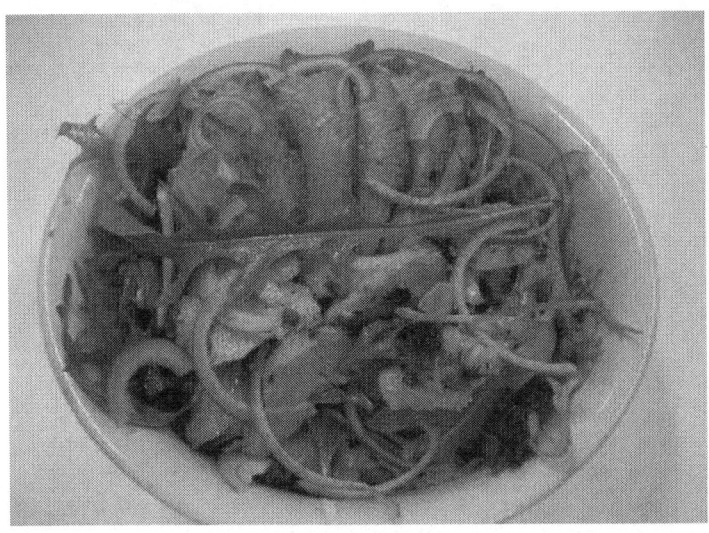

Tuna, Tomato, Eggs & Lettuce Salad

Serves 2

Ingredients - Allergies: SF, GF, DF, NF

- 1 cup tuna
- 2 boiled eggs, sliced
- 1 cup chopped tomato
- 1 cup lettuce

Dressing:
- 1 tbsp. olive oil or avocado oil
- 1 tbsp. fresh lemon juice
- pinch of black pepper
- pinch of sea salt

Instructions: Mix all ingredients.

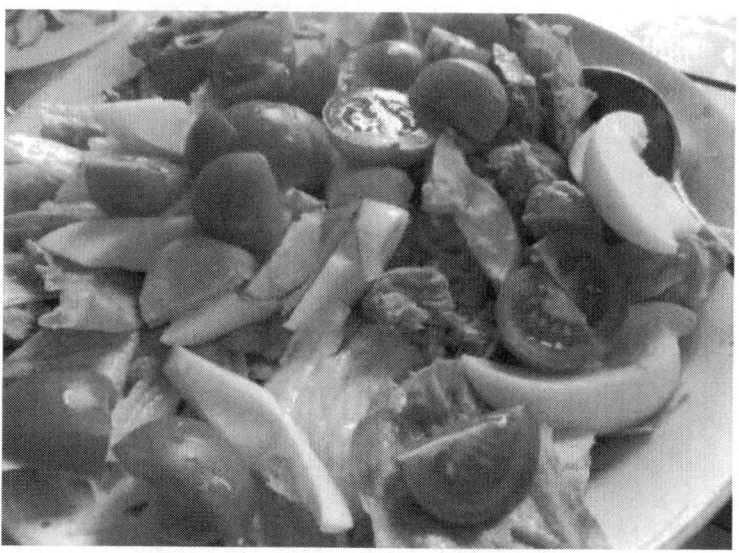

Soups

Cream of Broccoli Soup
Serves 4

Ingredients - Allergies: SF, GF, EF, NF

- 1 1/2 pounds broccoli, fresh
- 2 cups water
- 3/4 tsp. salt, pepper to taste
- 1/2 cup tapioca flour, mixed with 1 cup cold water
- 1/2 cup coconut cream
- 1/2 cup low-fat farmers cheese

Steam or boil broccoli until it gets tender.
Put 2 cups water and coconut cream in top of double boiler.
Add salt, cheese and pepper. Heat until cheese gets melted.
Add broccoli. Mix water and tapioca flour in a small bowl.
Stir tapioca mixture into cheese mixture in double boiler and heat until soup thickens.

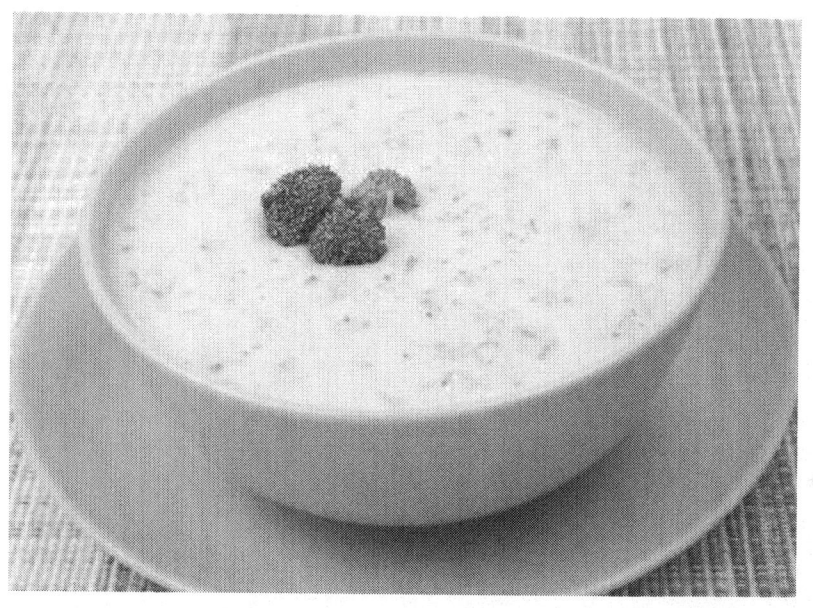

Lentil Soup

Serves 4-6

Ingredients - Allergies: SF, GF, DF, EF, NF
- 2 tbsp. olive oil or avocado oil
- 1 cup finely chopped onion
- 1/2 cup chopped carrot
- 1/2 cup chopped celery
- 2 teaspoons salt
- 1 pound lentils
- 1 cup chopped tomatoes
- 2 quarts chicken or vegetable broth
- 1/2 tsp. ground coriander & toasted cumin

Instructions

Place the olive oil into a large Dutch oven. Set over medium heat. Once hot, add the celery, onion, carrot and salt and do until the onions are translucent. Add the lentils, tomatoes, cumin, broth and coriander and stir to combine. Increase the heat and bring just to a boil. Reduce the heat, cover and simmer at a low until the lentils are tender (approx. 35 to 40 minutes). Puree with a bender to your preferred consistency (optional). Serve immediately.

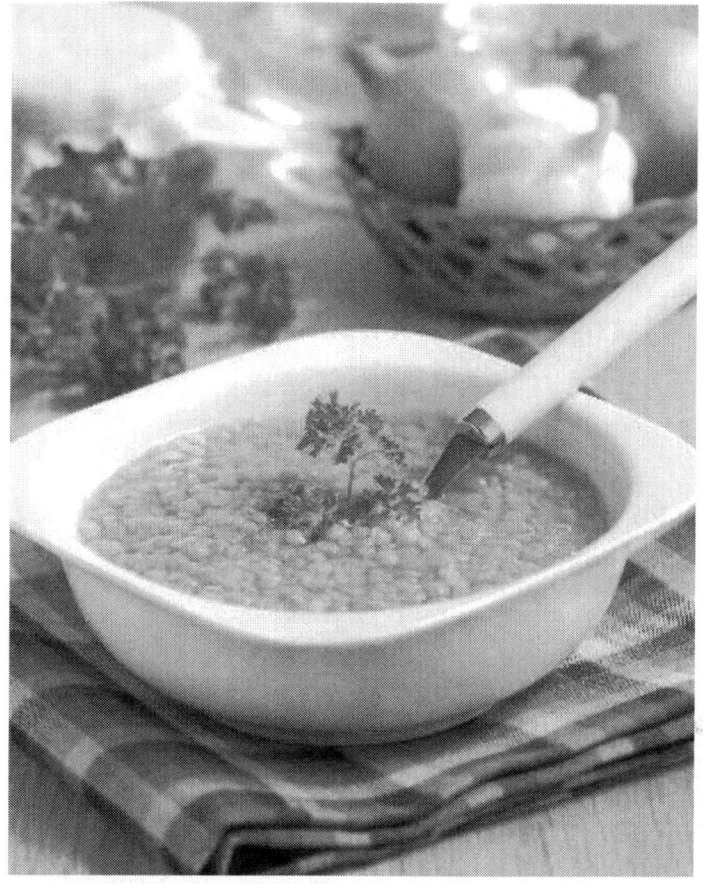

Cold Cucumber Avocado Soup
Serves 2-3

Ingredients - Allergies: SF, GF, EF, NF
- 1 cucumber peeled, seeded and cut into 2-inch chunks
- 1 avocado, peeled
- 2 chopped scallions
- 1 cup chicken broth
- 3/4 cup Greek low-fat yogurt
- 2 tbsp. lemon juice
- 1/2 tsp. ground pepper, or to taste

Garnish:
- Chopped chives, dill, mint, scallions or cucumber

Instructions
Combine the cucumber, avocado and scallions in a blender. Pulse until chopped.
Add yogurt, broth and lemon juice and continue until smooth.
Season with pepper and salt to taste and chill for 4 hours.
Taste for seasoning and garnish.

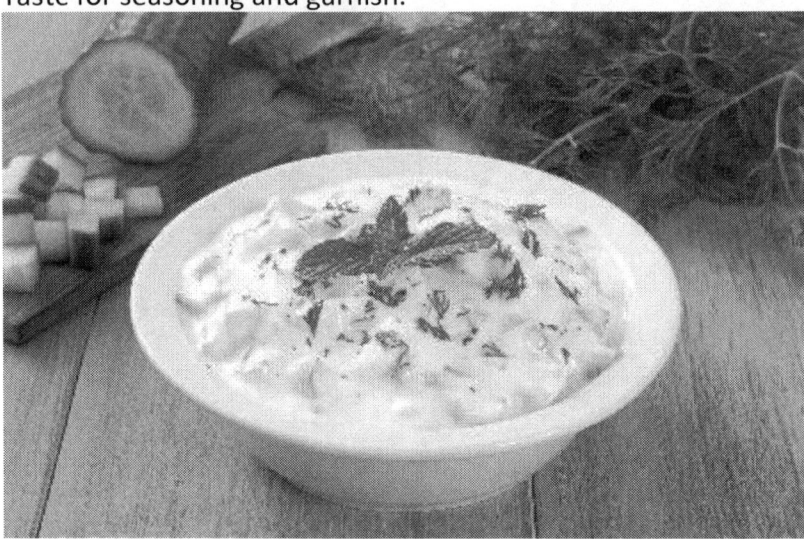

Bouillabaisse

Serves 6.

Ingredients - Allergies: SF, GF, DF, EF, NF

- 3 pounds of 3 different kinds of fish fillets
- 1/2 cup coconut oil
- 1-2 pounds of Oysters, clams, or mussels
- 1 cup cooked shrimp, crab, or lobster meat, or rock lobster tails
- 1 cup thinly sliced onions
- 4 Shallots or the white parts of 2 or 3 leeks, thinly sliced
- 2 cloves garlic, crushed
- 1 large tomato, chopped
- 1 sweet red pepper, chopped
- 4 stalks celery, thinly sliced
- 2-inch slice of fennel or 1 tsp. of fennel seed
- 3 sprigs fresh thyme or 3/4 tsp. dried thyme
- 1 bay leaf
- 2-3 whole cloves
- Zest of half an orange
- 1/2 tsp. saffron
- 2 teaspoons salt
- 1/4 tsp. ground black pepper
- 1 cup clam juice or fish broth
- 2 Tbps lemon juice
- 2/3 cup white wine

Instructions

In a large saucepan heat 1/4 cup of the coconut oil. When it is hot, add onions and shallots (or leeks). Sauté for a minute. Add crushed garlic, and sweet red pepper. Add celery, tomato, and fennel. Stir the vegetables until well coated. Add another 1/4 cup of coconut oil, bay leaf, thyme, cloves and the orange zest. Cook until the onion is golden. Cut fish fillets into 2-inch pieces. Add 2 cups of water and the pieces of fish to the vegetable mixture.

Bring to a boil, then reduce heat and let it simmer, uncovered, for about 10 minutes. Add clams, oysters or mussels (optional) and crabmeat, shrimp or lobster tails, cut into pieces. Add salt, saffron and pepper. Add lemon juice, clam juice, and white wine. Bring to a simmer again and cook for 5 minutes longer.

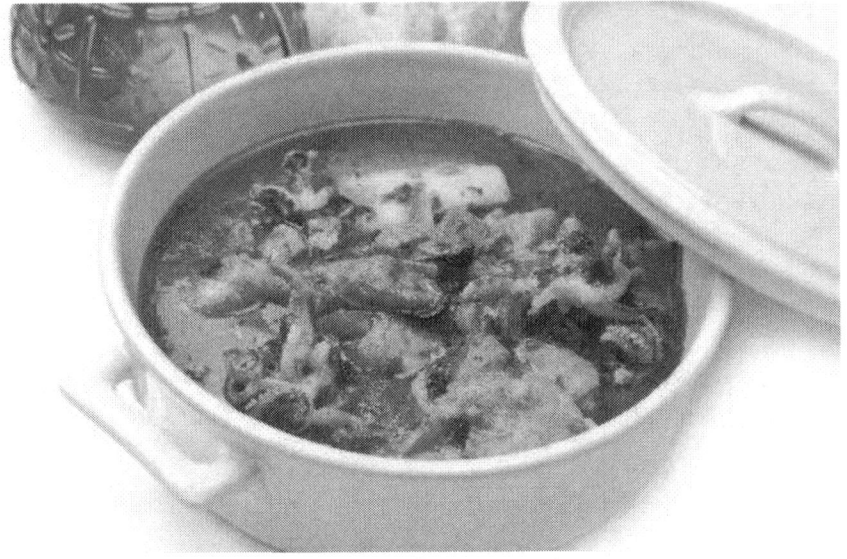

Gaspacho

Serves 4

Ingredients - Allergies: SF, GF, DF, EF, V, NF
- 1/2 cup of flax seeds meal
- 1kg tomatoes, diced
- 1 red pepper and 1 green pepper, diced
- 1 cucumber, peeled and diced
- 2 cloves of garlic, peeled and crushed
- 150ml extra virgin olive oil or avocado oil
- 2tbsp lemon juice
- Salt, to taste

Instructions
Mix the peppers, tomatoes and cucumber with the crushed garlic and olive oil in the bowl of a blender. Add flax meal to the mixture. Blend until smooth. Add salt and lemon juice to taste and stir well. Refrigerate until well chilled. Serve with black olives, hard-boiled egg, cilantro, mint or parsley.

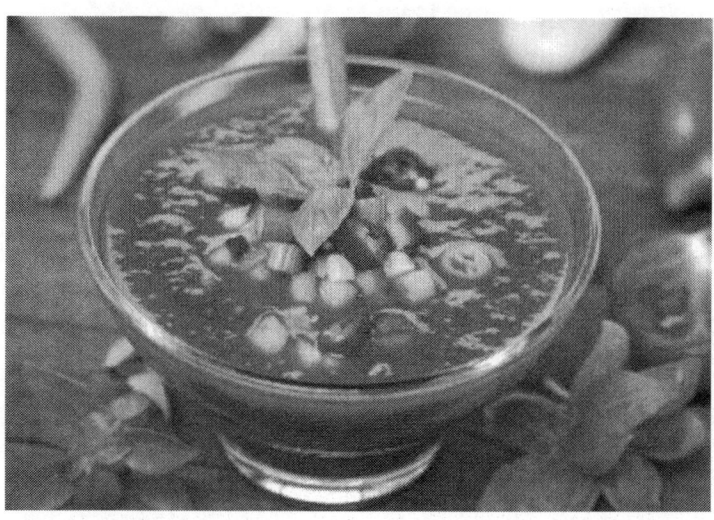

Italian Beef Soup

Serves 6

Ingredients - Allergies: SF, GF, DF, EF, NF

- 1 pound minced beef
- 1 clove garlic, minced
- 2 cups beef broth
- few large tomatoes
- 1 cup sliced carrots
- 2 cups cooked beans
- 2 small zucchini, cubed
- 2 cups spinach - rinsed and torn
- 1/4 tsp. black pepper
- 1/4 tsp. salt

Brown beef with garlic in a stockpot. Stir in broth, carrots and tomatoes. Season with salt and pepper. Reduce heat, cover, and simmer for 15 minutes.

Stir in beans with liquid and zucchini. Cover, and simmer until zucchini is tender. Remove from heat, add spinach and cover. Serve after 5 minutes.

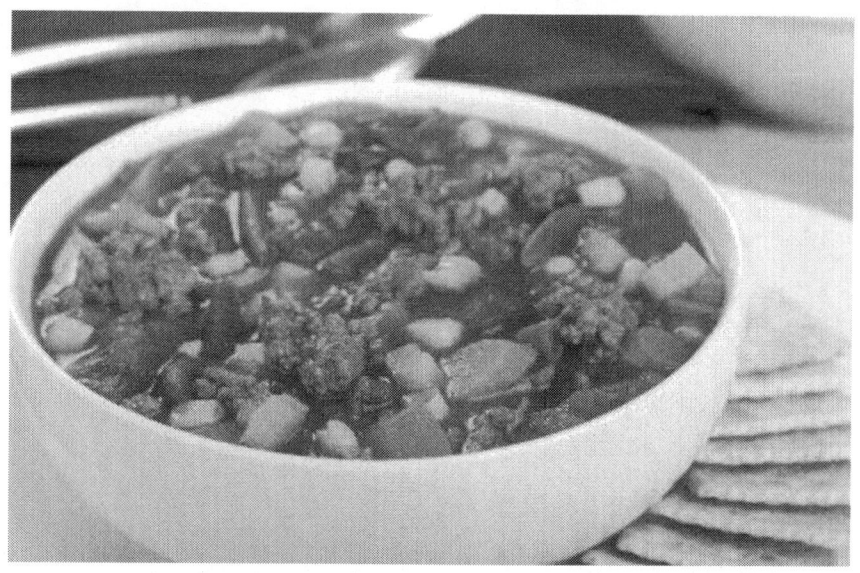

Creamy roasted mushroom

Serves 4

Ingredients - Allergies: SF, GF, DF, EF, V, NF

- 1 pound Portobello mushrooms, cut into 1inch pieces
- 1/2 pound shiitake mushrooms, stemmed
- 6 tbsp. olive oil or avocado oil
- 2 cups vegetable broth
- 1 1/2 tbsp. coconut oil
- 1 onion, chopped
- 3 garlic cloves, minced
- 3 tbsp. arrowroot flour
- 1 cup coconut cream
- 3/4 tsp. chopped thyme

Instructions

Heat oven to 400°F. Line one large baking sheets with foil. Spread mushrooms and drizzle some olive oil on them. Season with salt and pepper and toss. Cover with foil and bake them for half an hour. Uncover and continue baking 15 minutes more. Cool slightly. Mix one half of the mushrooms with one can of broth in a blender. Set aside.

Melt coconut oil in a large pot over high heat. Add onion and garlic and sauté until onion is translucent. Add flour and stir 2 minutes. Add cream, broth, and thyme. Stir in remaining cooked mushrooms and mushroom puree. Simmer over low heat until thickened (approx. 10 minutes). Season to taste with salt and pepper.

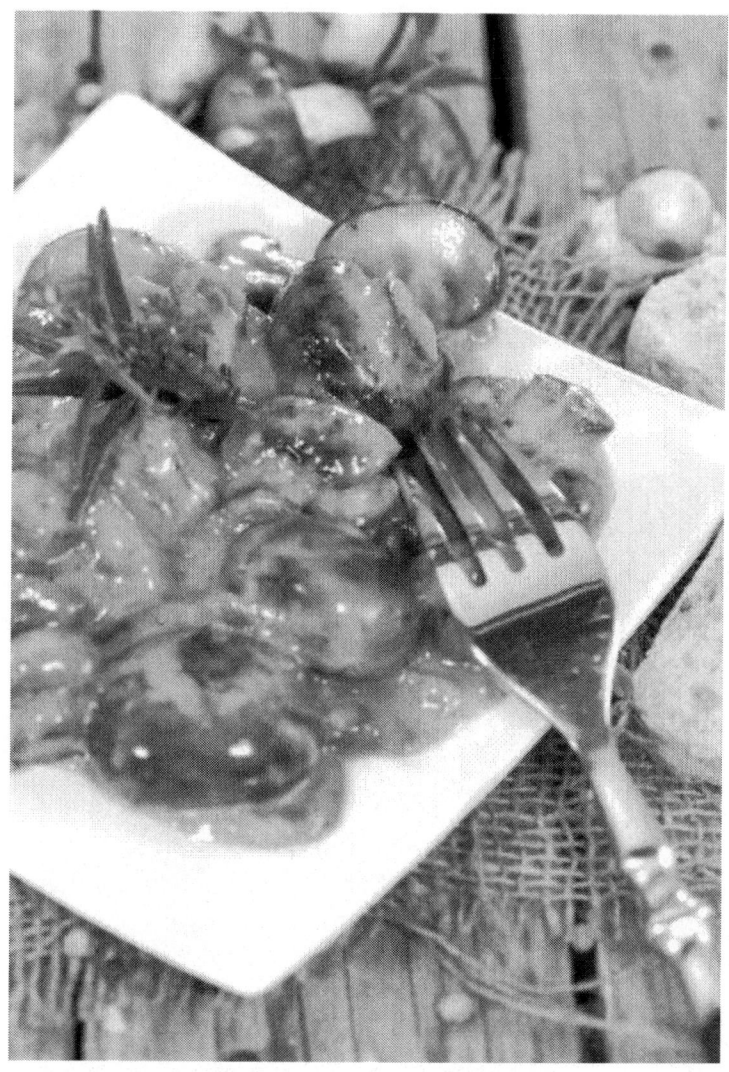

Black Bean Soup

Serves 6-8

Ingredients - Allergies: SF, GF, DF, EF, NF

- 1/4 cup coconut oil
- 1/4 cup Onion, Diced
- 1/4 cup Carrots, Diced
- 1/4 cup Green Bell Pepper, Diced
- 1 cup beef broth
- 3 pounds cooked Black Beans
- 1 tbsp. lemon juice
- 2 teaspoons Garlic
- 2 teaspoons Salt
- 1/2 tsp. Black Pepper, Ground
- 2 teaspoons Chili Powder
- 8 oz. pork
- 1 tbsp. tapioca flour
- 2 tbsp. Water

Instructions

Place coconut oil, onion, carrot, and bell pepper in a stock pot. Cook the veggies until tender. Bring broth to a boil. Add cooked beans, broth and the remaining ingredients (except tapioca flour and 2 tbsp. water) to the vegetables. Bring that mixture to a simmer and cook approximately 15 minutes. Puree 1 quart of the soup in a blender and put back into the pot. Combine the tapioca flour and 2 tbsp. water in a separate bowl. Add the tapioca flour mixture to the bean soup and bring to a boil for around 1 minute.

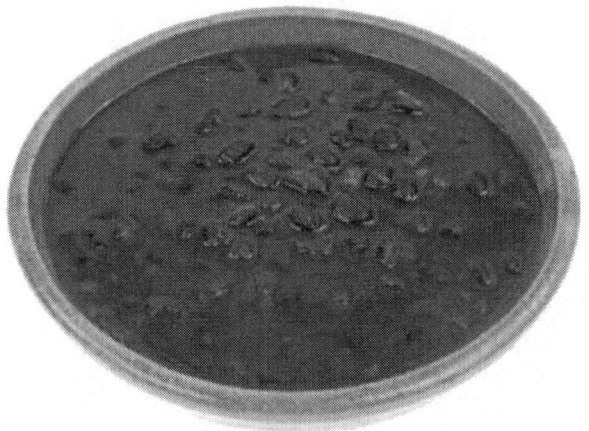

Squash soup

Serves 4-6

Ingredients - Allergies: SF, GF, DF, EF, V, NF

- 1 Squash
- 1 carrot, chopped
- 1 onion (diced)
- 3/4 – 1 cup coconut milk
- 1/4 – 1/2 cup water
- <u>olive</u> oil or <u>avocado</u> oil
- Salt
- Pepper
- Cinnamon
- Turmeric

Instructions

Cut the squash and spoon out the seeds. Cut it into large pieces and place on a baking sheet. Sprinkle with salt, olive oil, and pepper and bake at 375 degrees F until soft (approx. 1 hour). Let cool.

In the meantime, sauté the onions in olive oil (put it in a soup pot). Add the carrots. Add 3/4 cup coconut milk and 1/4 cup water after few minutes and let simmer. Scoop the squash out of its skin. Add it to the soup pot. Stir to combine the ingredients and let simmer a few minutes. Add more milk or water if needed. Season to taste with the salt, pepper and spices. Blend until smooth and creamy.

Sprinkle it with toasted pumpkin seeds.

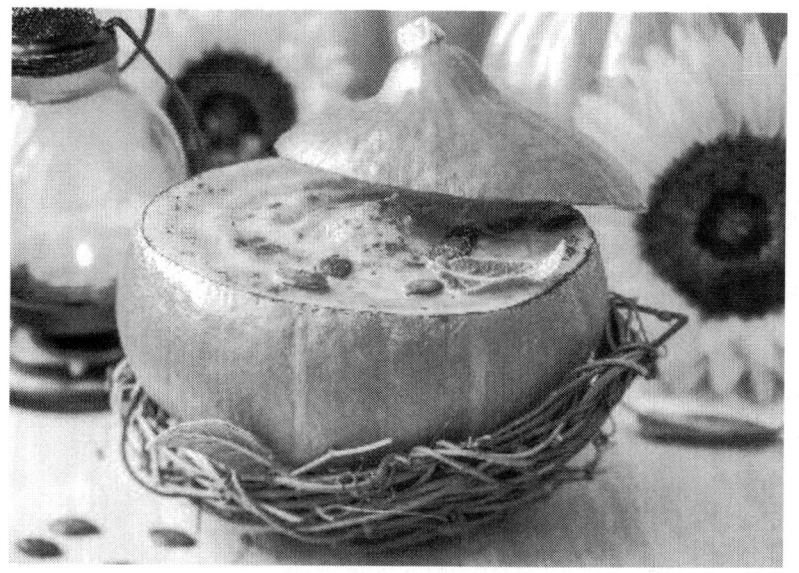

Kale White Bean Pork Soup

Serves 4-6

Ingredients - Allergies: SF, GF, DF, EF, NF

- 2 tbsp. each extra-virgin <u>olive</u> oil or <u>cumin</u> oil and <u>coconut</u> oil
- 3 tbsp. chili powder
- 1 tbsp. jalapeno hot sauce
- 2 pounds bone-in pork chops
- Salt
- 4 stalks celery, chopped
- 1 large white onion, chopped
- 3 cloves garlic, chopped
- 2 cups chicken broth
- 2 cups diced tomatoes
- 2 cups cooked white beans
- 6 cups packed Kale

Instructions

Preheat the broiler. Whisk hot sauce, 1 tbsp. olive oil and chili powder in a bowl. Season the pork chops with 1/2 tsp. salt. Rub chops with the spice mixture on both sides and place them on a rack set over a baking sheet. Set aside.

Heat 1 tbsp. coconut oil in a large pot over high heat. Add the celery, garlic, onion and the remaining 2 tbsp. chili powder. Cook until onions are translucent, stirring (approx. 8 minutes).

Add tomatoes and the chicken broth to the pot. Cook and stir occasionally until reduced by about one-third (approx. 7 minutes). Add the kale and the beans. Reduce the heat to medium, cover and cook until the kale is tender (approx. 7 minutes). Add up to 1/2 cup water if the mixture looks dry and season with salt.

In the meantime, broil the pork until browned (approx. 4 to 6 minutes). Flip and broil until cooked through. Serve with the kale and beans.

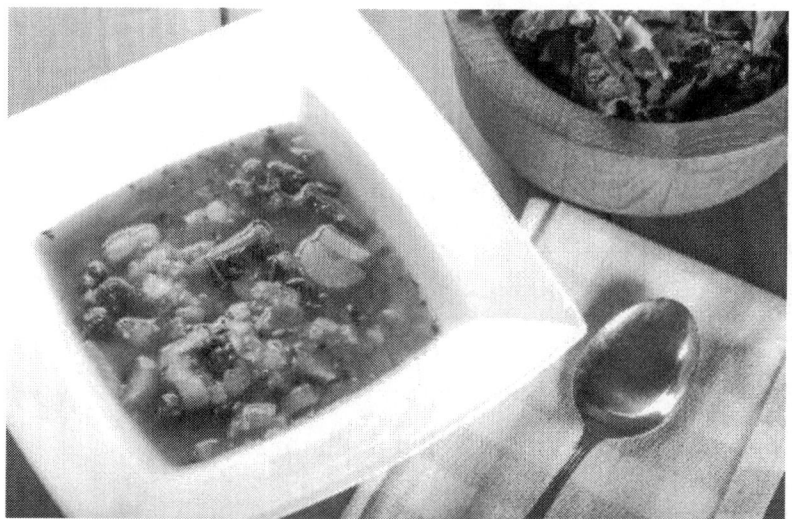

Avgolemono – Greek lemon chicken soup
Serves 4

Ingredients - Allergies: SF, GF, DF, EF, NF

- 4 cups chicken broth
- 1/4 cup uncooked quinoa
- salt and pepper
- 3 eggs
- 3 tbsp. lemon juice
- Handful fresh dill (chopped)
- shredded roasted chicken (optional)

Bring the broth to a boil in a saucepan. Add the quinoa and cook until tender. Season with the salt and pepper. Reduce heat to low & let simmer. In a separate bowl, whisk lemon juice and the eggs until smooth. Add about 1 cup of the hot broth into the egg/lemon mixture and whisk to combine.

Add the mixture back to the saucepan. Stir until the soup becomes opaque and thickens. Add dill, salt and pepper to taste & chicken if you have it, and serve.

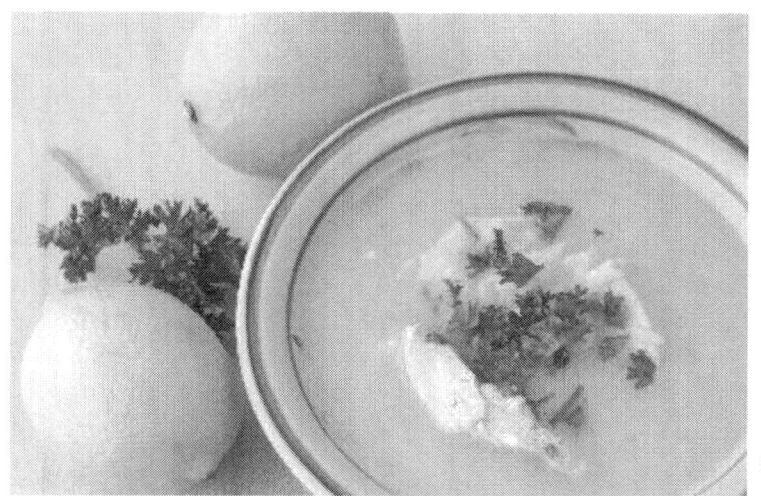

Egg-Drop Soup

Serves 4-6

Ingredients - Allergies: SF, GF, DF, NF

- 1 1/2 quarts chicken broth
- 2 tbsps. Tapioca flour, mixed in 1/4 cup cold water
- 2 eggs, slightly beaten with a fork
- 2 scallions, chopped, including green ends

Instructions

Bring broth to a boil. Slowly pour in the tapioca flour mixture while stirring the broth. The broth should thicken. Reduce heat and let it simmer. Mix in the eggs very slowly while stirring. As soon as the last drop of egg is in, turn off the heat. Serve with chopped scallions on top.

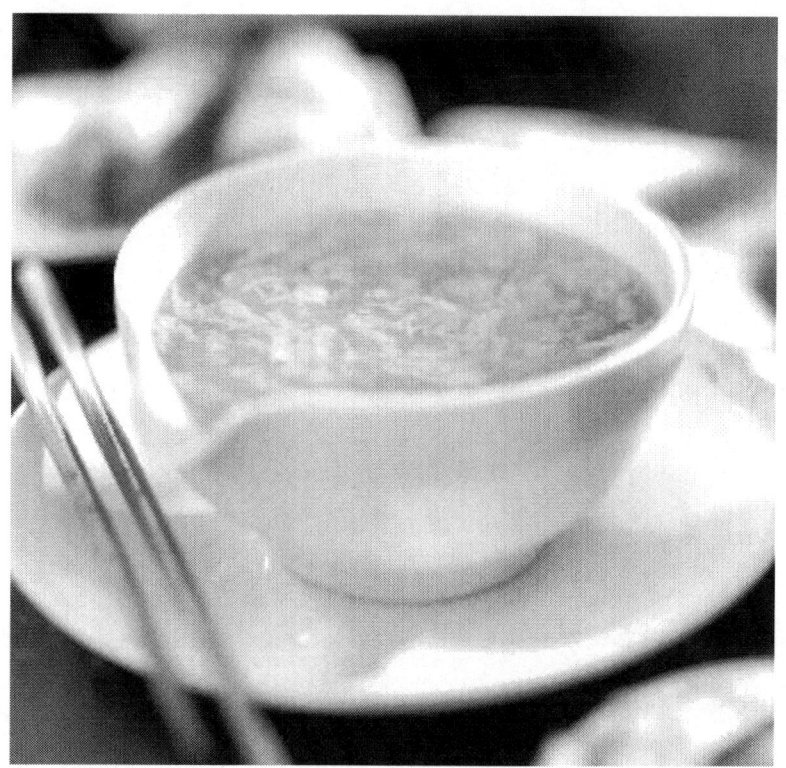

Creamy Tomato Basil Soup

Serves 6

Ingredients - Allergies: SF, GF, DF, EF, V, NF

- 4 tomatoes - peeled, seeded and diced
- 4 cups tomato juice*
- 14 leaves fresh basil
- 1 cup coconut cream
- salt to taste
- ground black pepper according to taste

Instructions

Combine tomatoes and tomato juice in stock pot. Simmer 30 minutes. Puree mixture with basil leaves in a processor. Put back in a stock pot and add coconut cream. Add salt and pepper to taste.

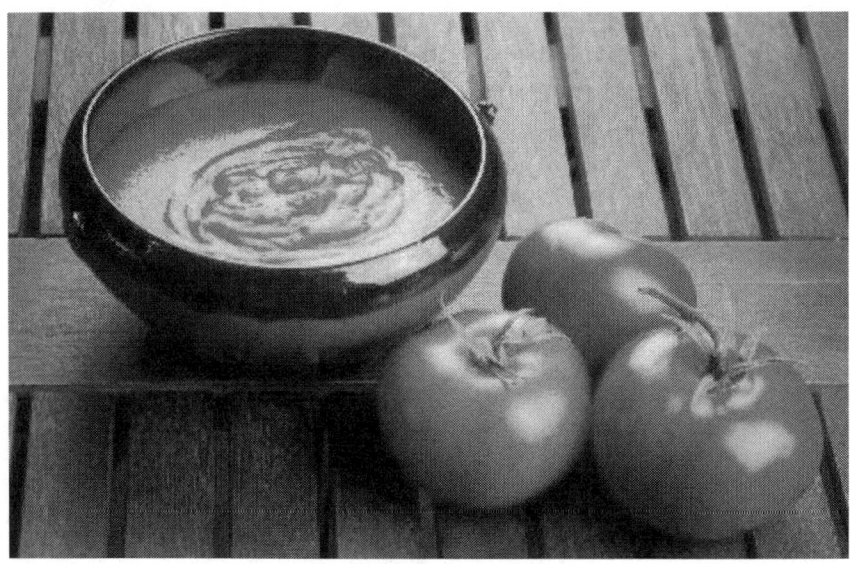

Minestrone

Serves 8-10

Ingredients - Allergies: SF, GF, DF, EF, NF

- 3 tbsp. coconut oil
- 3 cloves garlic, chopped
- 2 onions, chopped
- 2 cups chopped celery
- 5 carrots, sliced
- 2 cups chicken broth
- 2 cups water
- 4 cups tomato sauce
- 1/2 oz. red wine (optional)
- 1 cup cooked kidney beans
- 2 cups green beans
- 2 cups baby spinach, rinsed
- 3 zucchinis, quartered and sliced
- 1 tbsp. chopped oregano
- 2 tbsp. chopped basil
- salt and pepper to taste
- 1 tbsp. olive oil or cumin oil

Instructions

Heat coconut oil over medium heat in a stock pot, and sauté garlic for few minutes. Add onion and sauté for few more minutes. Add celery and carrots and sauté for 2 minutes.
Add chicken broth, tomato sauce and water and bring to boil, stirring frequently. Add red wine at this point. Reduce heat to low. Add kidney beans, zucchini, green beans, spinach leaves, oregano,

basil, salt and pepper. Simmer for 30 to 40 minutes.

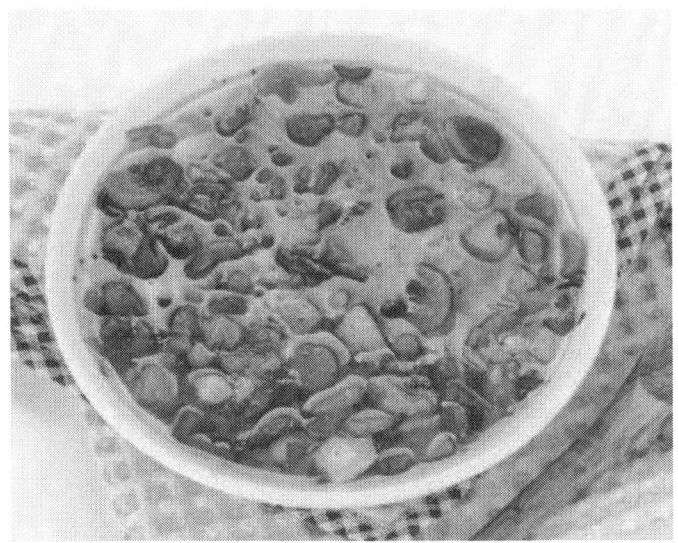

Grilled Meats & Salad

Chicken and Large Fiber Loaded Salad with Italian Dressing

Serves 1 - Allergies: SF, GF, EF, NF

• 6oz. of Chicken (or turkey), skinless, boneless grilled or prepared in the skillet.

• Large mixed spinach and lettuce salad with Italian Dressing and half a tsp of mustard. Salad can be as large as you want, but use half a cup of the dressing.

• Salad with Yogurt Dressing would have 80 calories more (330 calories total)

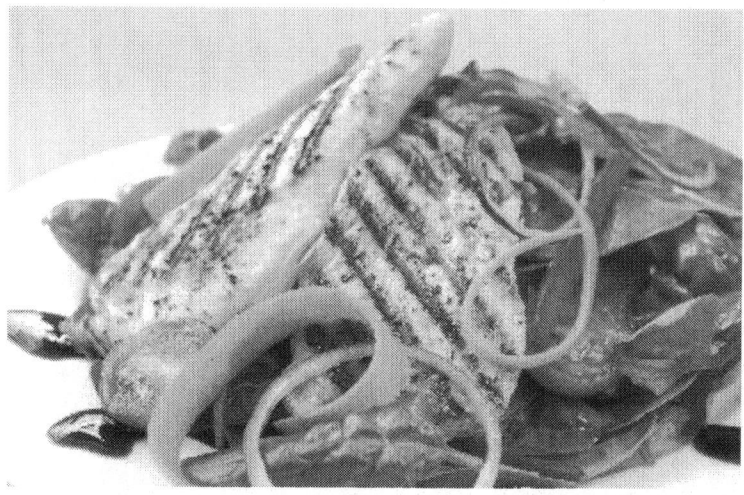

Nutrition Facts

Serving Size 247 g

Amount Per Serving

Calories 252　　　Calories from Fat 122

	% Daily Value*
Total Fat 13.6g	**21%**
Saturated Fat 2.0g	**10%**
Trans Fat 0.0g	
Cholesterol 63mg	**21%**
Sodium 99mg	**4%**
Potassium 831mg	**24%**
Total Carbohydrates 5.1g	**2%**
Dietary Fiber 2.4g	**10%**
Sugars 2.4g	
Protein 29.3g	

Vitamin A 60%　•　Vitamin C 57%
Calcium 11%　•　Iron 11%

Nutrition Grade B+

* Based on a 2000 calorie diet

Salmon with Large Fiber Loaded Salad with Italian Dressing

Serves 1 - Allergies: SF, GF, DF, EF, NF

- 4oz. of Salmon grilled or prepared in the skillet.

- Large mixed spinach and lettuce salad with "Italian Dressing" and some thyme sprinkled on top of it. Salad can be as large as you want, but use the prescribed amount of the dressing.

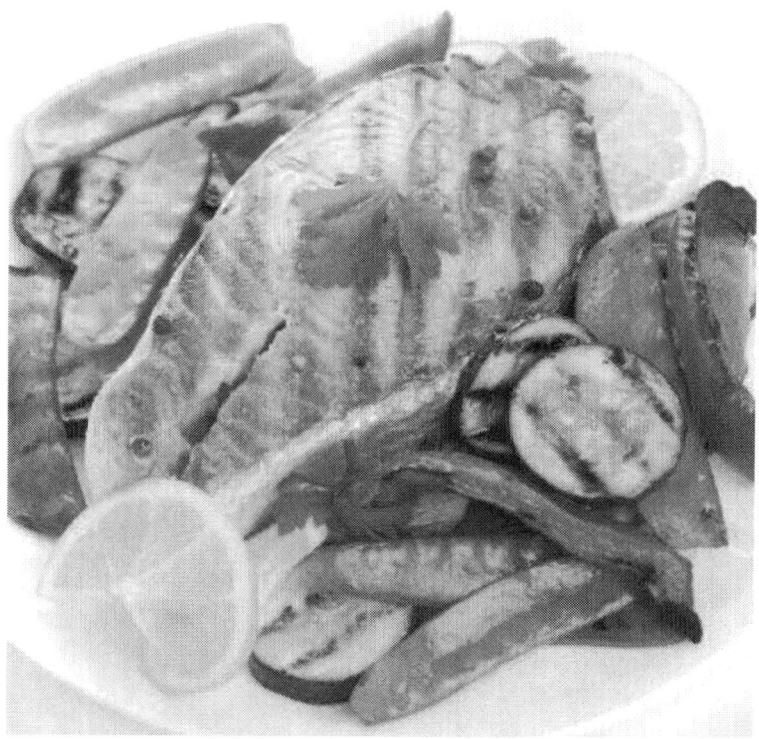

Herb Crusted Salmon

Serves 1 - Allergies: SF, GF, DF, EF, NF

Rub some tarragon, chives and parsley over 4 oz. salmon and add some salt and pepper. Heat the pan with 1 tsp of coconut oil to medium high and place the salmon, skin-side up in the pan. Cook until golden brown on 1 side, about 4 minutes. Turn the fish over and cook until it feels firm to the touch. Salmon is done when it flakes easily with a fork. Serve with a lemon wedge.

- Large mixed spinach and lettuce salad with "Italian Dressing" and some thyme sprinkled on top of it. Salad can be as large as you want, but use the prescribed amount of the dressing.

Nutrition Facts

Serving Size 247 g

Amount Per Serving

Calories 252	Calories from Fat 122
	% Daily Value*
Total Fat 13.6g	**21%**
Saturated Fat 2.0g	**10%**
Trans Fat 0.0g	
Cholesterol 63mg	**21%**
Sodium 99mg	**4%**
Potassium 831mg	**24%**
Total Carbohydrates 5.1g	**2%**
Dietary Fiber 2.4g	**10%**
Sugars 2.4g	
Protein 29.3g	
Vitamin A 60% •	Vitamin C 57%
Calcium 11% •	Iron 11%

Nutrition Grade B+

* Based on a 2000 calorie diet

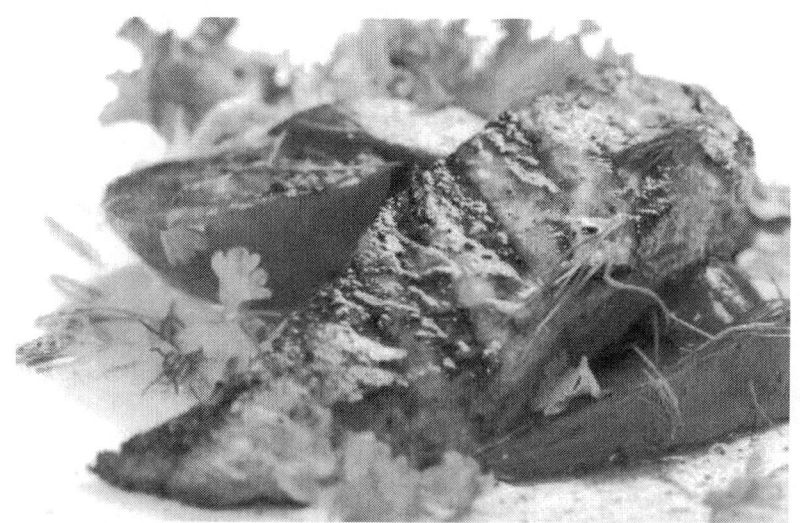

Ground Beef Patty with Large Fiber Loaded Salad with Yogurt Dressing

Serves 1 - Allergies: SF, GF, EF, NF

- 5oz. lean ground beef patty grilled or prepared in the skillet.
- Large mixed spinach and shredded cabbage salad with Yogurt Dressing. Salad can be as large as you want, but use half a cup of a dressing.

Nutrition Facts

Serving Size 247 g

Amount Per Serving

Calories 328	Calories from Fat 123
	% Daily Value*
Total Fat 13.7g	21%
Saturated Fat 4.0g	20%
Cholesterol 127mg	42%
Sodium 130mg	5%
Potassium 857mg	24%
Total Carbohydrates 5.1g	2%
Dietary Fiber 2.4g	10%
Sugars 2.4g	
Protein 44.8g	

Vitamin A 58%	•	Vitamin C 57%
Calcium 6%	•	Iron 155%

Nutrition Grade A
* Based on a 2000 calorie diet

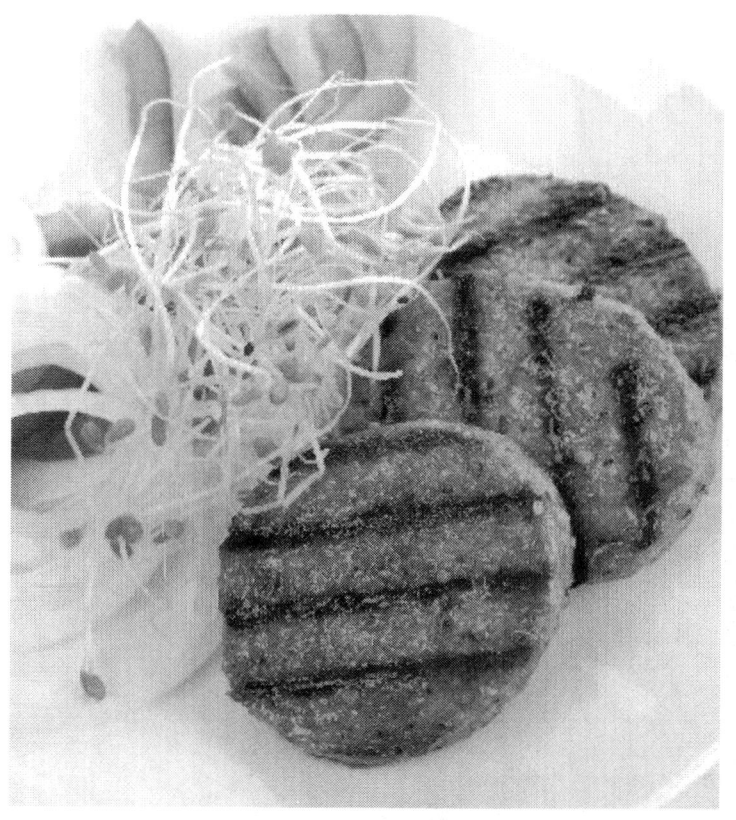

Lean Pork with Fiber Loaded Salad with Yogurt Dressing

Serves 1 - Allergies: SF, GF, EF, NF

- 5oz. of lean Pork Tenderloin grilled or prepared in the skillet.
- Large mixed spinach and shredded cabbage salad with Yogurt Dressing and half a tsp of mustard. Salad can be as large as you want, but use half a cup of the dressing.

Nutrition Facts

Serving Size 275 g

Amount Per Serving

Calories 231	Calories from Fat 71
	% Daily Value*
Total Fat 7.9g	12%
Saturated Fat 1.5g	7%
Trans Fat 0.0g	
Cholesterol 99mg	33%
Sodium 249mg	10%
Potassium 818mg	23%
Total Carbohydrates 5.1g	2%
Dietary Fiber 2.4g	10%
Sugars 2.4g	
Protein 33.6g	
Vitamin A 58%	Vitamin C 57%
Calcium 6%	Iron 15%

Nutrition Grade B-

* Based on a 2000 calorie diet

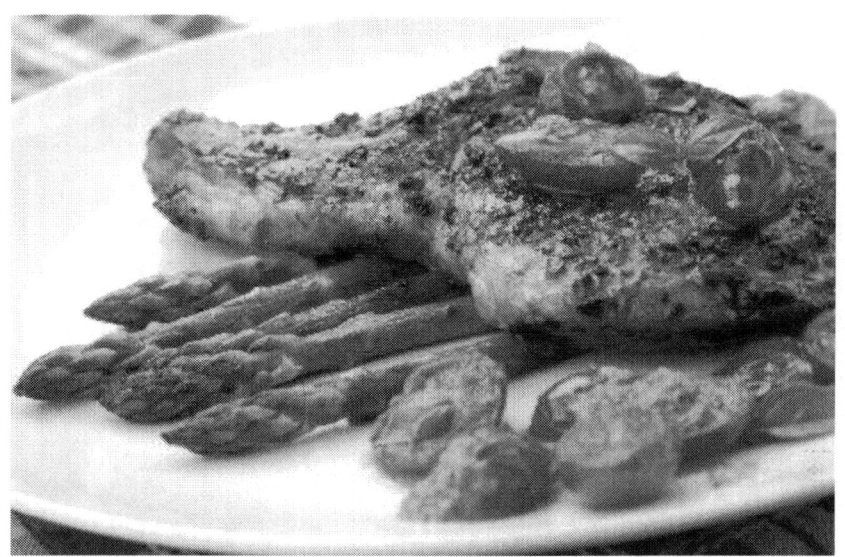

Caribbean Chicken salad

Serves 2

Ingredients - Allergies: SF, GF, DF, EF, NF

- 2 boneless skinless chicken breasts

Marinade
- 1/2 cup fish sauce
- 2 tomatoes (seeded and chopped)
- 1/2 cup chopped onion
- 2 tsps. jalapeno chilies (minced)
- 2 tsps. chopped cilantro fresh

Lucuma powder *Lime Dressing:*
- 1/4 cup mustard
- 1/4 cup lucuma powder
- 1 tbsp coconut oil
- 1 1/2 tbsps. lemon juice
- 1 1/2 tsps. lime juice
- 3/4 lb mixed greens

Instructions

Blend all the marinade ingredients in a small bowl with a hand blender. Cover and chill. Marinate the chicken for at least two hours in the fridge. Grill the chicken for few minutes per side or until done.

Serve the greens into 2 large salad bowls.
Slice the chicken into thin strips. Divide among bowls.
Pour the dressing aside and serve with the salads.

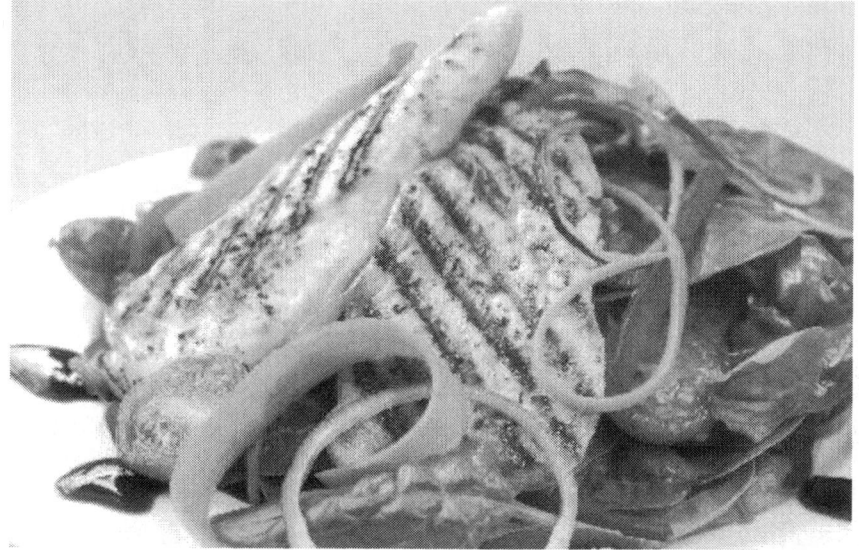

Tuna with Large Fiber Loaded Salad with Italian Dressing

Serves 1 - Allergies: SF, GF, DF, EF, NF

- 6 oz. can of Tuna, drained.

- Large mixed spinach and green onion salad with Italian Dressing and half a tsp of mustard. Salad can be as large as you want, but use only the prescribed amount of dressing. You may use fish sauce instead of salt.

Nutrition Facts

Serving Size 155 g

Amount Per Serving

Calories 275	Calories from Fat 134
	% Daily Value*
Total Fat 14.8g	**23%**
Saturated Fat 2.7g	**13%**
Cholesterol 37mg	**12%**
Sodium 83mg	**3%**
Potassium 574mg	**16%**
Total Carbohydrates 1.7g	**1%**
Dietary Fiber 0.9g	**4%**
Protein 32.8g	

Vitamin A 58%	•	Vitamin C 14%
Calcium 4%	•	Iron 10%

Nutrition Grade B+

* Based on a 2000 calorie diet

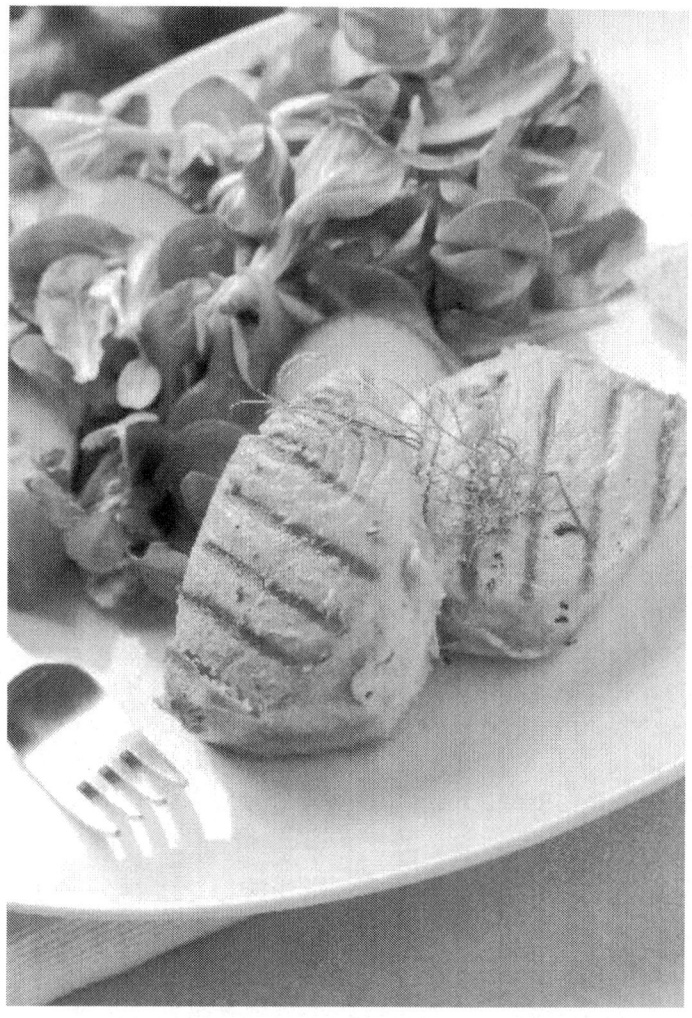

Stews, Chilies and Curries

Stuffed Peppers with beans
Serves 2

Ingredients - Allergies: SF, GF, DF, EF, V, NF

2 large red or green bell peppers
1 cup stewed tomatoes
1/3 cup brown rice
2 tbsp. hot water
2 green onions
8 ounces cooked black beans
1/4 tsp. crushed red pepper flakes

Instructions

Discard seeds and membrane from peppers. Place cut-side down and cover. Bake at 375F for 15 minutes.
While the peppers are cooking, cook tomatoes, rice and water for 15 minutes. In the meantime, thinly slice green onions.
Stir beans, green onions, and pepper flakes into tomato mixture. Cook for 10 minutes more. Drain peppers. Turn cut-side up. Spoon beans mixture evenly into peppers and bake in the oven for 5-10 minutes.

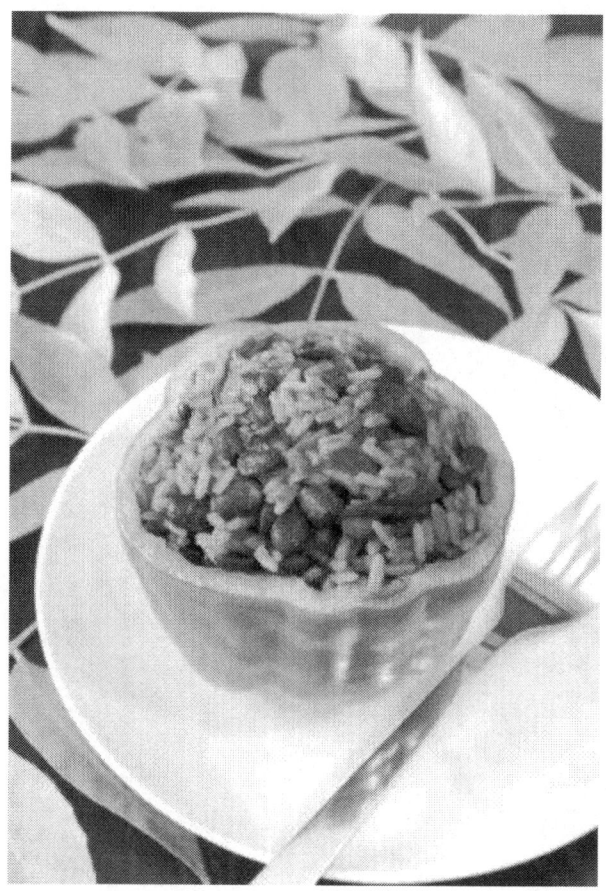

Vegetarian Chili

Serves 4-6

Ingredients - Allergies: SF, GF, DF, EF, V, NF

1 tbsp. coconut oil
1 cup chopped onions
3/4 cup chopped carrots
3 cloves garlic, minced
1 cup chopped green bell pepper
1 cup chopped red bell pepper
3/4 cup chopped celery
1 tbsp. chili powder
1-1/2 cups chopped mushrooms
3 cups chopped tomatoes
2 cups cooked kidney beans
1 tbsp. ground cumin
1-1/2 teaspoons oregano
1-1/2 teaspoons crushed basil leaves

Instructions

Heat coconut oil in a large saucepan and add onions, carrots and garlic; sauté until tender. Stir in green pepper, red pepper, celery and chili powder.
Cook, stirring often, until vegetables are tender, about 6 minutes. To the vegetables add mushrooms; cook 4 minutes. Stir in tomatoes, kidney beans, corn, cumin, oregano and basil. Bring to a boil. Reduce heat to medium. Cover & simmer for 20 minutes, stirring occasionally.

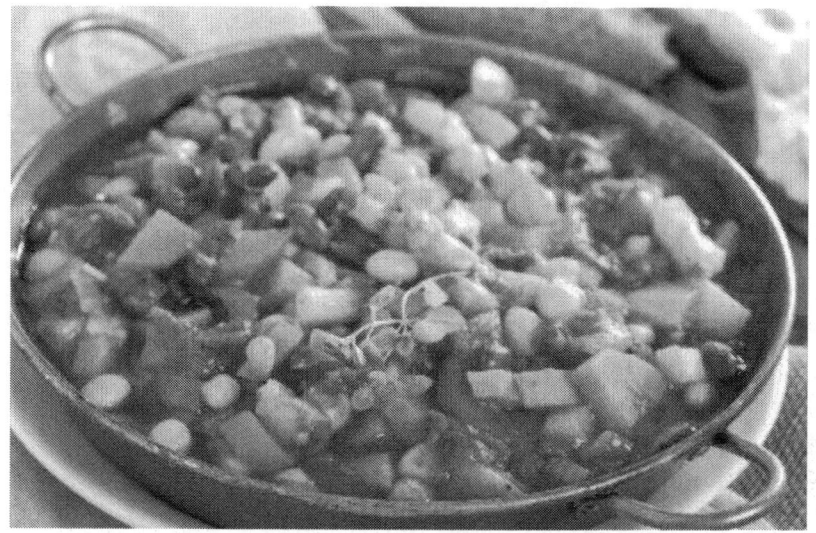

Lentil Stew

Recipe is for 4 servings, but you might want to adjust to 2 servings (eat one, freeze one)

Ingredients - Allergies: SF, GF, DF, EF, NF

- 1 cup dry lentils
- 3 1/2 cups chicken broth
- few tomatoes
- 1 medium potato chopped + 1/2 cup chopped carrot
- 1/2 cup chopped onion + 1/2 cup chopped celery (optional)
- few sprigs of parsley and basil + 1 garlic clove (minced)
- 1 pound of cubed lean pork or beef + pepper to taste

Nutrition Facts

Serving Size 456 g

Amount Per Serving

Calories 453	Calories from Fat 79
	% Daily Value*
Total Fat 8.8g	**14%**
Saturated Fat 3.0g	**15%**
Trans Fat 0.0g	
Cholesterol 101mg	**34%**
Sodium 684mg	**29%**
Potassium 1394mg	**40%**
Total Carbohydrates 39.4g	**13%**
Dietary Fiber 16.8g	**67%**
Sugars 4.8g	
Protein 51.7g	
Vitamin A 13%	Vitamin C 28%
Calcium 5%	Iron 148%

Nutrition Grade A

* Based on a 2000 calorie diet

You can eat a salad of your choice with this stew.

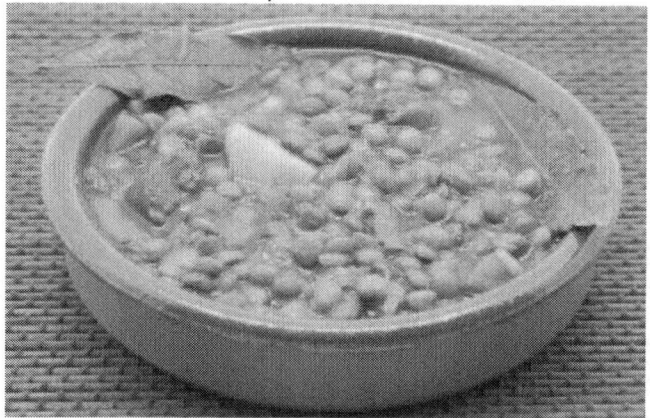

Braised Green Peas with Beef

Serves 1

Ingredients - Allergies: SF, GF, DF, EF, NF

- 1 cup fresh or frozen green peas
- 1 onion, finely chopped
- 2 cloves of garlic, thinly sliced and 1/2 inch of peeled/sliced fresh ginger (if you like)
- 1/2 tsp. red pepper flakes, or to taste
- 1 tomato, roughly chopped
- 1 chopped carrot
- 1 tbsp. coconut oil
- 1/2 cup chicken broth
- 4 oz. cubed beef
- Salt and ground black pepper

Heat the coconut oil in a skillet over medium heat. Sauté the onion, garlic and ginger until they are soft. Add the red pepper, carrot, and tomatoes and sauté until the tomato begins to soften. Add in the green peas. Add 4 oz. cubed lean beef. Add in the broth and simmer over medium heat. Cover and cook until the peas are tender. Season to taste with salt and pepper.

Nutrition Facts

Serving Size 497 g

Amount Per Serving

Calories 387 — Calories from Fat 156

	% Daily Value*
Total Fat 17.3g	**27%**
Saturated Fat 5.9g	**30%**
Trans Fat 0.0g	
Cholesterol 75mg	**25%**
Sodium 497mg	**21%**
Potassium 657mg	**19%**
Total Carbohydrates 24.8g	**8%**
Dietary Fiber 7.8g	**31%**
Sugars 10.7g	
Protein 35.9g	

Vitamin A 32% • Vitamin C 100%
Calcium 4% • Iron 44%

Nutrition Grade B

* Based on a 2000 calorie diet

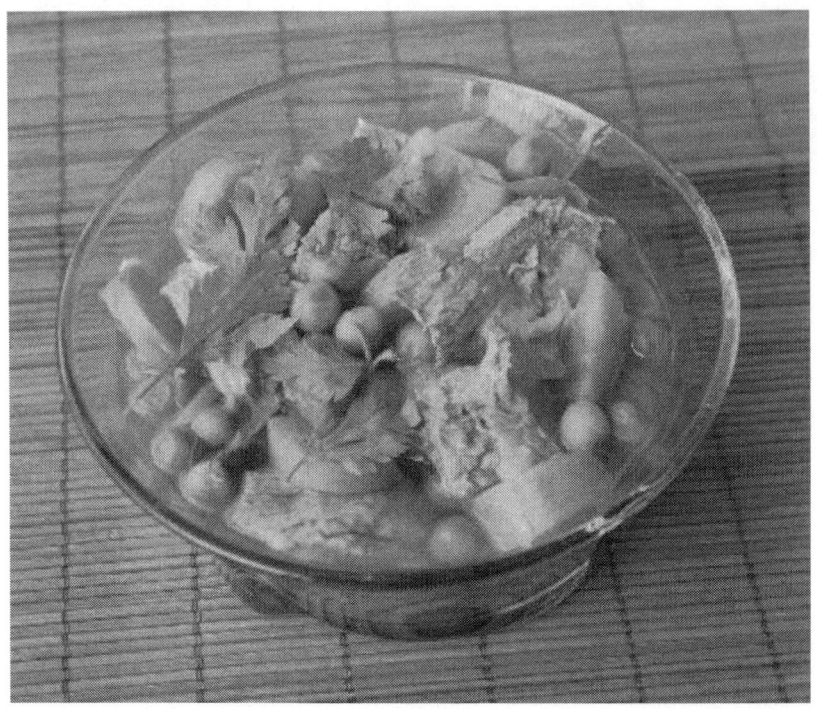

White Chicken Chili
Serves: 5

Ingredients - Allergies: SF, GF, DF, EF, NF

- 4 large boneless, skinless chicken breasts
- 2 green bell peppers
- 1 large yellow onion
- 1 jalapeno
- 1/2 cup diced green chilies (optional)
- 1/2 cup of spring onions
- 1.5 tbsp. coconut oil
- 3 cups cooked white beans
- 3.5 cups chicken or vegetable broth
- 1 tsp. ground cumin
- 1/4 tsp. cayenne pepper
- salt to taste

Instructions

Bring a pot of water to boil. Add the chicken breasts & cook until cooked through. Drain water and allow chicken to cool. When cool, shred and set aside.

Dice the bell peppers, jalapeno and onion. Melt the coconut oil in a pot over high heat. Add the peppers and onions and sauté until soft, approx. 8-10 minutes.

Add the broth, beans, chicken and spices to the pot. Stir and bring to a low boil. Cover & simmer for 25-30 minutes.

Simmer for 10 more minutes and stir occasionally. Remove from heat. Let stand for 10 minutes to thicken. Top with cilantro.

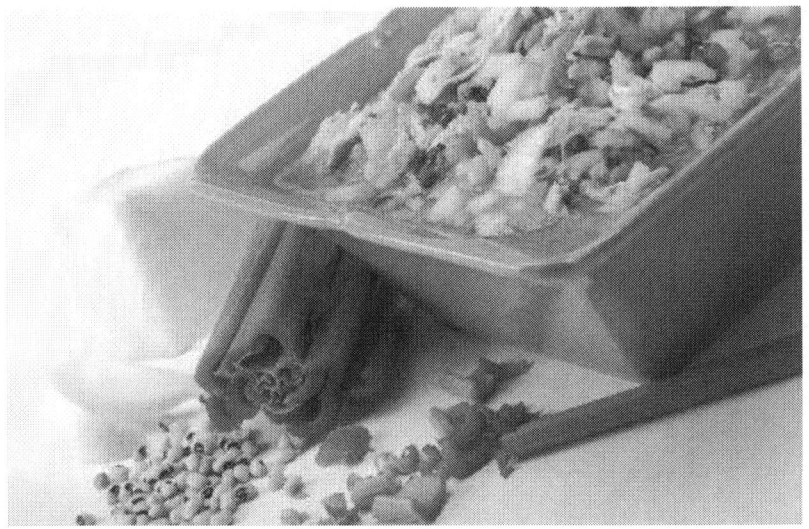

Kale Pork

Serves 4

Ingredients - Allergies: SF, GF, DF, EF, NF

- 1 tbsp. coconut oil
- 1 pound cubed pork tenderloin
- 3/4 tsp. salt
- 1 medium onion, finely chopped
- 4 cloves garlic, minced
- 2 teaspoons paprika
- 1/4 tsp. crushed red pepper (optional)
- 1 cup white wine
- 4 plum tomatoes, chopped
- 4 cups chicken broth
- 1 bunch kale, chopped
- 2 cups cooked white beans

Instructions

Heat coconut oil in a pot over medium heat. Add pork, season with salt and cook until no longer pink. Transfer to a plate and leave juices in the pot.

Add onion to the pot and cook until turns translucent. Add paprika, garlic and crushed red pepper and cook about 30 seconds. Add tomatoes and wine, increase heat and stir to scrape up any browned bits. Add broth. Bring to a boil.

Add kale and stir until it wilts. Lower the heat and simmer, until the kale is tender. Stir in beans, pork and pork juices. Simmer for 2 more minutes.

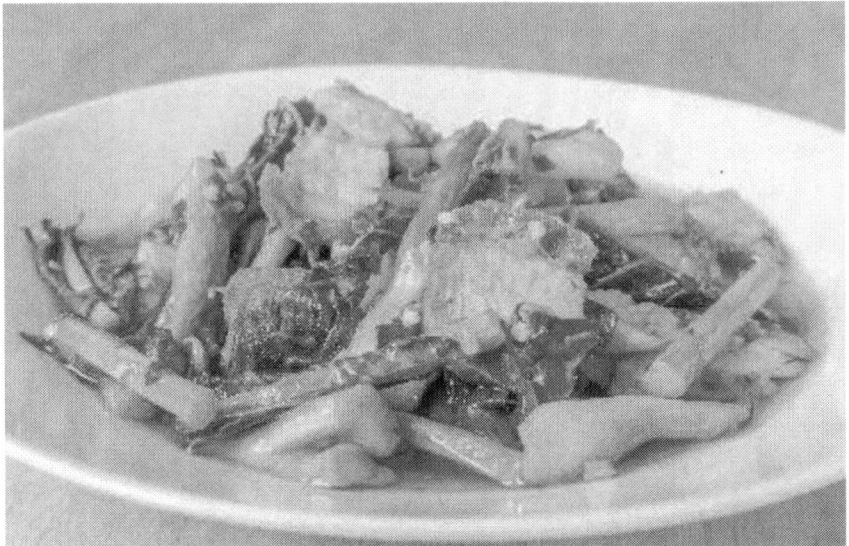

30-Minute Squash Cauliflower and Green Peppers Coconut Curry

Serves: 6

Ingredients - Allergies: SF, GF, DF, EF, V, NF

- Curry Paste
- 3 cups peeled, chopped squash
- 2 cups thick coconut milk
- 3 tbsp. coconut oil
- 2 tbsp. lucuma powder
- 2 pounds tomatoes
- 1 and 1/4 cup brown rice, uncooked
- 1 cup chopped Cauliflower
- 1 cup chopped Green Peppers
- Cilantro for topping

Instructions

Cook brown rice. Set aside.

Make Curry Paste. Pour the coconut milk into the skillet and mix the curry and lucuma powder into the coconut milk. Add the cauliflower, squash, and green peppers. Cover and simmer until squash is tender. Remove from heat and let stand for 10 minutes. The sauce will thicken.

Serve the curry over brown rice. Add chopped cilantro before serving.

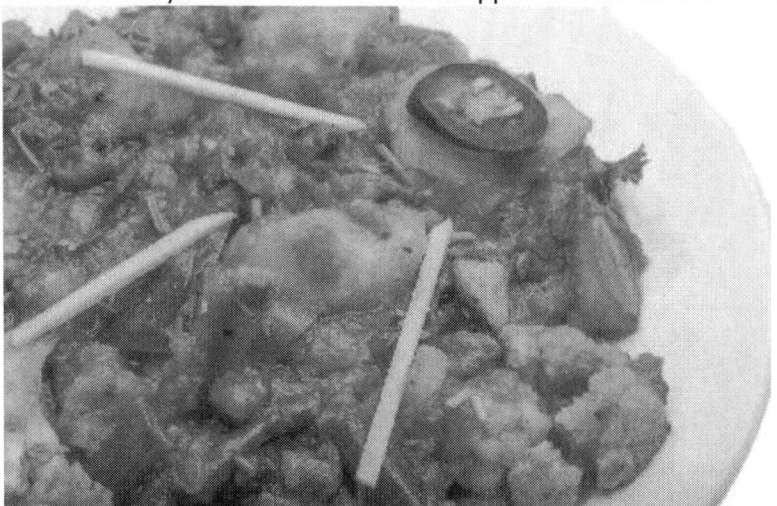

Crockpot Red Curry Lamb

Serves: 16

Ingredients - Allergies: SF, GF, DF, EF, NF

- 3 pounds cubed lamb meat
- Curry Paste *
- 4 cups tomato paste
- 1 tsp. salt plus more to taste
- 1/2 cup coconut milk or cream

Instructions

Make the Curry Paste. Add lamb and the curry paste in a crockpot. Pour one cup of tomato paste over the lamb. Add 2 cups of water to the crockpot. Stir, cover and cook on high for 2 hours or low for 4-5 hours. Taste and season with salt.

Stir in the coconut milk and sprinkle with cilantro before serving. Serve over brown rice or naan bread.

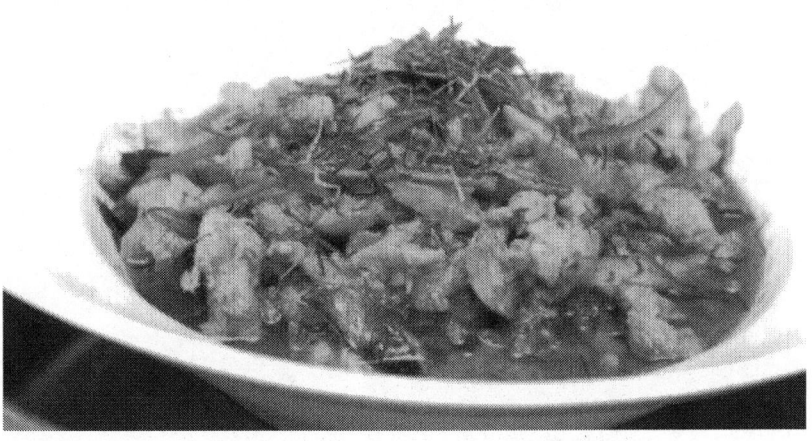

Easy Lentil Dhal

Serves: 6

Ingredients - Allergies: SF, GF, DF, EF, V, NF

- 2 1/2 cups lentils
- 5-6 cups of water
- Curry Paste *
- 1/2 cup coconut milk
- 1/3 cup water
- 1/2 teaspoons salt + 1/4 tsp. black pepper
- lime juice
- Cilantro and spring onions for garnish

Instructions

Bring the water to a boil in a large pot. Add lentils and cook uncovered for 10 minutes, stirring frequently. Remove from heat. Stir in remaining ingredients. Season with salt and herbs for garnish.

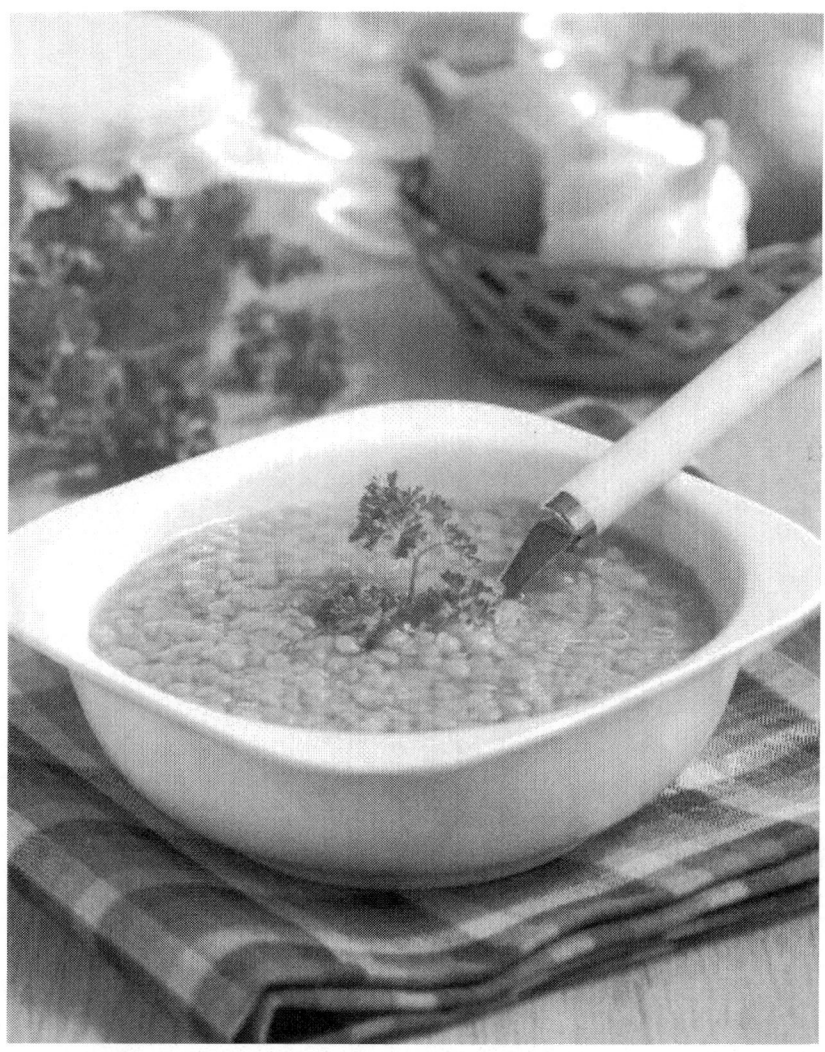

Gumbo

8 servings

Ingredients - Allergies: SF, GF, DF, EF, NF

- 1 pound medium shrimp peeled
- 1/2 pound skinless, boneless chicken breasts, cut bite size
- 1/2 cup coconut oil
- 3/4 cup almond flour
- 2 cups chopped onions
- 1 cup chopped celery
- 1 cup chopped green pepper
- 1 tsp. ground cumin
- 1 tbsp. minced fresh garlic
- 1 tsp. fresh thyme chopped
- 1/2 tsp. red pepper
- 6 cups chicken broth
- 2 cups diced tomatoes
- 3 cups sliced okra
- 1/2 cup fresh parsley chopped
- 2 bay leaves
- 1 tsp. hot sauce

Instructions

Sauté' chicken on high heat until brown in a large pot. Remove and set aside. Chop onions, celery, and green pepper and set aside.

Place oil and flour in pot. Stir well and brown to make a roux. When roux is done add chopped vegetables. Sauté on low heat for 10 minutes.

Slowly add chicken broth stirring constantly.

Add chicken and all other ingredients except the okra, shrimp and parsley, which will be saved for the end.

Cover and simmer on low for half an hour. Remove lid and cook for half an hour more, stirring occasionally.

Add shrimp, okra and parsley. Continue to cook on low heat uncovered for 15 minutes.

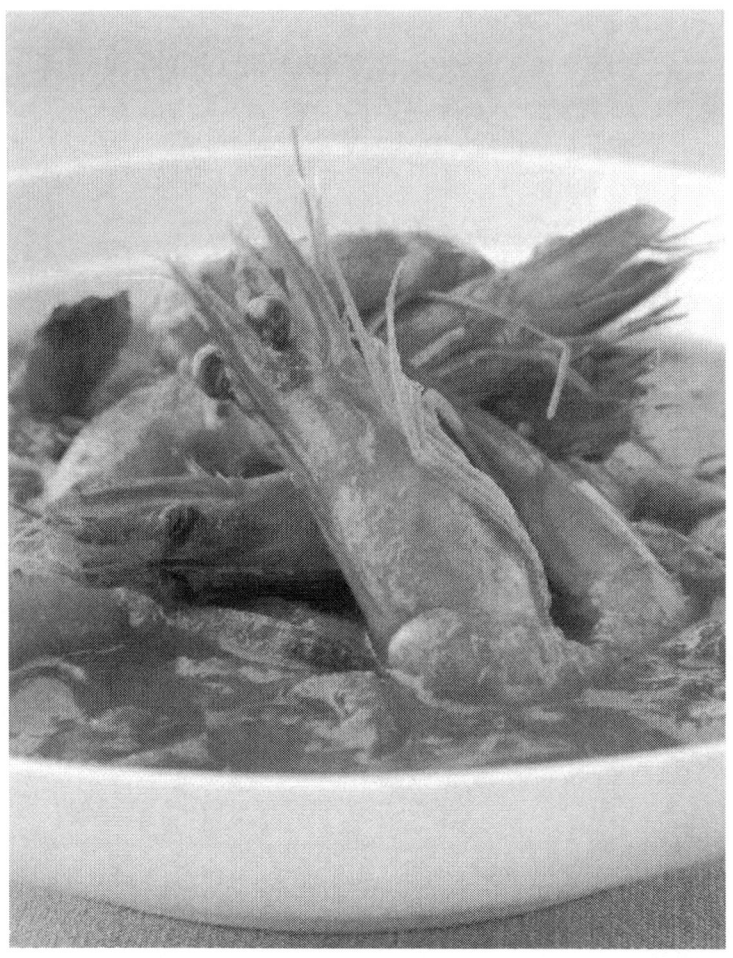

Chickpea Curry

Serves 4

Ingredients - Allergies: SF, GF, DF, EF, V, NF

- Curry Paste
- 4 cups cooked chickpeas
- 1 cup chopped cilantro

Instructions

Make Curry Paste. Mix in chickpeas and their liquid. Continue to cook. Stir until all ingredients are blended. Remove from heat. Stir in cilantro just before serving, reserving 1 tbsp. for garnish.

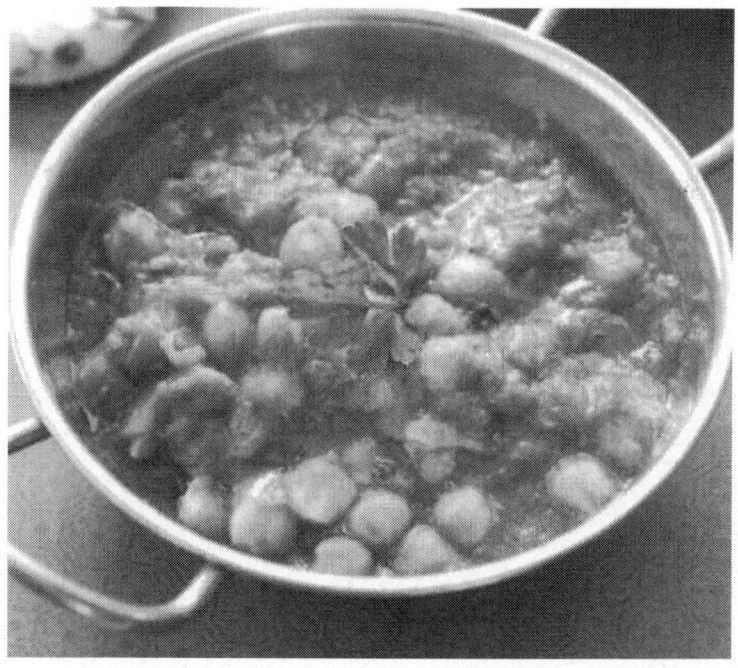

Red Curry Chicken

Serves: 6

Ingredients - Allergies: SF, GF, DF, EF, NF

- 2 cups cubed chicken meat
- Curry Paste
- 2 cups tomato paste
- 1/4 cup coconut milk or cream
- Cilantro for garnishing
- Brown rice for serving

Instructions

Make Curry Paste. Add the tomato paste; stir and simmer until smooth. Add the chicken and the cream. Stir to combine. Simmer for 20 minutes. Serve with brown rice and cilantro.

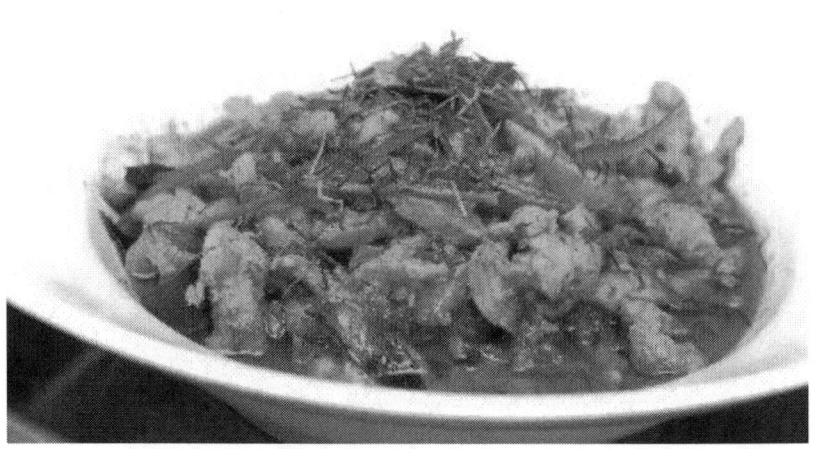

Braised Green Beans with Pork

Serves 1

Ingredients - Allergies: SF, GF, DF, EF, NF

- 1cup fresh or frozen green beans
- 1 onion, finely chopped
- 2 cloves of garlic, thinly sliced
- 1/2 inch of peeled/sliced fresh ginger
- 1/2 tsp. red pepper flakes, or to taste
- 1 tomato, roughly chopped
- 1 tbsp. coconut oil
- 1/2 cup chicken broth
- Salt and ground black pepper
- 1/4 lemon, cut into wedges, to serve
- 5 oz. lean pork

Instructions

Cut each bean in half. Heat the coconut oil in a skillet over medium heat. Sauté the onion, garlic and ginger over medium heat until they are soft. Add the red pepper and tomatoes and sauté until the tomato begins to break down. Stir in the green beans. Add 5 oz. cubed lean pork. Add broth and bring to a simmer over medium heat. Cover and cook until the beans are tender. Season to taste with salt and pepper. Serve with lemon wedge on the side.

Nutrition Facts

Serving Size 574 g

Amount Per Serving

Calories 316	Calories from Fat 39
	% Daily Value*
Total Fat 4.3g	**7%**
Saturated Fat 1.1g	**6%**
Trans Fat 0.0g	
Cholesterol 82mg	**27%**
Sodium 1156mg	**48%**
Potassium 1314mg	**38%**
Total Carbohydrates 34.6g	**12%**
Dietary Fiber 8.8g	**35%**
Sugars 8.8g	
Protein 34.5g	

Vitamin A 33%	•	Vitamin C 81%
Calcium 9%	•	Iron 30%

Nutrition Grade A

* Based on a 2000 calorie diet

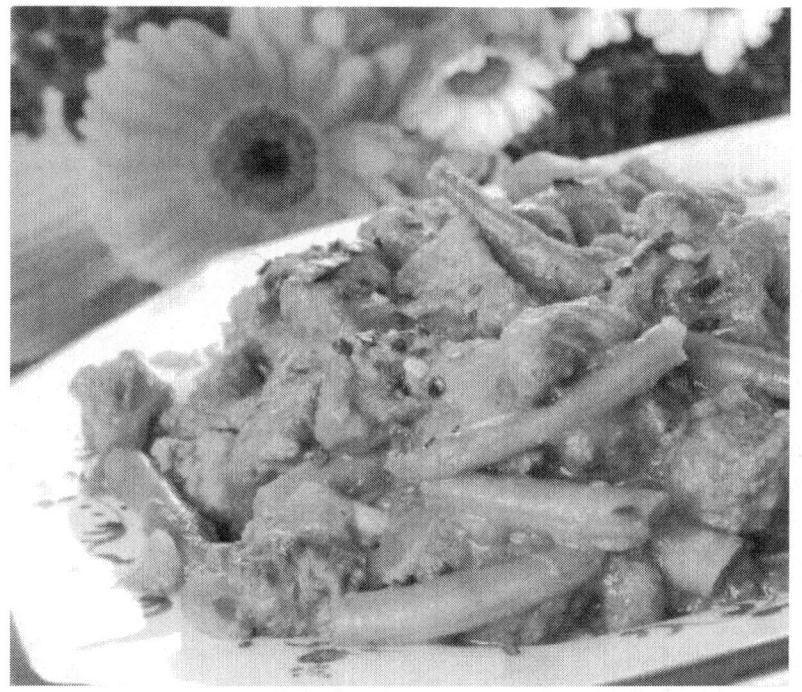

Ratatouille

Serves 4-6

Ingredients - Allergies: SF, GF, DF, EF, V, NF

- 2 large eggplants
- 3 medium zucchinis
- 2 medium onions
- 2 red or green peppers
- 4 large tomatoes
- 2 cloves garlic, crushed
- 4 tbsp. coconut oil
- 1 tbsp. fresh basil
- Salt and freshly milled black pepper

Instructions

Cut eggplant and zucchini into 1 inch slices. Then cut each slice in half. Salt them and leave them for one hour. The salt will draw out the bitterness.

Chop peppers and onions. Skin the tomatoes by boiling them for few minutes. Then quarter them, take out the seeds and chop the flesh. Fry garlic and the onions in the coconut oil in a saucepan for a 10 minutes. Add the peppers. Dry the eggplant and zucchini and add them to the saucepan. Add the basil, salt and pepper. Stir and simmer for half an hour.

Add the tomato flesh, check the seasoning and cook for an additional 15 minutes with the lid off.

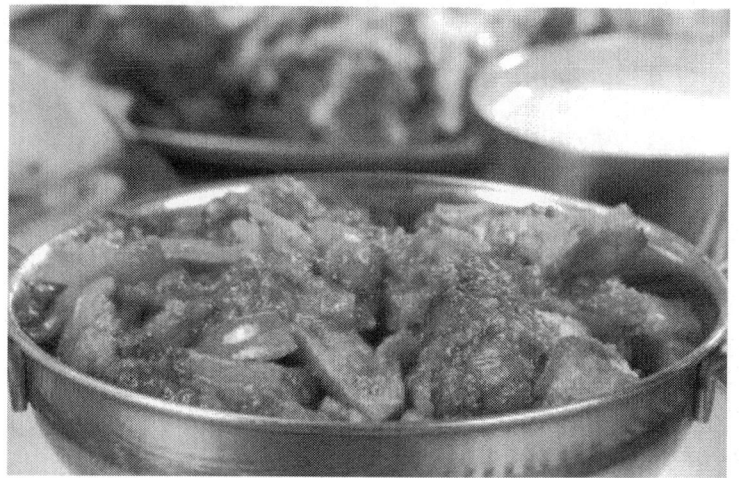

Barbecued Beef

Serves 8

Ingredients - Allergies: SF, GF, DF, EF, NF

- 1-1/2 cups tomato paste
- 1/4 cup lemon juice
- 2 tbsp. mustard
- 1/2 tsp. salt
- 1 chopped carrot
- 1/4 tsp. ground black pepper
- 1/2 tsp. minced garlic
- 4 pounds boneless chuck roast

Instructions

In a large bowl, combine tomato paste, lemon juice and mustard. Stir in salt, pepper and garlic.
Place chuck roast and carrot in a slow cooker. Pour tomato mixture over chuck roast. Cover, & cook on low for 7 to 9 hours. Remove chuck roast from slow cooker, shred with a fork, and return to the slow cooker. Stir meat to evenly coat with sauce. Continue cooking approximately 1 hour.

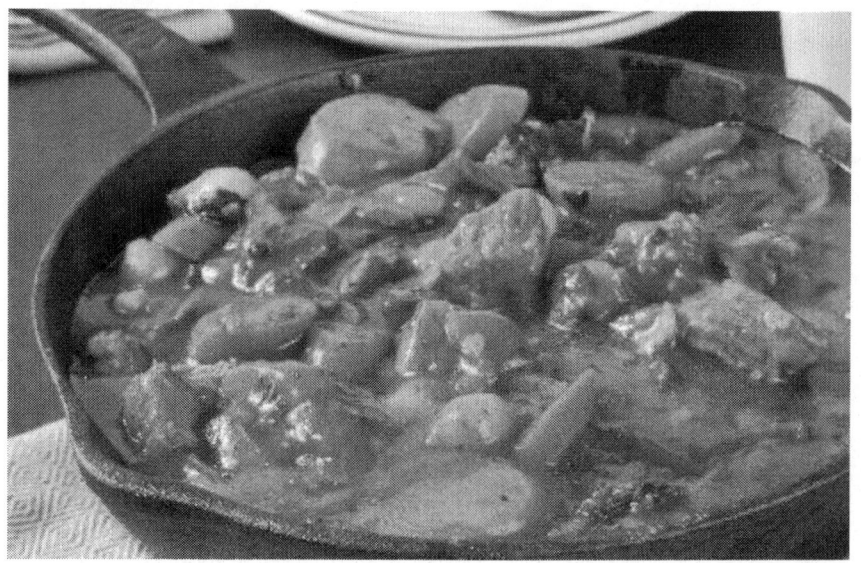

Beef Tenderloin with Roasted Shallots

Serves 4-6

Ingredients - Allergies: SF, GF, DF, EF

- 3/4 pound shallots, halved lengthwise and peeled
- 1-1/2 tbsp. olive oil or avocado oil
- salt and pepper to taste
- 3 cups beef broth
- 3/4 cup red wine
- 1-1/2 teaspoons tomato paste
- 2 pounds beef tenderloin roast, trimmed
- 1 tsp. dried thyme
- 3 tbsp. coconut oil
- 1 tbsp. almond flour

Instructions

Heat oven to 375 degrees F. Toss shallots with olive oil to coat in a baking pan and season with salt and pepper. Roast until shallots are tender, stirring occasionally, about half an hour.
Combine wine and beef broth in a sauce pan and bring to a boil. Cook over high heat. Volume should be reduced by half. Add in tomato paste. Set aside.
Pat beef dry and sprinkle with salt and thyme and pepper. Add beef to pan oiled with coconut oil. Brown on all sides over high heat.
Put pan back to the oven. Roast beef about half an hour for medium rare. Transfer beef to platter. Cover loosely with foil.
Place pan on stove top and add broth mixture. Bring to boil and stir to scrape up any browned bits. Transfer to a different saucepan, and bring to simmer. Mix 1 1/2 tbsp. coconut oil and

flour in small bowl and mix. Whisk into broth, and simmer until sauce thickens. Stir in roasted shallots. Season with salt and pepper.

Cut beef into 1/2 inch thick slices. Spoon some sauce over.

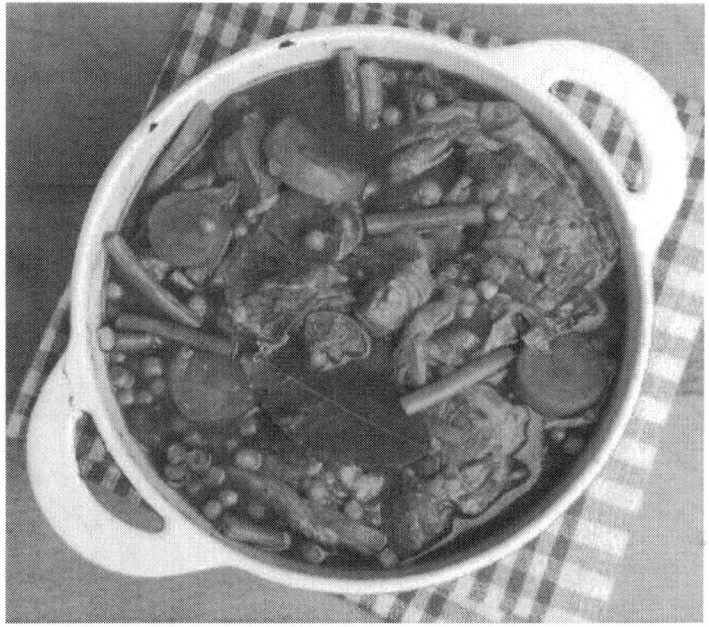

Chili

Serves 6

Ingredients - Allergies: SF, GF, DF, EF, NF

- 2 tbsp. coconut oil
- 2 onions, chopped
- 3 cloves garlic, minced
- 1 pound ground beef
- 3/4 pound beef sirloin, cubed
- 2 cups diced tomatoes
- 1 cup strong brewed coffee
- 1 cup tomato paste
- 2 cups beef broth
- 1 tbsp. cumin seeds
- 1 tbsp. unsweetened cocoa powder
- 1 tsp. dried oregano
- 1 tsp. ground cayenne pepper
- 1 tsp. ground coriander
- 1 tsp. salt
- 6 cups cooked kidney beans
- 4 fresh hot chili peppers, chopped

Instructions

Heat oil in a saucepan over medium/high heat. Cook garlic, onions, sirloin and ground beef in oil until the meat is browned and the onions are translucent.
Mix in the diced tomatoes, coffee, tomato paste and beef broth. Season with oregano, cumin, cocoa powder, cayenne pepper, coriander and salt. Stir in hot chile peppers and 3 cups of the beans. Reduce heat to low, and simmer for two hours.

Stir in the 3 remaining cups of beans. Simmer for another 30 minutes.

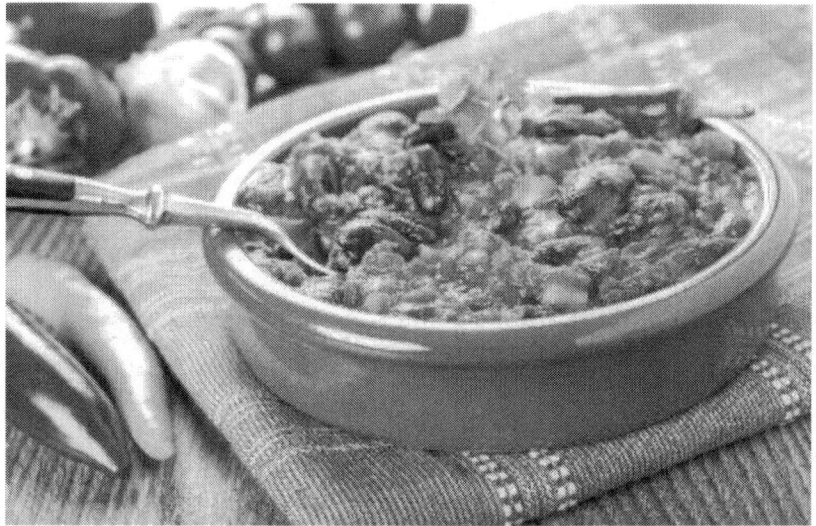

Glazed Meatloaf

Serves 4

Ingredients - Allergies: SF, GF, DF, NF

- 1/2 cup tomato paste
- 1/4 cup lemon juice, divided
- 1 tsp. mustard powder
- 2 pounds ground beef
- 1 cup flax seeds meal
- 1/4 cup chopped onion
- 1 egg, beaten

Instructions

Heat oven to 350 degrees F. Combine mustard, tomato paste, 1 tbsp. lemon juice in a small bowl.

Combine onion, ground beef, flax, egg and remaining lemon juice in a separate larger bowl. And add 1/3 of the tomato paste mixture from the smaller bowl. Mix all well and place in a loaf pan.

Bake at 350 degrees F for one hour. Drain any excess fat and coat with remaining tomato paste mixture. Bake for 10 more minutes.

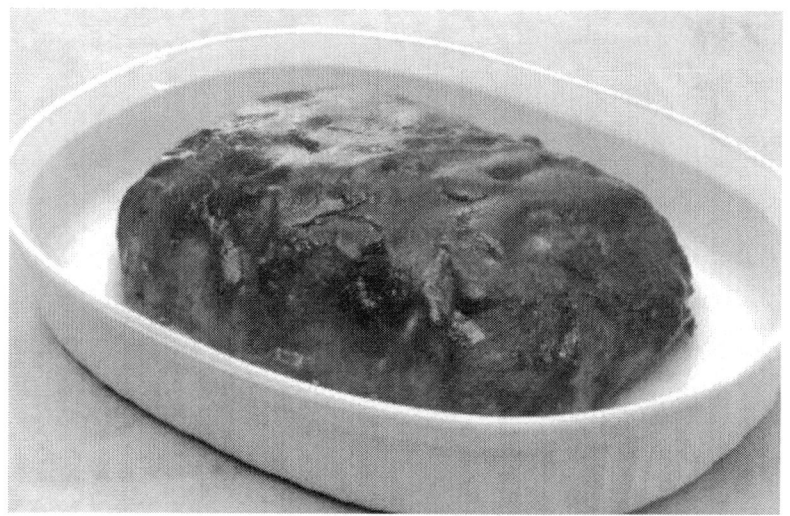

Eggplant Lasagna

Serves 4-6

Ingredients - Allergies: SF, GF, NF

- 2 large eggplants, peeled and sliced lengthwise into strips
- coconut oil
- salt and pepper

Meat Sauce

- 1 1/2 lbs ground sirloin or 1 1/2 lbs turkey breast
- 2 tbsp. coconut oil
- 2 onions, chopped
- 3 cloves chopped garlic
- 1 red pepper, chopped
- 1 (16 ounce) package sliced mushrooms
- 1 tbsp. of oregano, basil and thyme each
- 1 tsp. fennel seed (optional)
- salt and pepper
- 1 tsp. red pepper flakes (optional)
- 1 cup chopped spinach
- 2 cups tomato sauce
- 1 cup diced tomatoes

Cheese Mixture

- 2 cups low-fat farmers cheese
- 2 eggs
- 3 green onions, chopped

- 1 cup shredded low-fat mozzarella cheese (optional)

Instructions

Heat oven to 425 degrees.

Oil cookie sheet and arrange eggplant slice. Sprinkle with salt and pepper. Bake slices five minutes on each side. Lower oven temp to 375.

Brown onion, meat and garlic in coconut oil for 5 minutes. Add mushrooms and red pepper, and cook for 5 minutes. Add tomatoes, spinach and spices and simmer for 5-10 minutes.

Blend farmers' cheese, egg and onion mixture. Spread one third of meat sauce in bottom of a glass pan. Layer one half of eggplant slices and one half farmers' cheese. Repeat. Add last layer of sauce and then mozzarella on top.

Cover with foil. Bake at 375 degrees for one hour. Remove foil and bake until cheese is browned. Let it rest 10 minutes before serving.

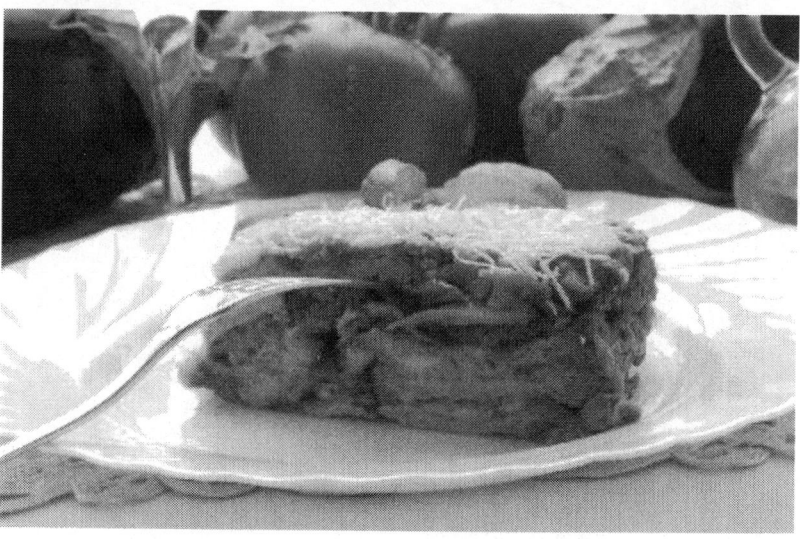

Stuffed Eggplant

Serves – one half of eggplant per person

Allergies: SF, GF, DF, EF, NF

Rinse the eggplants. Cut off a slice from one end. Make a wide slit and salt them. Deseed tomatoes. Chop them finely. Cut the onions in thin slices. Chop the garlic cloves. Place them in a frying pan with coconut oil. Add the tomatoes, salt parsley, cumin, pepper, hot peppers and ground beef. Sauté for 10 minutes.

Squeeze eggplants, so the bitter juice goes out. Fill the wide slit with the ground beef mix. Pour the remaining mix over. Heat the oven to 375F in the meantime. Place eggplants a baking pan. Sprinkle them with olive oil, lemon juice and 1 cup of water. Cover the pan with a foil.

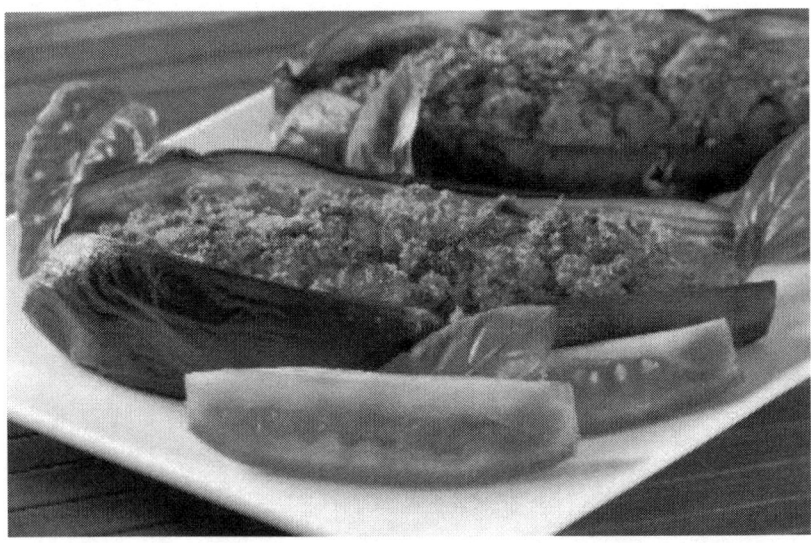

Stuffed Red Peppers with Beef
Serves 4-6

Ingredients - Allergies: SF, GF, DF, EF, NF

- 6 red bell peppers
- salt to taste
- 1 pound ground beef
- 1/3 cup chopped onion
- salt and pepper to taste
- 2 cups chopped tomatoes
- 1/2 cup uncooked brown rice or quinoa
- 1/2 cup water
- 2 cups tomato soup
- water as needed

Instructions

Bring a pot of salted water to a boil. Cut the tops off the peppers. Remove the seeds. Cook peppers in boiling water for 5 minutes and drain.
Sprinkle salt inside each pepper, and set aside.
In a skillet, sauté onions and beef until beef is browned. Drain off excess fat. Season with salt and pepper. Stir in rice, tomatoes and 1/2 cup water. Cover, and simmer until rice is tender. Remove from heat. Stir in the cheese.
Heat the oven to 350 degrees F. Stuff each pepper with the rice and beef mixture. Place peppers open side up in a baking dish. Combine tomato soup with just enough water to make the soup a gravy consistency in a separate bowl. Pour over the peppers.
Bake covered for 25 to 35 minutes.

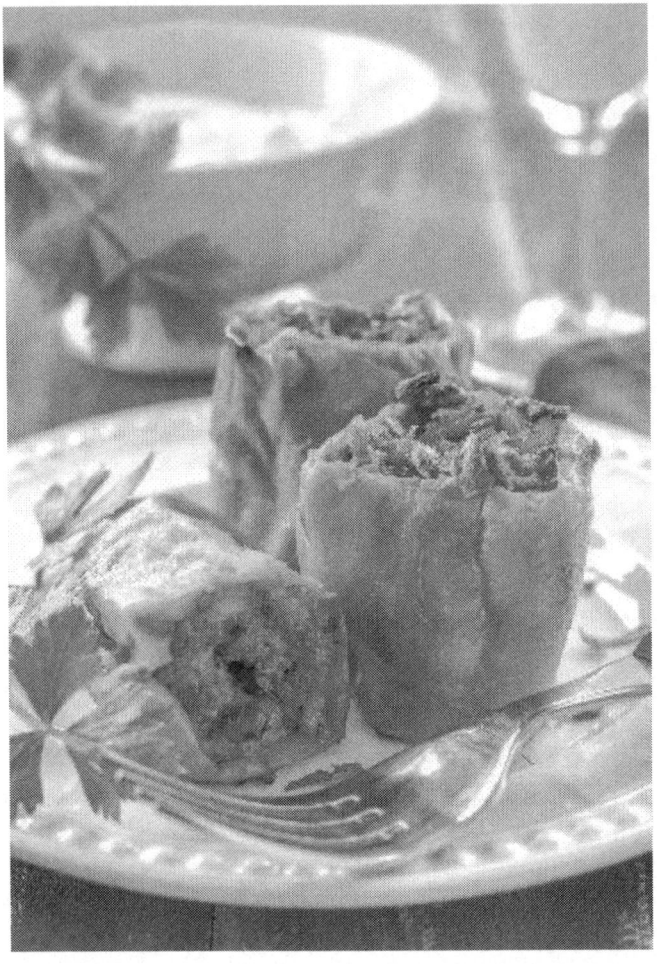

Superfoods Goulash

Serves 4-6

Ingredients - Allergies: SF, GF, DF, EF, NF

- 3 cups cauliflower
- 1 pound ground beef
- 1 medium onion, chopped
- salt to taste
- ground black pepper according to taste
- garlic to taste
- 2 cups cooked kidney beans
- 1 cup tomato paste

Brown the ground beef and onion in a skillet, over medium heat. Drain off the fat. Add garlic, salt and pepper to taste.
Stir in the cauliflower, kidney beans and tomato paste. Cook until cauliflower is done.

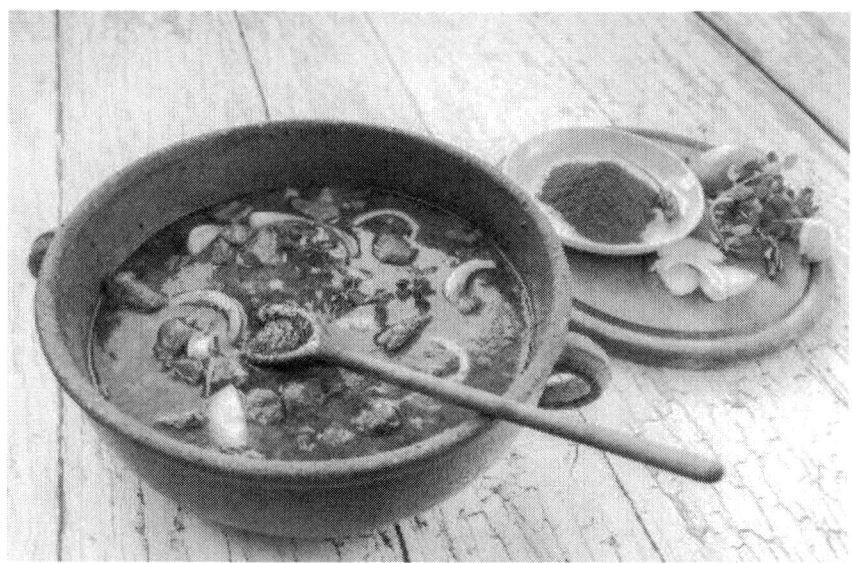

Frijoles Charros

Serves 4-6

Ingredients - Allergies: SF, GF, DF, EF, NF

- 1 pound dry pinto beans
- 5 cloves garlic, chopped
- 1 tsp. salt
- 1/2 pound pork, diced
- 1 onion, chopped & 2 fresh tomatoes, diced
- few sliced sliced jalapeno peppers
- 1/3 cup chopped cilantro

Instructions

Place pinto beans in a slow cooker. Cover with water. Mix in garlic and salt. Cover, and cook 1 hour on High.

Cook the pork in a skillet over medium/high heat until brown. Drain the fat. Place onion in the skillet. Cook until tender. Mix in jalapenos and tomatoes. Cook until heated through. Transfer to the slow cooker and stir into the beans. Continue cooking for 4 hours on Low. Mix in cilantro about half an hour before the end of the cook time.

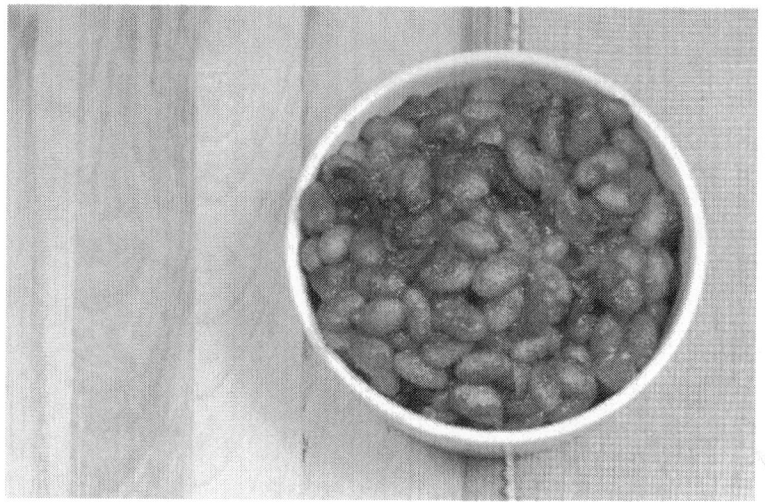

Chicken Cacciatore
Serves 8

Ingredients - Allergies: SF, GF, DF, EF, NF

- 4 pounds of chicken thighs, with skin on
- 2 Tbsp. extra virgin olive oil or avocado oil
- Salt
- 1 sliced onion
- 1/3 cup red wine
- 1 sliced red or green bell pepper
- 8 ounces sliced cremini mushrooms
- 2 sliced garlic cloves
- 3 cups peeled and chopped tomatoes
- 1/2 tsp. ground black pepper
- 1 tsp. dry oregano
- 1 tsp. dry thyme
- 1 sprig fresh rosemary
- 1 tbsp. fresh parsley

Instructions

Pat the chicken on all sides with salt. Heat the olive oil in a skillet on medium. Brown few chicken pieces skin side down in the pan (don't overcrowd) for 5 minutes, then turn. Set aside. Make sure you have 2 tbsp. of the rendered fat left.

Add the onions, mushrooms and bell peppers to the pan. Increase the heat to medium high. Cook until the onions are tender, stirring, about 10 minutes. Add the garlic and cook a minute more.

Add the wine. Scrape up any browned bits and simmer until the wine is reduced by half. Add the tomatoes, pepper, oregano, thyme and a tsp. of salt. Simmer uncovered for maybe 5 more minutes. Put the chicken pieces on top of the tomatoes, skin side up. Lower the heat. Cover the skillet with the lid slightly ajar.

Cook the chicken on a low simmer. Turning and baste from time to time. Add rosemary and cook until the meat is tender, about 30 to 40 minutes. Garnish with parsley.

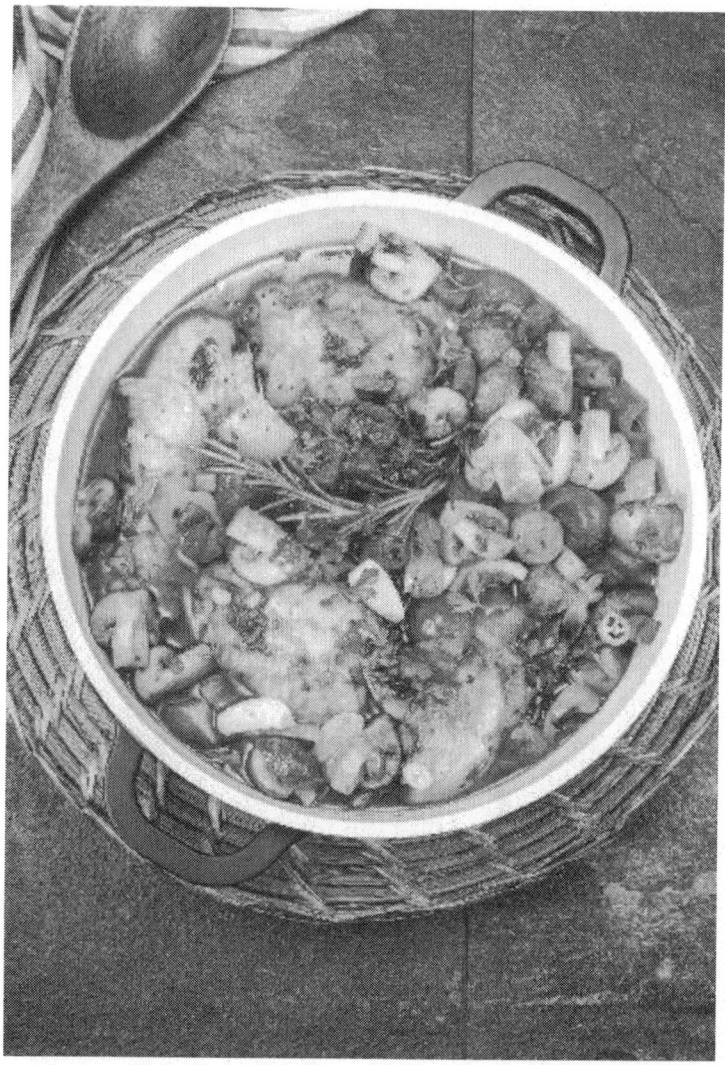

Cabbage Stewed with Meat

Serves 8

Ingredients - Allergies: SF, GF, DF, EF, NF

- 1-1/2 pounds ground beef
- 1 cup beef stock
- 1 chopped onion
- 1 bay leaf
- 1/4 tsp. pepper
- 2 sliced celery ribs
- 4 cups shredded cabbage
- 1 carrot, sliced
- 1 cup tomato paste
- 1/4 tsp. salt

Instructions

Brown ground meat in a pot. Add beef stock, onion, pepper and bay leaf. Cover and simmer until tender (approx.. 30 minutes). Add celery, cabbage and carrot.

Cover and simmer until vegetables are tender. Mix in tomato paste and seasoning blend. Simmer uncovered for 20 minutes.

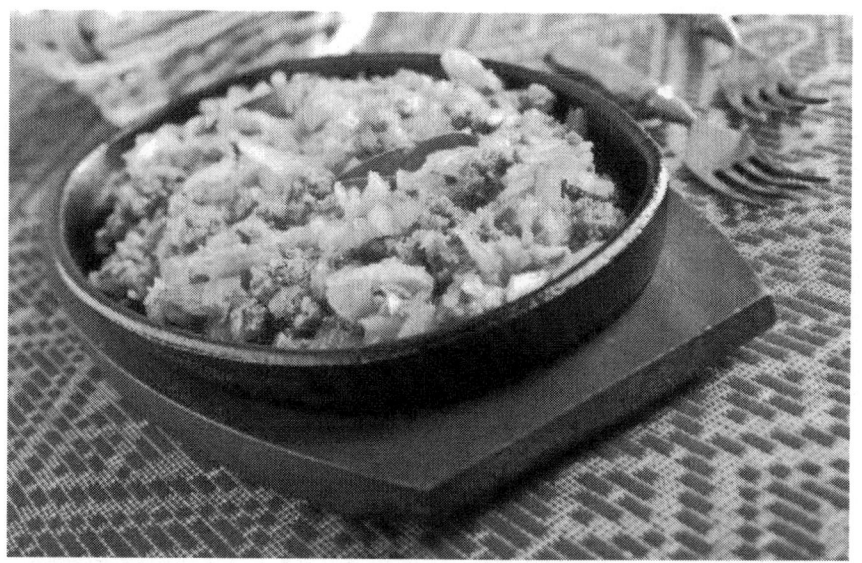

Beef Stew with Peas and Carrots
Serves 8

Ingredients - Allergies: SF, GF, DF, EF, NF

- 1-1/2 cups chopped carrots
- 1 cup chopped onions
- 2 tbsp. coconut oil
- 1-1/2 cups green peas
- 4 cups beef stock
- 1/2 tsp. salt
- 1/4 tsp. ground black pepper
- 1/2 tsp. minced garlic
- 4 pounds boneless chuck roast

Instructions

Cook the onions in coconut oil on medium until they are tender (few minutes). Add all other ingredients and stir. Cover & cook on low heat for 2 hours. Mix almond flour with some cold water, add to the stew & cook for another minute.

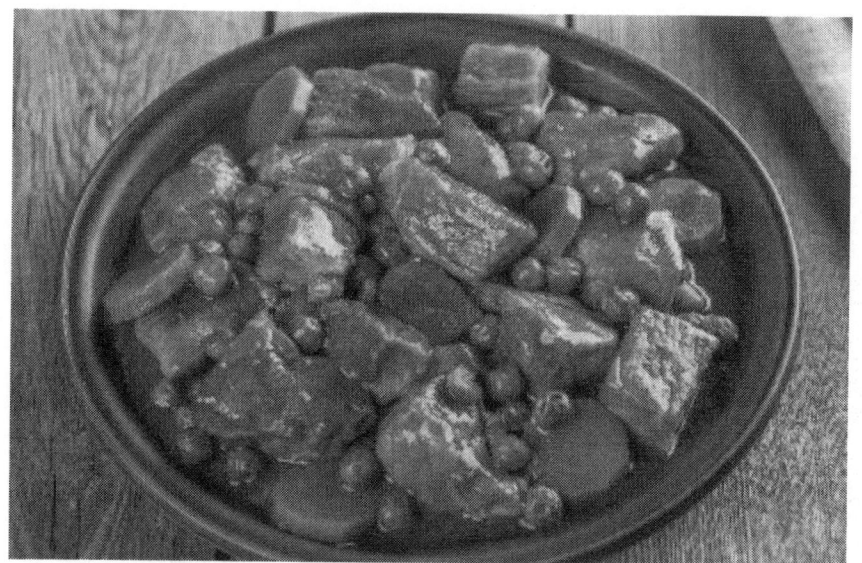

Green Chicken Stew

Serves 6-8

Ingredients - Allergies: SF, GF, DF, EF, NF

- 1-1/2 cups broccoli florets
- 1 cup chopped celery stalks
- 1 cup sliced leeks
- 2 tbsp. coconut oil
- 1-1/2 cups green peas
- 2 cups chicken stock
- 1/2 tsp. salt
- 1/4 tsp. ground black pepper
- 1/2 tsp. minced garlic
- 4 pounds boneless skinless chicken pieces

Instructions

Cook the leeks in coconut oil on medium until they are tender (few minutes). Add all other ingredients and stir. Cover & cook on low heat for 1 hour. Mix almond flour with some cold water, add to the stew & cook for another minute.

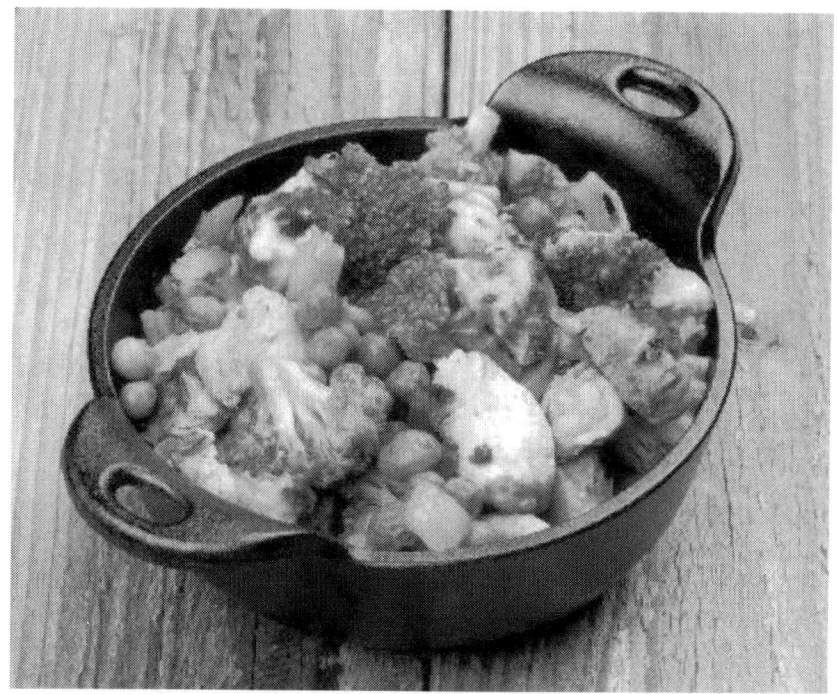

Irish Stew

Serves 8

Ingredients - Allergies: SF, GF, DF, EF, NF

- 2 chopped onions
- 2 Tbsp. coconut oil
- 1 sprig dried thyme
- 2 1/2 pounds chopped meat from lamb neck
- 6 chopped carrots
- 2 tbsp. brown rice
- 5 cups chicken stock
- Salt
- Ground black pepper
- 1 bouquet garni (thyme, parsley and bay leaf)
- 2 chopped sweet potatoes
- 1 bunch chopped parsley
- 1 bunch chives

Instructions

Cook the onions in coconut oil on medium until they are tender. Add the dried thyme and lamb and stir. Add brown rice, carrots and chicken stock. Add salt, pepper and bouquet garni. Cover & cook on low heat for 2 hours. Place sweet potatoes on top of the stew and cook for 30 minutes until the meat is falling apart.

Garnish with parsley and chives.

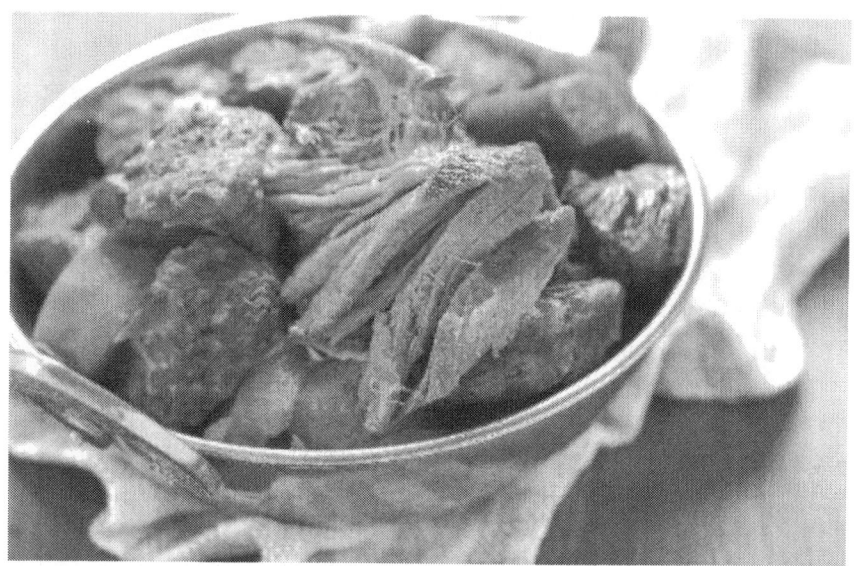

Hungarian Pea Stew

Serves 8

Ingredients - Allergies: SF, GF, DF, EF, NF

- 6 cups green peas
- 1 pound cubed pork
- 2 tbsp olive oil or avocado oil
- 3 1/2 tbsp almond flour
- 2 tbsp chopped parsley
- 1 cup water
- 1/2 tsp salt
- 1 cup coconut milk
- 1 tsp lucuma powder

Instructions

Simmer the pork and green peas in the olive oil over medium heat until almost tender (approx. 10 minutes)

Add salt, chopped parsley, lucuma powder and almond flour, & cook for another minute.

Add water then milk and stir.

Cook for another 4 minutes over low heat, stirring occasionally.

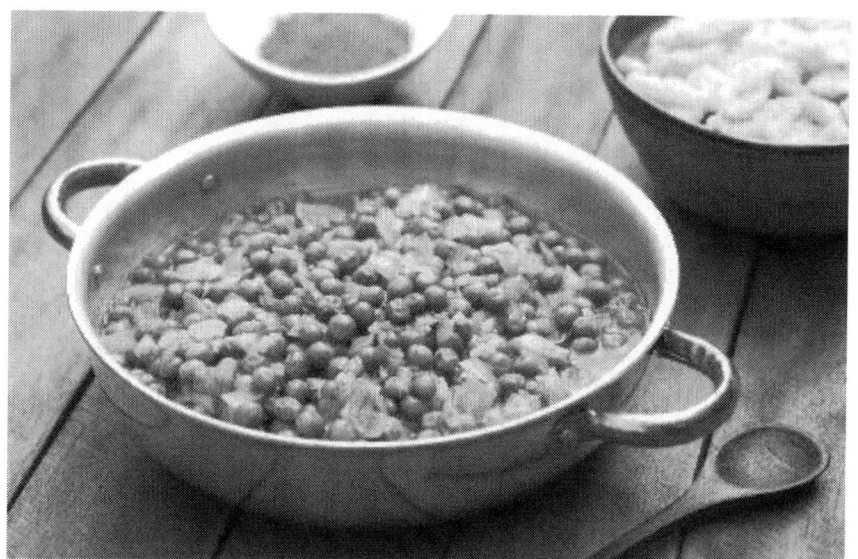

Chicken Tikka Masala
Serves 8

Ingredients - Allergies: SF, GF, DF, EF, NF

- 5 pounds chicken pieces, skinless, bone in
  3 tbsp. toasted paprika
  3 tbsp. toasted ground cumin
  1 tsp. cayenne pepper
  2 tbsp. toasted ground coriander seed
  2 tsp. ground turmeric
  12 chopped cloves garlic
  3 tbsp. chopped fresh ginger
  2 cups yogurt
  3/4 cup lemon juice (4 to 6 lemons)
  1 tsp. sea salt
  4 tbsp. coconut oil
  1 sliced onion
  4 cups chopped tomatoes
  1/2 cup chopped cilantro
  1 cup coconut cream

Instructions

Score chicken deeply at 1-inch intervals with a knife. Place chicken in a large baking dish.

Combine coriander, cumin, paprika, turmeric, and cayenne in a bowl and mix. Set aside 3 tbsp. of this spice mixture. Combine remaining 6 tbsp. spice mixture with 8 cloves garlic garlic, yogurt, 2 tbsp. ginger, 1/4 cup salt and 1/2 cup lemon juice in a large bowl and combine. Pour marinade over chicken pieces and coat every surface (use hands). Refrigerate and marinate between 4 and 8 hours, turning occasionally.

Heat coconut oil in a large pot over medium-high heat and add remaining garlic and ginger. Add onions. Cook about 10 minutes, stirring occasionally. Add reserved spice mixture and cook until fragrant, about half a minute. Scrape up any browned bits from bottom of pan and add tomatoes and half of cilantro. Simmer for 15 minutes. Let cool slightly and puree.

Stir in coconut cream and remaining one quarter cup lemon juice. Season to taste with salt and set aside until chicken is cooked.

Cook chicken on a grill or under a broiler.

Remove chicken from bone and cut into rough bite-sized chunks. Add chicken chunks to pot of sauce. Bring to a simmer over medium heat and cook about 10 minutes.

Sprinkle with remaining cilantro and serve with brown rice or grilled naan.

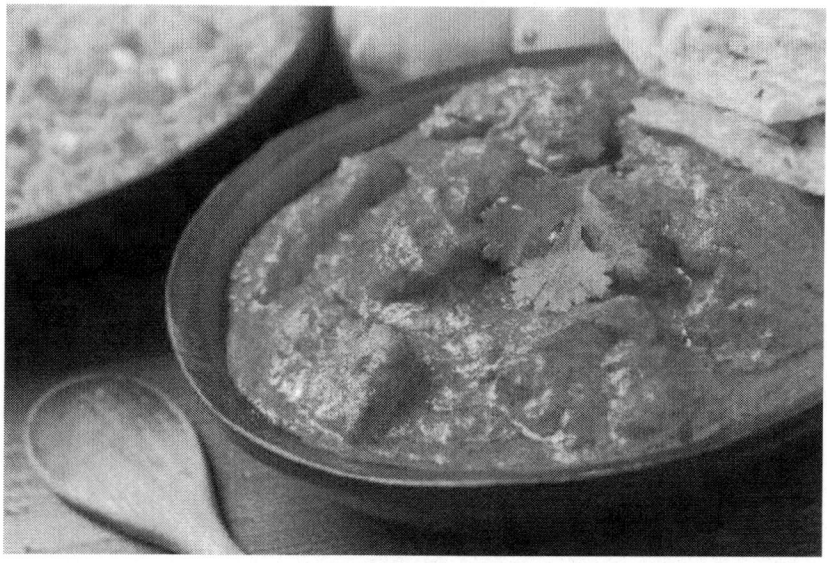

Greek Beef Stew (Stifado)
Serves 8

Ingredients - Allergies: SF, GF, DF, EF, NF

- 4 large pieces of veal or beef osso bucco
- 20 whole shallots, peeled
- 3 bay leaves
- 8 garlic cloves
- 3 sprigs rosemary
- 6 whole pimento
- 5 whole cloves
- 1/2 tsp ground nutmeg
- 1/2 cup olive oil or avocado oil
- 1/3 cup apple cider vinegar
- 1 tbsp. salt
- 2 cups tomato paste
- 1/4 tsp black pepper

Instructions

Mix vinegar and tomato paste and set aside. Place the meat, shallots, garlic and all spices in the pot.

Add the tomato paste, oil and vinegar. Cover the pot, bring to low boil and simmer on low for 2 hours. Do not open and stir, just shake the pot occasionally.

Serve with brown rice or maybe quinoa.

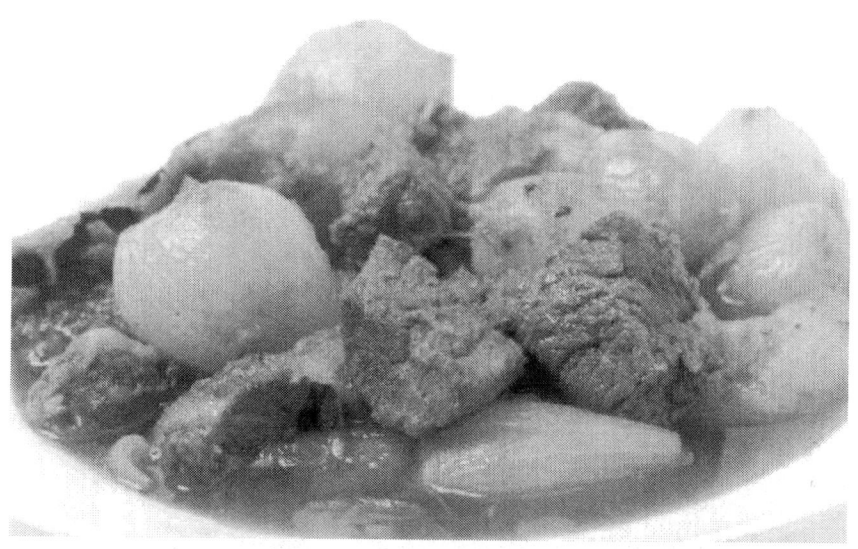

Beef, Parsnip, Celery Stew

Serves 8

Ingredients - Allergies: SF, GF, DF, EF, NF

- 2 1/2 pounds cubed beef meat
- 2 chopped onions
- 6 chopped carrots
- 2 Tbsp. coconut oil
- 1 sprig dried thyme
- 2 chopped parsnips
- 2 tbsp. brown rice
- 4 cups beef stock
- Salt
- Ground black pepper
- 1 bouquet garni (thyme, parsley and bay leaf)
- 1 bunch chopped parsley
- 1 bunch chives

Instructions

Put all ingredients in the slow cooker & cook on low for 8 hours.

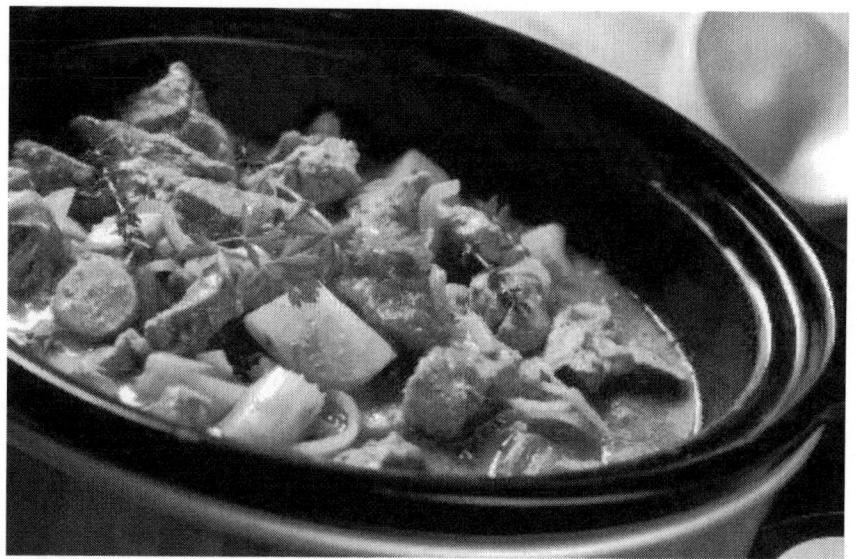

Chicken Mushrooms & Olives Stew

Serves 6

Ingredients - Allergies: SF, GF, DF, EF, NF

- 4 pounds chicken with skin on
- 1-1/2 cups chopped carrots
- 1 cup chopped onions
- 2 tbsp. coconut oil
- 1 cup sliced mushrooms
- 1/2 cup chopped celery
- 1 cup black olives
- 1/2 tsp. salt
- 1/4 tsp. ground black pepper
- 1/2 tsp. minced garlic
- ½ cup fresh parsley

Instructions

Put all ingredients in the crockpot, cover & cook on low 6 hours.

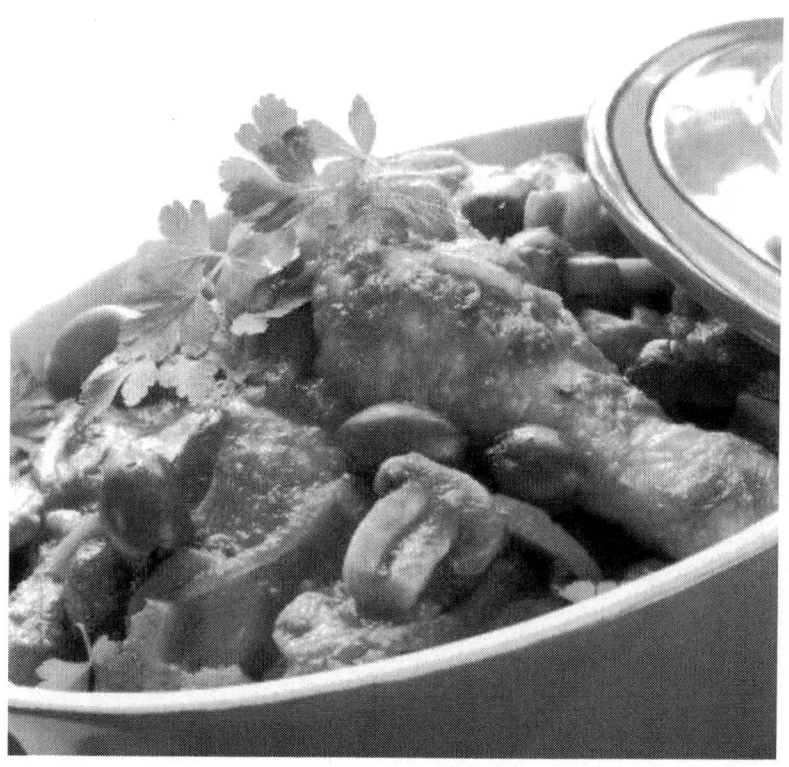

Chicken Pasanda Curry

Serves: 6

Ingredients - Allergies: SF, GF, DF, EF, NF

- 2 cups cubed chicken meat
- Curry Paste, but go low on the heat
- 2 cups tomato paste
- 1/2 cup coconut milk or cream
- Cilantro for garnishing

Instructions

Make Curry Paste. Add the tomato paste, chicken and the cream. Stir to combine, add to crockpot & cook on low for 3 hours.

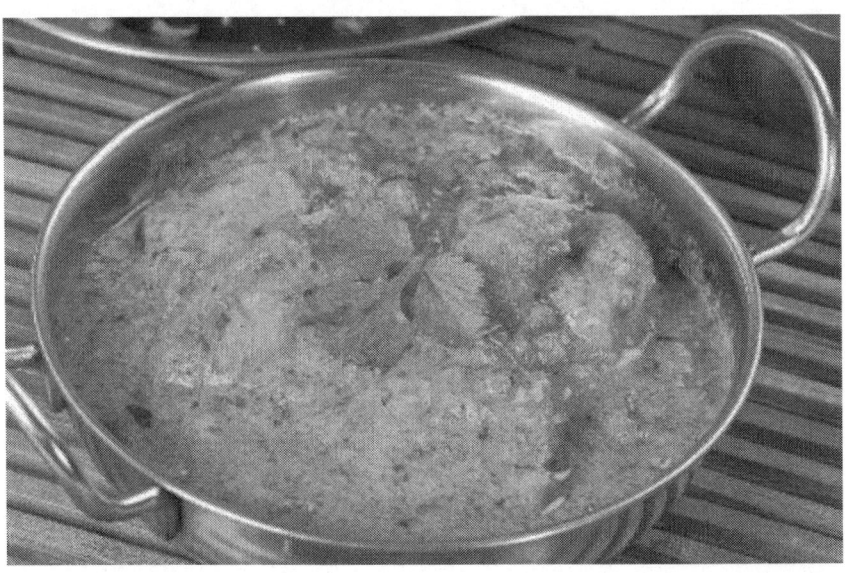

Osso Bucco & Garlic Stew
Serves 6-8

Ingredients - Allergies: SF, GF, DF, EF, NF

- 10 cloves garlic
- 2 cups chopped onions
- 1 cup chopped carrot
- 1 cup chopped celery
- 2 tbsp. coconut oil
- 2 cups beef stock
- 1/2 tsp. salt
- 1/4 tsp. ground black pepper
- 1 tsp. chopped parsley
- 4 pounds osso bucco

Instructions

Put all ingredients in the slow cooker & cook on low for 8 hours.

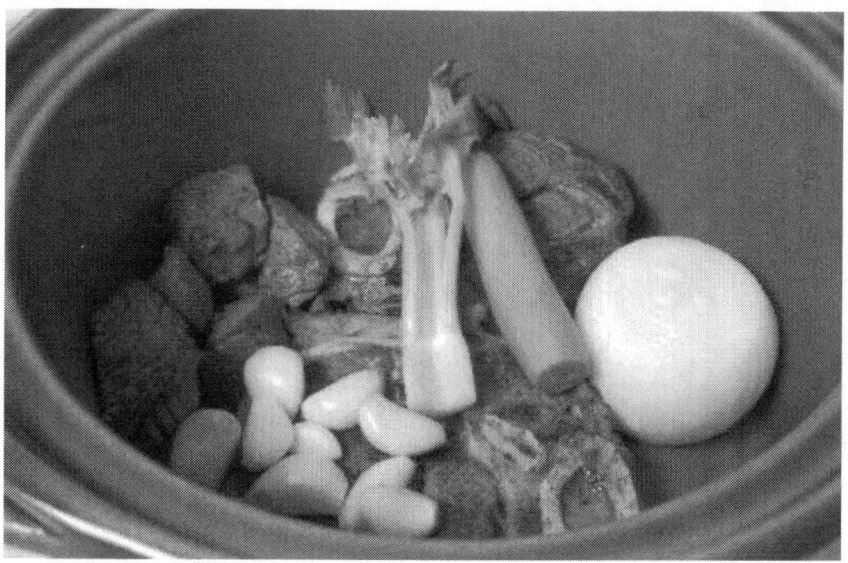

Beef Meatballs with White Beans
Serves 8

Ingredients - Allergies: SF, GF, DF, EF, NF

- 2 pounds baked meatballs (see recipe in bonus chapter)
- 2 Tbsp. coconut oil
- 1 sprig dried thyme
- 1 sprig dried thyme
- 2 cups uncooked white navy beans
- 4 cups beef stock
- Salt
- Ground black pepper
- 1 cup chopped onions
- 1 bunch chopped parsley
- 1 cup chopped carrots

Instructions

Add all ingredients but meatballs and cook on high for 4 hours. Add meatballs & cook on low for 2 hours more. Garnish with parsley.

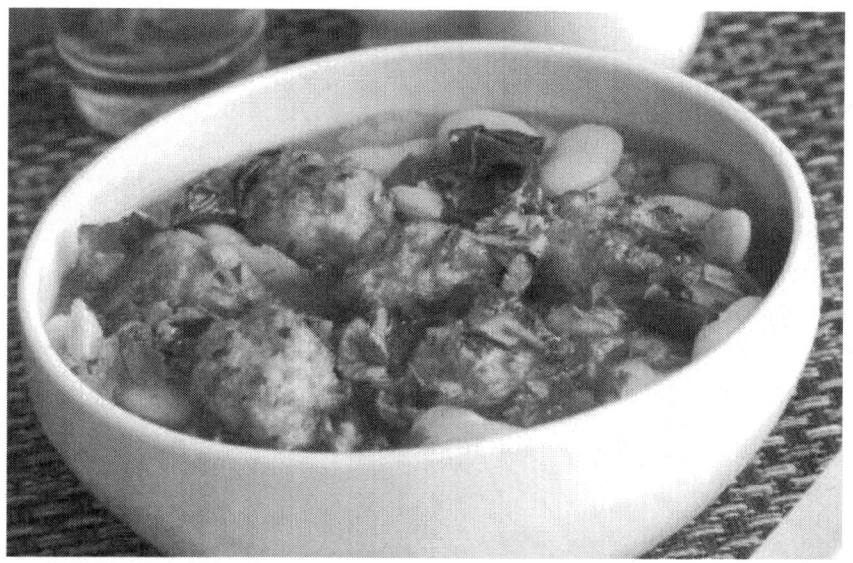

Duck Stew

Serves 8

Ingredients - Allergies: SF, GF, DF, EF, NF

- 2 Tbsp. olive oil
- 2 pound chopped duck meat (1/2 inch wide)
- 1/2 pound duck liver, sliced
- 1 cup chopped carrot
- 1 cup chopped celery
- 1 cup chopped onions
- 3 garlic cloves, chopped
- 2 cups chicken broth
- 1 cup sliced shiitake mushrooms
- 1/2 cup cilantro

Instructions

Put all ingredients in the slow cooker & cook on low for 4 Hrs.

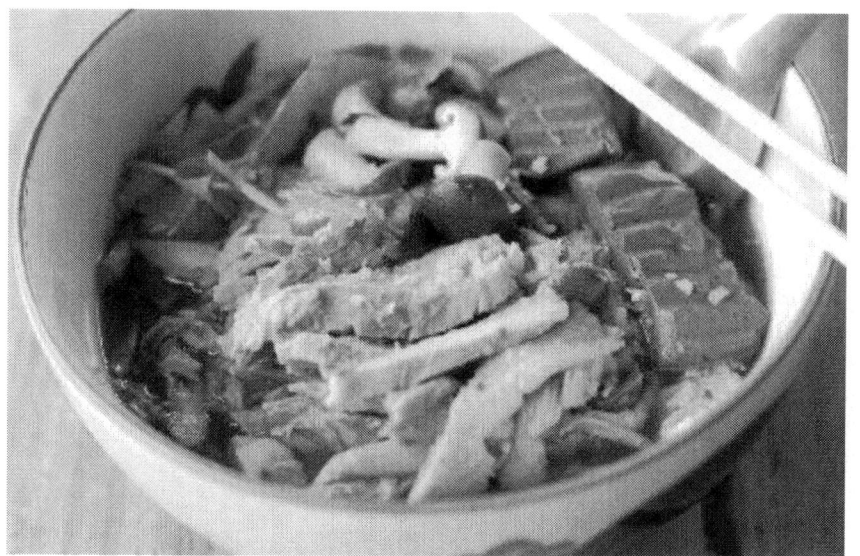

Pork, Celery and Basil Stew

Serves 8

Ingredients - Allergies: SF, GF, DF, EF, NF

- 1 cup chopped onions
- 2 Tbsp. coconut oil
- 2 1/2 pounds chopped pork meat
- 4 chopped carrots
- 2 cups beef stock
- 1 cup red wine (optional)
- Salt
- Ground black pepper
- 1 bunch chopped parsley
- 1 cup chopped celery
- 1/2 cup fresh basil

Instructions

Add all ingredients to slow cooker & cook on low for 8 hours.

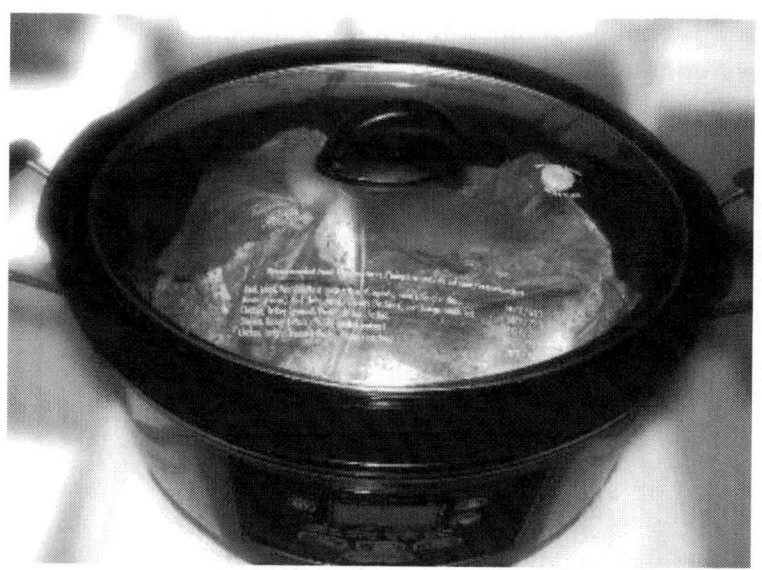

Meat Stew with Red Beans
Serves 8

Ingredients - Allergies: SF, GF, DF, EF, NF

- 3 tbsp. olive oil or avocado oil
- 1/2 chopped onion
- 1 lb lean cubed stewing beef
- 2 tsp. ground cumin
- 2 tsp. ground turmeric (optional)
- 1/2 tsp. ground cinnamon (optional)
- 2 1/2 cups water
- 5 tbsp. chopped fresh parsley
- 3 tbsp. snipped chives
- 2 cups cooked kidney beans
- 1 lemon, juice of
- 1 tbsp. almond flour
- salt and black pepper

Instructions

Sauté the onion in a pan with two tablespoons of the ive oil until tender.

Add beef and cook until meat is browned on all sides. Stir in turmeric, cinnamon (both optional) and cumin and cook for one minute. Add water and bring to a boil.

Cover and simmer over low heat for 45 minutes. Stir occasionally. Sauté parsley and chives with the remaining 1 tbsp. of olive oil for about 2 minutes and add this mixture to the beef. Add kidney beans and lemon juice and season with salt and pepper.

Stir in one tbsp. of almond flour mixed with a bit of water to thicken the stew. Simmer uncovered for half an hour until meat gets tender. Serve with brown rice.

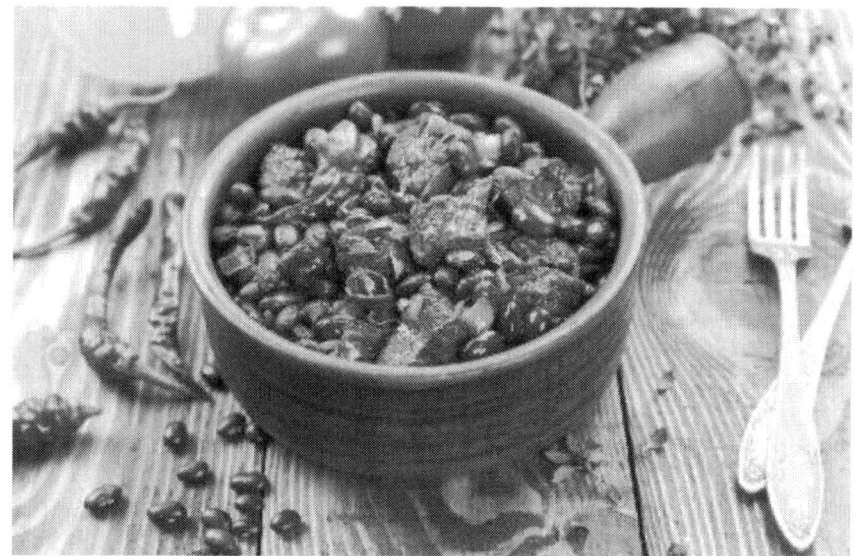

Vegetarian Garbanzo Chili

Serves 8

Ingredients - Allergies: SF, GF, DF, EF, NF

- 2 chopped onions
- 2 Tbsp. coconut oil
- 3 large tomatoes, chopped
- 1 cup dry beans (kidney, black, pinto)
- 1 cup garbanzo beans
- 4 chopped carrots
- a few chopped jalapeno peppers (watch for the heat)
- 4 cups beef stock
- Salt
- Ground black pepper
- 1 bunch chopped spring onions

Instructions

Put all ingredients in the slow cooker & cook on low for 4 Hrs.

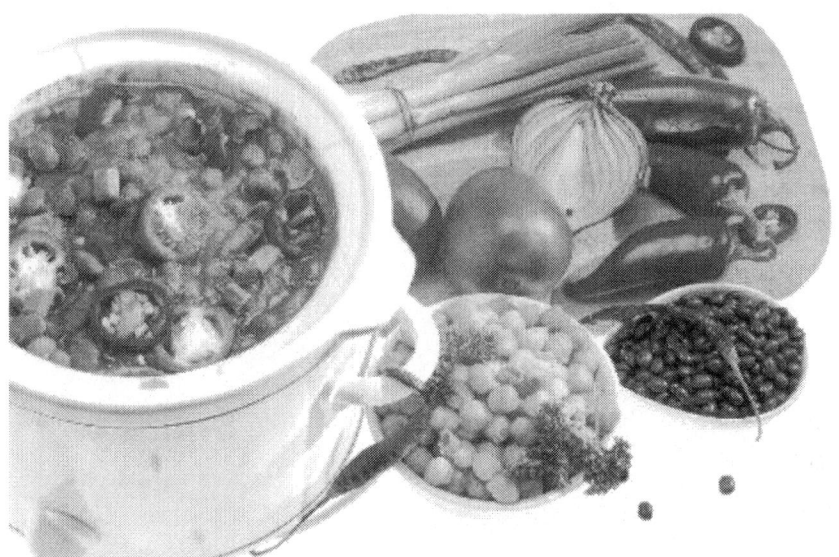

Red Peppers Pork Curry

Serves 8

Ingredients - Allergies: SF, GF, DF, EF, NF

- 3 cups sliced red peppers
- 2 cups chopped onions
- 2 tbsp. coconut oil
- 1 cup curry paste*
- 4 pounds chopped pork meat

Instructions

Put ingredients in the slow cooker. Cover, & cook on low for 7 to 9 hours.

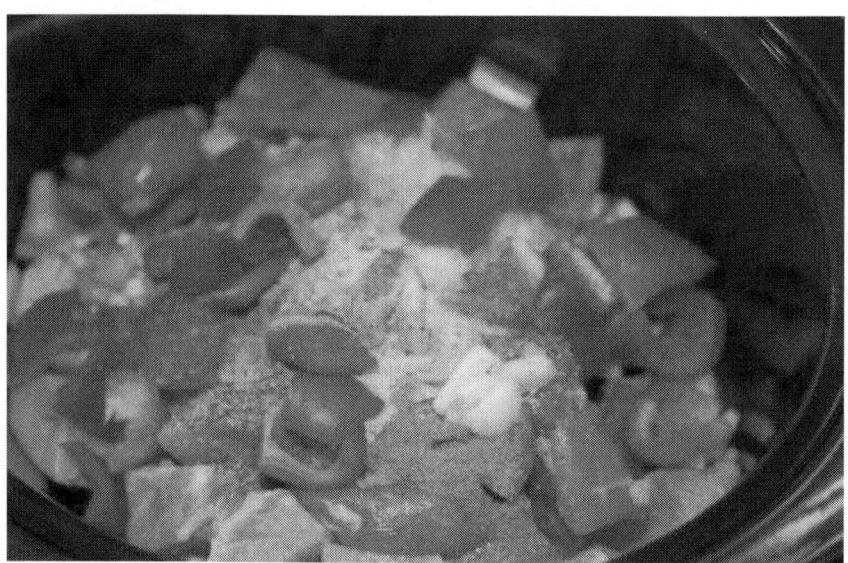

Beef Ratatouille

Serves 8

Ingredients - Allergies: SF, GF, DF, EF, NF

- 1-1/2 cups sliced zucchini
- 1 cup chopped onions
- 1-1/2 cups sliced eggplant
- 1-1/2 cups sliced red peppers (or tomato)
- 2 tbsp. coconut oil
- 2 tbsp. chopped garlic
- 2 tsp. salt and 1 tsp. ground pepper
- 4 pounds cubed beef

Instructions

Put ingredients in the slow cooker. Cover, & cook on low for 7 to 9 hours.

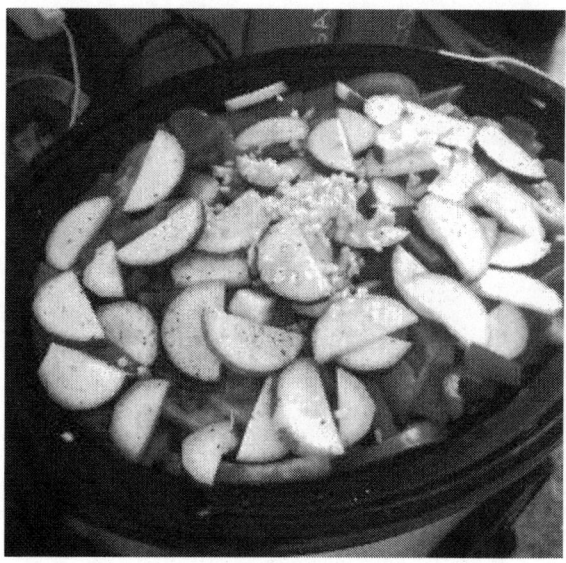

Chicken, Green Peas and Red Peppers Stew

Serves 8

Ingredients - Allergies: SF, GF, DF, EF, NF

- 1-1/2 cups green peas
- 1 cup chopped onions
- 1-1/2 cups sliced red peppers
- 2 tbsp. coconut oil
- 2 cups chicken broth
- 2 tsp. salt and 1 tsp. ground pepper
- 4 pounds cubed chicken

Instructions

Put ingredients in the slow cooker. Cover, & cook on low for 7 to 9 hours.

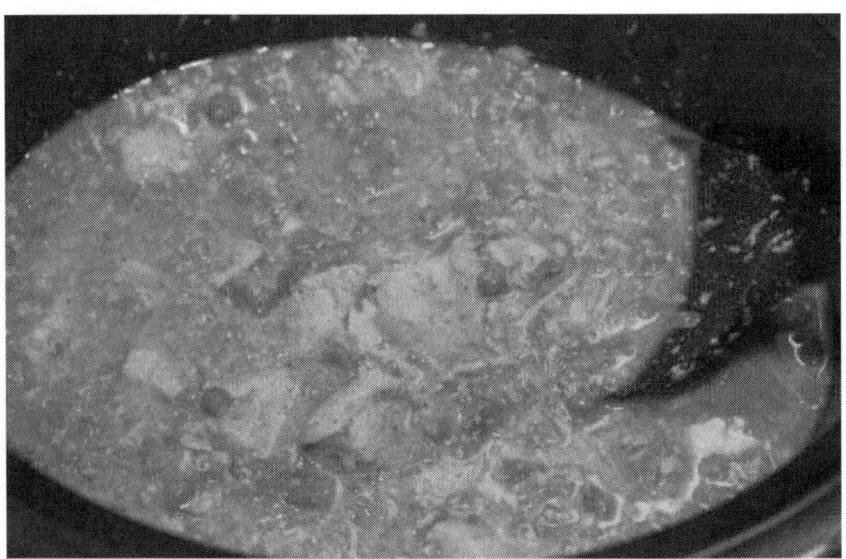

Crock Pot Turkey Roast Mediterranean style
Serves 8

Ingredients - Allergies: SF, GF, DF, EF, NF

- 1/2 cup Kalamata olives
- 1/2 cup chopped sun dried tomatoes
- 1 cup chicken broth
- 3 garlic cloves, minced
- 2 cups chopped onions
- 2 tbsp. coconut oil
- 4 pounds turkey breast
- Rub thyme, salt and ground black pepper.

Instructions

Put ingredients in the slow cooker. Cover, & cook on low for 7 to 9 hours.

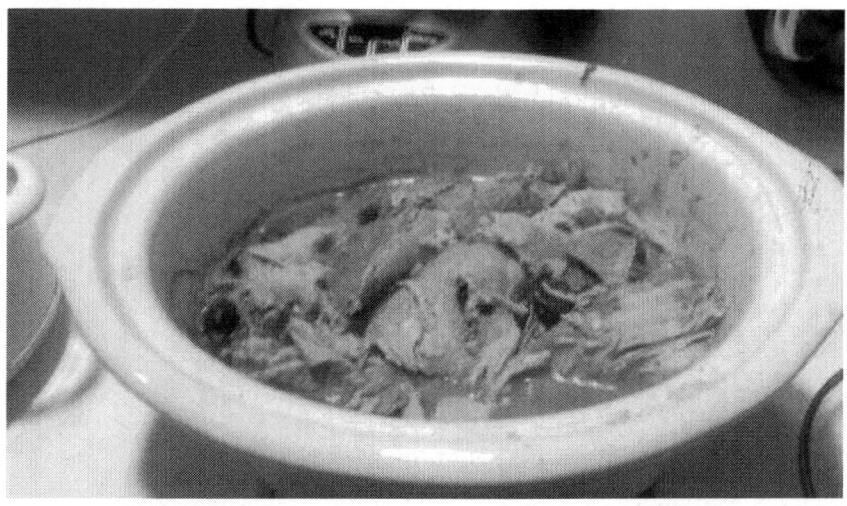

Slow Cooker Pot Roast

Serves 8

Ingredients - Allergies: SF, GF, DF, EF, NF

- 1 cup sliced celery
- 1 cup chopped carrot
- 3 cups beef broth
- 1 cup red wine (optional) & 3 garlic cloves (optional)
- 1 cup chopped onions
- 2 tbsp. coconut oil
- 4 pounds beef chuck roast
- Rub thyme, salt and ground black pepper. Add 1 bay leaf.

Instructions

Put ingredients in the slow cooker. Cover, & cook on low for 7 to 9 hours.

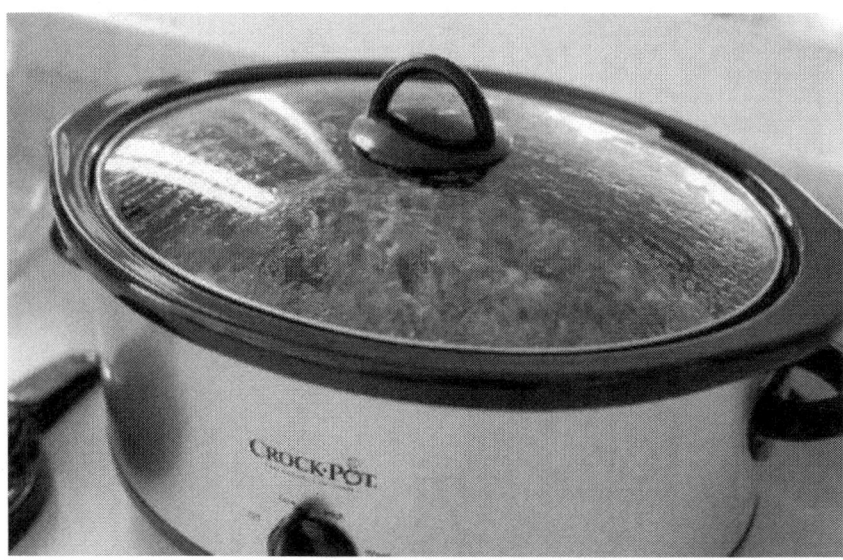

Crock Pot Whole Chicken

Serves 8

Ingredients - Allergies: SF, GF, DF, EF, NF

- 1 cup sliced celery
- 1 cup chopped carrot
- 1 cup chopped parsnip (optional)
- 2 cups chopped onions
- 2 tbsp. coconut oil
- 1 whole chicken with skin on
- Rub paprika, salt and ground black pepper on the chicken skin and inside. Optionally add lemon quarters inside.

Instructions

Put veggies in the slow cooker and place chicken on top. Cover, & cook on low for 7 to 9 hours.

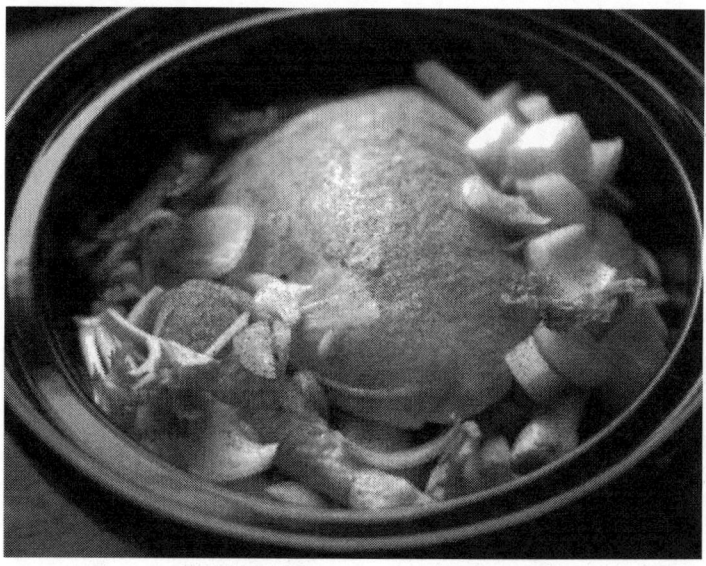

Beef, Leeks & Mushrooms Stew
Serves 8

Ingredients - Allergies: SF, GF, DF, EF, NF

- 2 cups chopped carrots
- 1 cup chopped onions
- 2 tbsp. coconut oil
- 1 cup chopped leeks
- Salt & ground black pepper according to taste
- 1 cup sliced mushrooms
- 1 cup sliced tomatoes
- 4 pounds beef meat cut into stripes

Instructions

Put ingredients in the slow cooker. Cover, & cook on low for 7 to 9 hours.

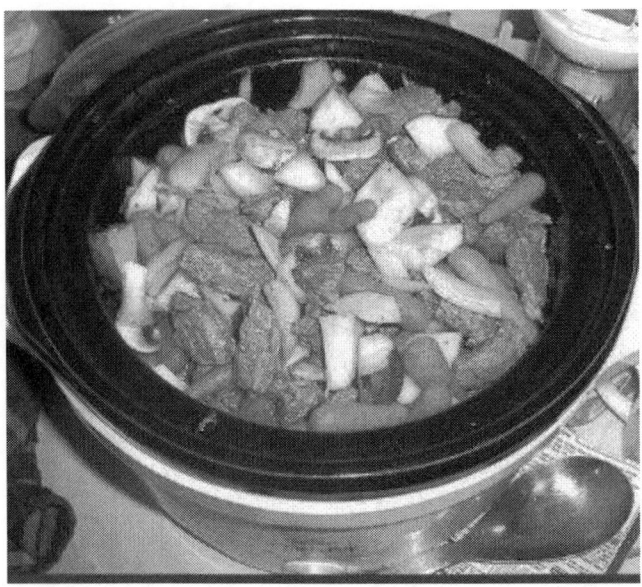

Chicken, Garlic & Tomato Stew

Serves 8

Ingredients - Allergies: SF, GF, DF, EF, NF

- 3 cups tomatoes
- 2 cups chopped onions
- 2 tbsp. coconut oil
- 1 garlic bulb, cut across
- Salt, ground black pepper and ground cumin to taste
- 1 Tbsp. minced garlic
- 4 pounds chicken breast meat cut into stripes

Instructions

Put ingredients in the slow cooker. Cover, & cook on low for 7 to 9 hours.

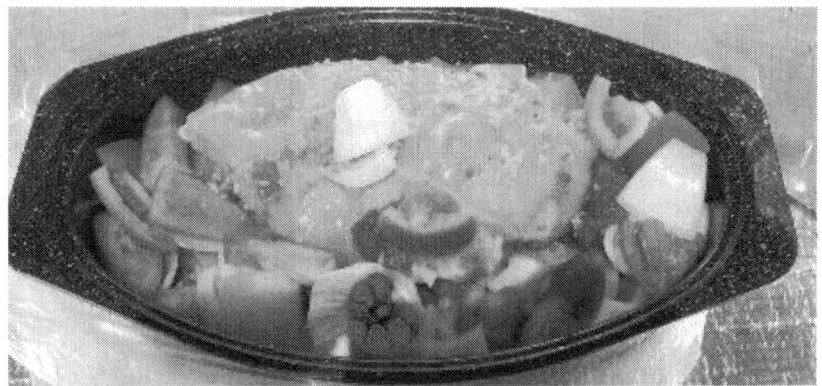

Minced Pork, Tomato & Red Peppers Stew
Serves 8

Ingredients - Allergies: SF, GF, DF, EF, NF

- 3 cups quartered tomatoes
- 1 cup chopped onions
- 2 tbsp. coconut oil
- 2 cups chopped red peppers
- Salt, ground black pepper and ground cumin to taste
- 1 cup shredded carrots
- 4 pounds minced pork meat

Instructions

Put ingredients in the slow cooker. Cover, & cook on low for 7 to 9 hours.

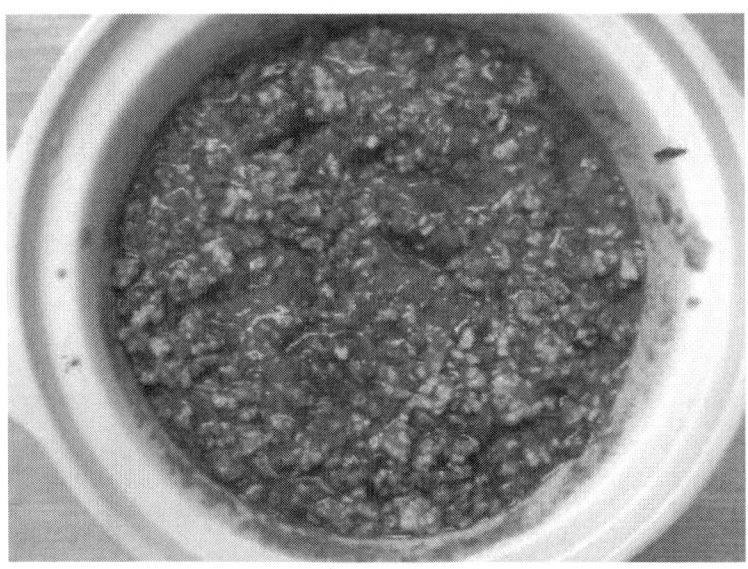

Beef, Eggplant, Celery & Peppers Stew

Serves 8

Ingredients - Allergies: SF, GF, DF, EF, NF

- 1 cup cubed eggplant
- 2 cups chopped onions
- 2 tbsp. coconut oil
- 1 cup sliced celery
- Salt, ground black pepper according to taste
- 1 cup sliced red peppers
- 4 pounds beef meat cut into stripes

Instructions

Put ingredients in the slow cooker. Cover, & cook on low for 7 to 9 hours.

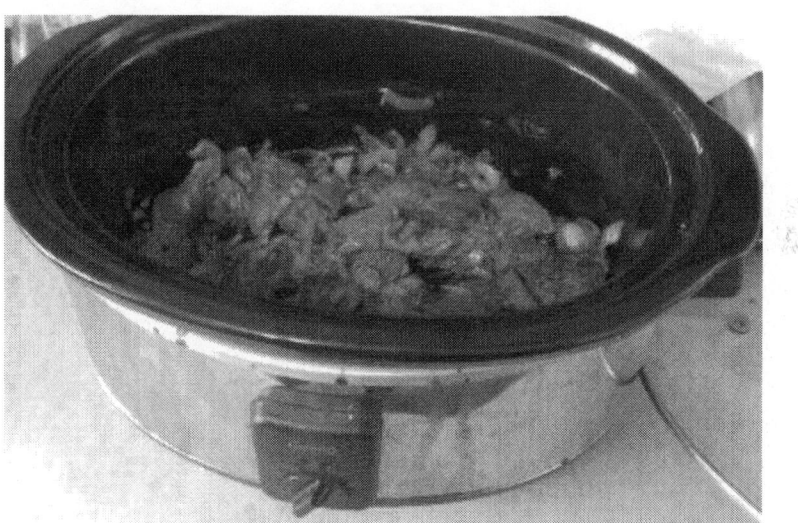

Chicken & Onion Stew

Serves 8

Ingredients - Allergies: SF, GF, DF, EF, NF

- 1 cup sliced mushrooms
- 6 large onions, quartered
- 2 tbsp. coconut oil
- Salt, ground black pepper according to taste
- 2 cups chicken stock
- 4 pounds chicken drumsticks with skin on

Instructions

Put ingredients in the slow cooker. Cover, & cook on low for 7 to 9 hours.

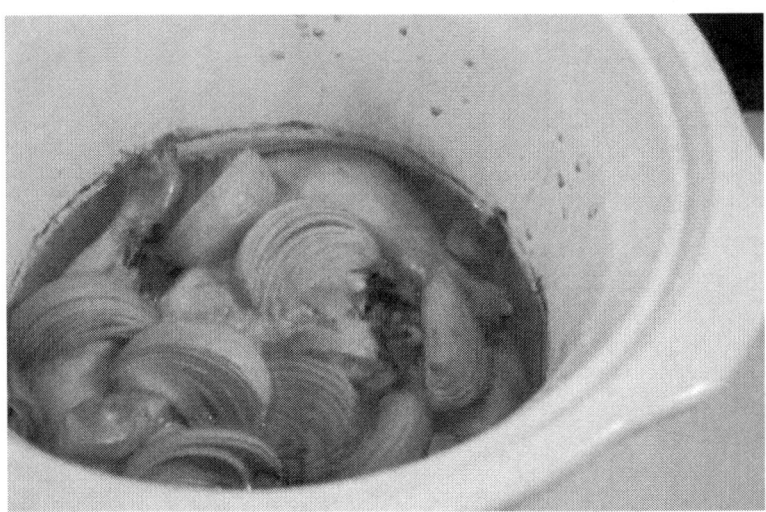

Leeks, Mushrooms & Pork Neck Meat
Serves 8

Ingredients - Allergies: SF, GF, DF, EF, NF

- 2 cups mushrooms, sliced
- 2 cups chopped leeks
- 2 tbsp. coconut oil
- Salt, ground black pepper and ground cumin to taste
- 2 bay leaves & 2 Tbsp. chopped garlic
- 4 cups beef stock
- ¼ cup sesame seeds
- ¼ cup chopped spring onions
- 4 pounds pork neck meat

Instructions

Put all ingredients in the slow cooker except spring onions and sesame seeds. Cover, & cook on low for 9 hours. Sprinkle with chopped spring onions and sesame seeds.

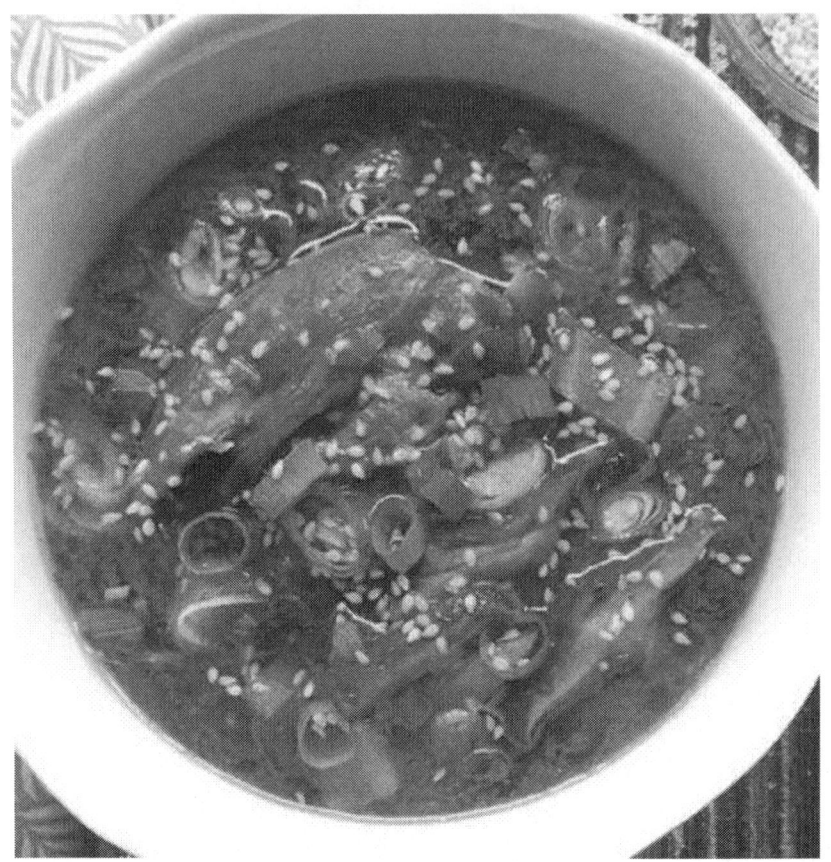

Beef, Beet, Carrots & Onions

Serves 8

Ingredients - Allergies: SF, GF, DF, EF, NF

- 2 cups julienned carrots
- 2 medium beets, peeled and sliced
- 2 cups chopped onions
- 2 tbsp. coconut oil
- Salt, ground black pepper according to taste
- 2 cups beef stock
- 4 pounds cubed beef
- 2 Tbsp. minced garlic.

Instructions

Put ingredients in the slow cooker. Cover, & cook on low for 8 hours.

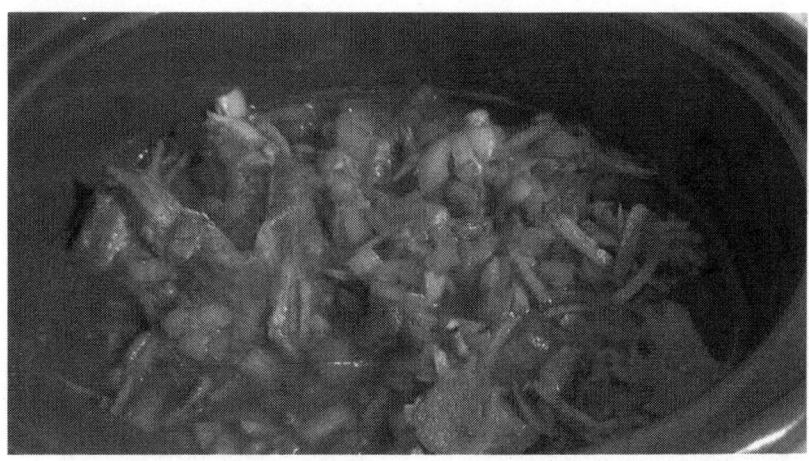

Broccoli, Pork & Peppers

Serves 8

Ingredients - Allergies: SF, GF, DF, EF, NF

- 2 cup sliced yellow and orange peppers
- 1 cup chopped onions
- 2 tbsp. coconut oil
- Salt, ground black pepper according to taste
- 1 cup beef stock
- 2 pounds pork chops
- 2 pounds pork neck
- 2 Tbsp. minced garlic.
- 2 cups broccoli florets

Instructions

Put ingredients in the slow cooker. Cover, & cook on low for 8 hours.

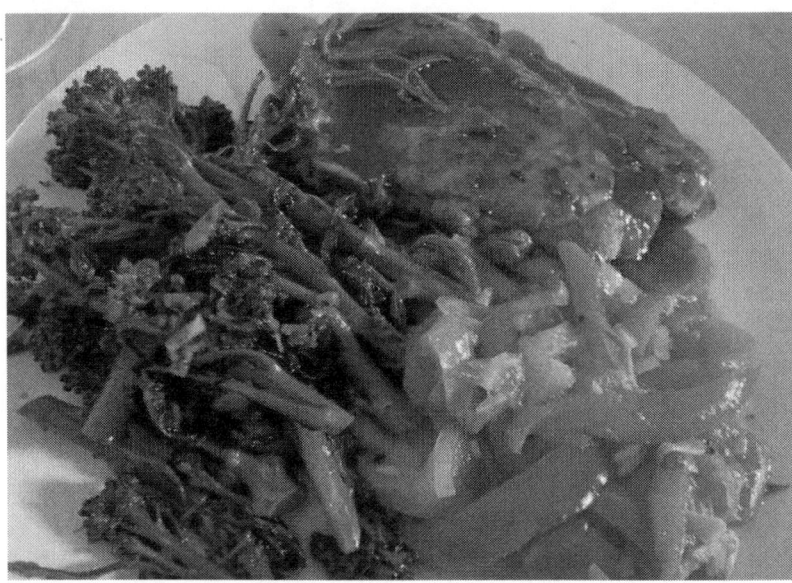

Haitian Chicken Broccoli

Serves 8

Ingredients - Allergies: SF, GF, DF, EF, NF

- 2 cup broccoli florets
- 2 cups chopped onions
- 2 tbsp. coconut oil
- Salt, ground black pepper according to taste
- 3 cups chicken stock
- 4 pounds cubed chicken meat
- 1 tsp. dried red pepper flakes (to taste).
- 4 whole cloves (discard after cooking)
- 2 Tbsp. minced garlic
- 1 Tbsp. apple vinegar

Instructions

Put ingredients in the slow cooker. Cover, & cook on low for 8 hours.

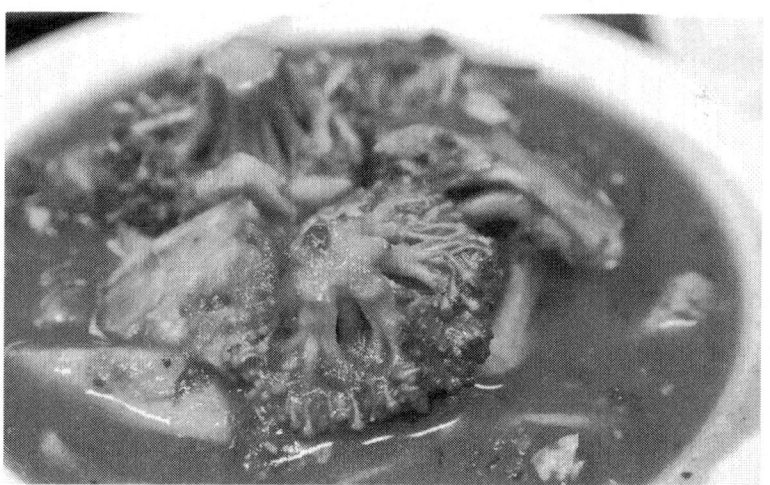

Leeks, Cauliflower, Chicken & Carrot

Serves 8

Ingredients - Allergies: SF, GF, DF, EF, NF

- 3 cups sliced leeks
- 2 cups carrot
- 2 tbsp. coconut oil
- Salt, ground black pepper according to taste
- 2 cups chicken stock
- 4 pounds cubed chicken meat
- 2 Tbsp. minced ginger & 2 Tbsp. minced garlic.
- 2 sticks celery, chopped

Instructions

Put ingredients in the slow cooker. Cover, & cook on low for 8 hours.

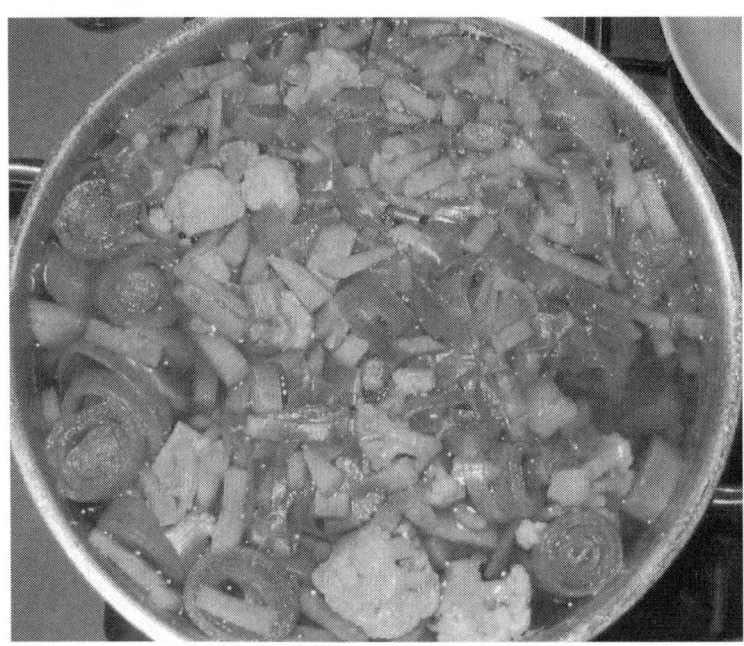

Okra & Pork Stew

Serves 8

Ingredients - Allergies: SF, GF, DF, EF, NF

- 3 cups sliced okra
- 2 cups chopped onions
- 2 tbsp. coconut oil
- Salt, ground black pepper according to taste
- 2 cups beef stock
- 4 pounds pork neck meat
- 5 cloves garlic, halved lengthwise
- 2 sticks celery, chopped

Instructions

Put ingredients in the slow cooker. Cover, & cook on low for 8 hours.

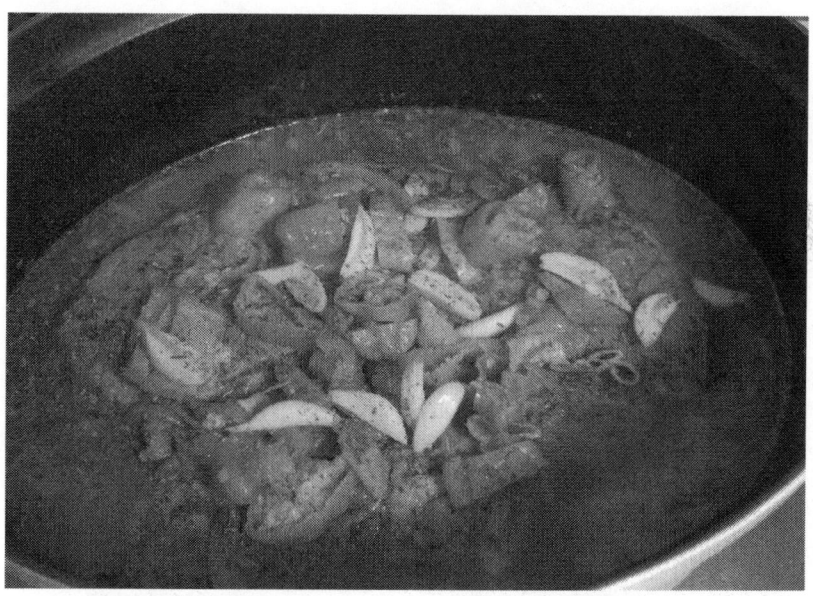

Chicken, Black Beans and Cauliflower
Serves 8

Ingredients - Allergies: SF, GF, DF, EF, NF

- 2 cups cauliflower
- 1 cup black beans
- 2 cups chopped onions & 3 carrots - chopped
- 2 tbsp. coconut oil
- Salt, ground black pepper according to taste
- 3 cups chicken stock
- 4 pounds dark chicken meat
- 2 Tbsp. minced garlic & 1 tsp. ground cumin

Instructions

Put ingredients in the slow cooker. Cover, & cook on low for 8 hours.

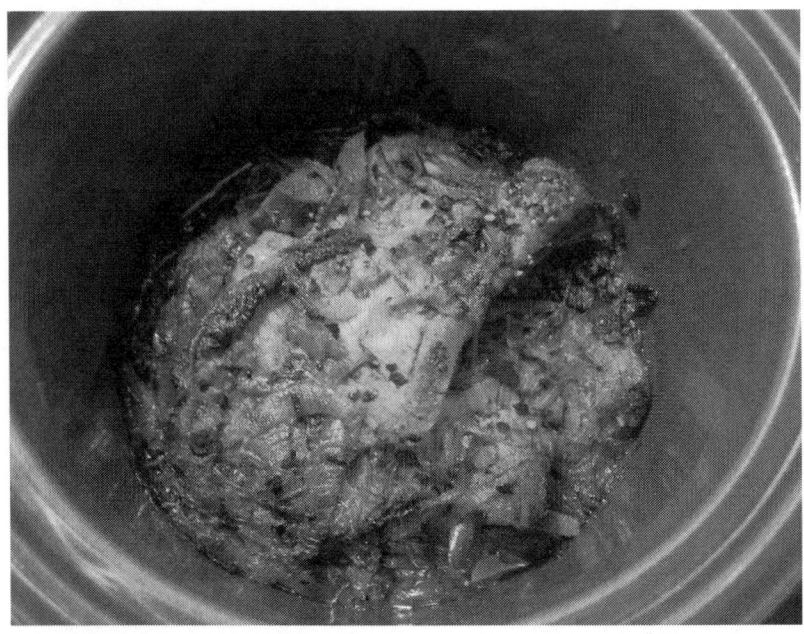

Celery, Carrots & Cauliflower Pork
Serves 8

Ingredients - Allergies: SF, GF, DF, EF, NF

- 2 cup sliced celery
- 2 cups chopped onions
- 2 tbsp. coconut oil
- Salt, ground black pepper according to taste
- 2 cups beef stock
- 4 pounds cubed pork meat
- 2 cups chopped carrots
- 2 cups chopped cauliflower
- 2 Tbsp. minced garlic & 3-4 bay leaves (discard after cooking).

Instructions

Put ingredients in the slow cooker. Cover, & cook on low for 8 hours.

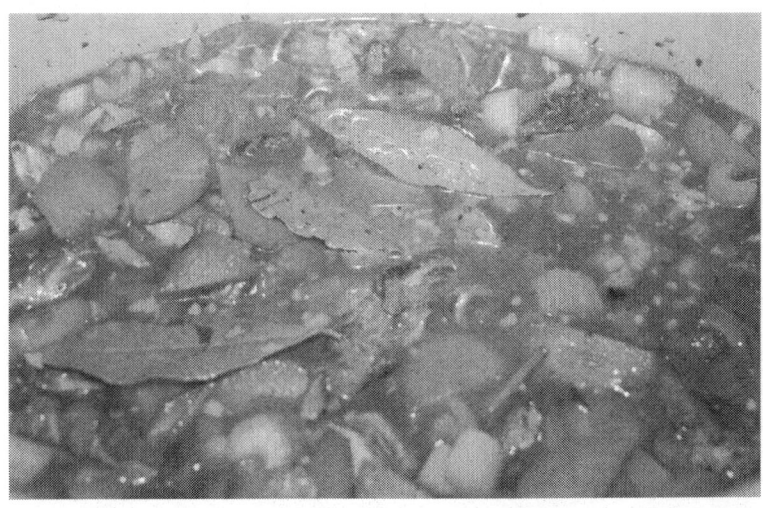

Slow Cooked Carnitas

Serves 8

Ingredients - Allergies: SF, GF, DF, EF, NF

- 2 cups chopped onions
- 2 tbsp. coconut oil
- Salt, ground black pepper according to taste
- 2 pounds pork shoulder
- 2 pounds pork neck
- 1 Jalapeno pepper, chopped (to taste).
- 2 Tbsp. minced garlic.
- 1 Tbsp. ground cumin.

Instructions

Put ingredients in the slow cooker. Cover, & cook on low for 8 hours.

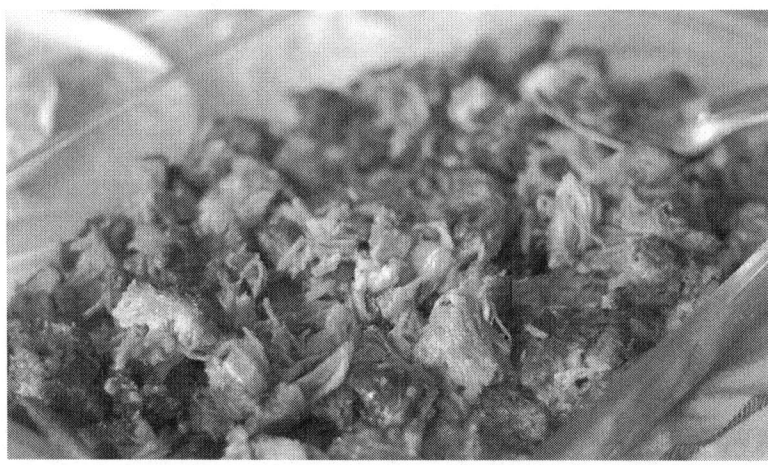

Beef & Apple
Serves 8

Ingredients - Allergies: SF, GF, DF, EF, NF

- 2 cups chopped carrots
- 2 cups chopped onions
- 2 tbsp. coconut oil
- Salt, ground black pepper according to taste
- 2 cups beef stock mixed with 4 Tbsp. almond flour
- 4 pounds cubed beef
- 1 lime - juice.
- 2 Tbsp. minced garlic.
- 6 large sour apples, cored and cut in 8 pieces

Instructions

Put ingredients in the slow cooker. Cover, & cook on low for 8 hours.

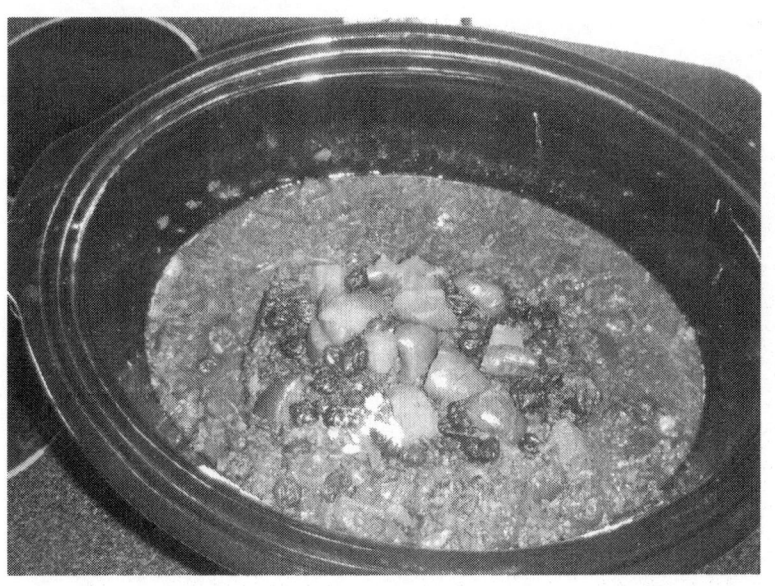

Bigos - Polish Pork, Venison & Cabbage Stew
Serves 8

Ingredients - Allergies: SF, GF, DF, EF, NF

- 1 cup chopped onions
- 2 tbsp. coconut oil
- Salt, ground black pepper according to taste
- 2 pound pork shoulder meat, cubed
- 2 pounds venison meat, cubed
- 3 cups shredded cabbage
- 2 Tbsp. minced garlic
- 1 Tbsp. ground paprika

Instructions

Put ingredients in the slow cooker. Cover, & cook on low for 8 hours.

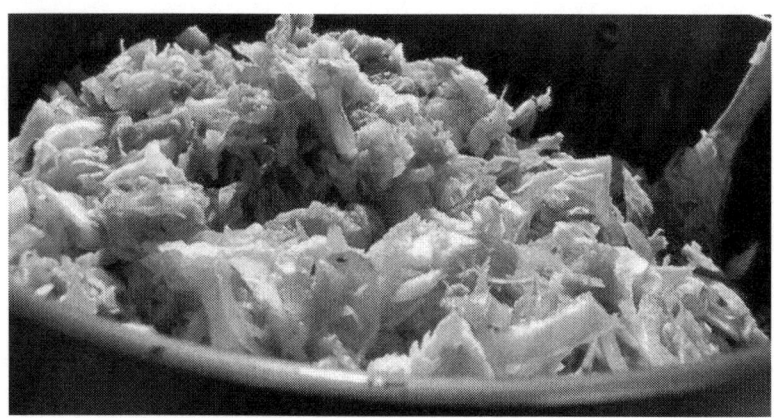

Cumin Lamb

Serves 8

Ingredients - Allergies: SF, GF, DF, EF, NF

- 2 cups chopped onions
- 2 tbsp. coconut oil
- Salt, ground black pepper according to taste
- 4 pounds lamb meat, cubed
- 1 cup parsley
- 1 cup sesame seeds
- 2 Tbsp. minced garlic
- 3 Tbsp. ground cumin

Instructions

Put ingredients in the slow cooker. Cover, & cook on low for 8 hours.

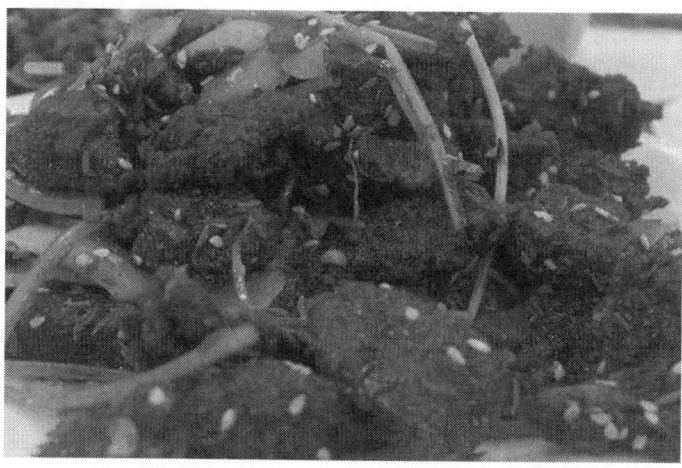

Mexican Lamb Chili

Serves 6

Ingredients - Allergies: SF, GF, DF, EF, NF

- 2 tbsp. coconut oil
- 2 onions, chopped
- 3 cloves garlic, minced
- 3 pounds cubed lamb meat
- 1 cup corn
- 1 cup tomato paste
- 2 cups beef broth
- 2 tbsp. cumin seeds
- 1 tsp. ground cayenne pepper
- 1 tsp. ground coriander
- 1 tsp. salt
- 3 cups cooked kidney beans
- 2-3 fresh hot chili peppers, chopped

Instructions

Put ingredients in the slow cooker. Cover, & cook on low for 8 hours.

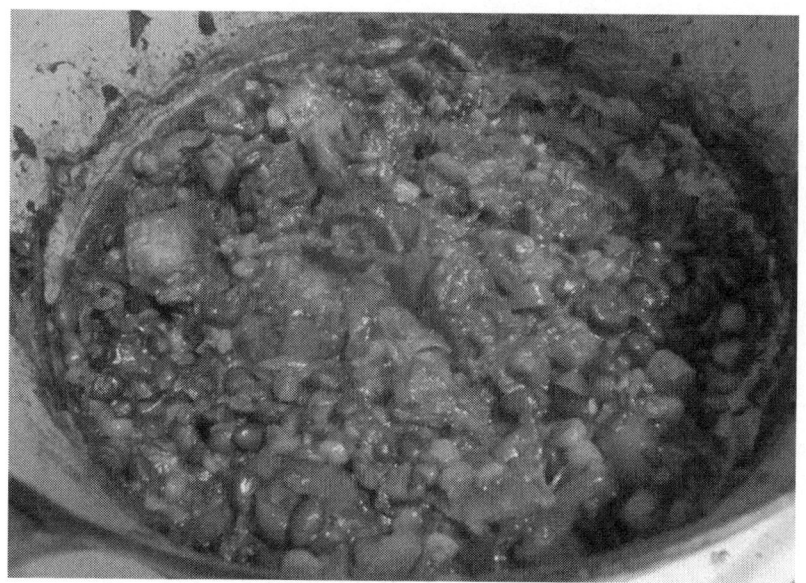

Moroccan Lamb, Tomato Sauce & Green Peppers Stew
Serves 8

Ingredients - Allergies: SF, GF, DF, EF, NF

- 2 cups chopped onions
- 2 tbsp. coconut oil
- Salt, ground black pepper according to taste
- 4 pounds lamb meat, cubed
- 2 cups tomato paste
- 3 cups green peppers
- 2 Tbsp. minced garlic.
- 2 Tbsp. ground cumin.

Instructions

Put ingredients in the slow cooker. Cover, & cook on low for 8 hours.

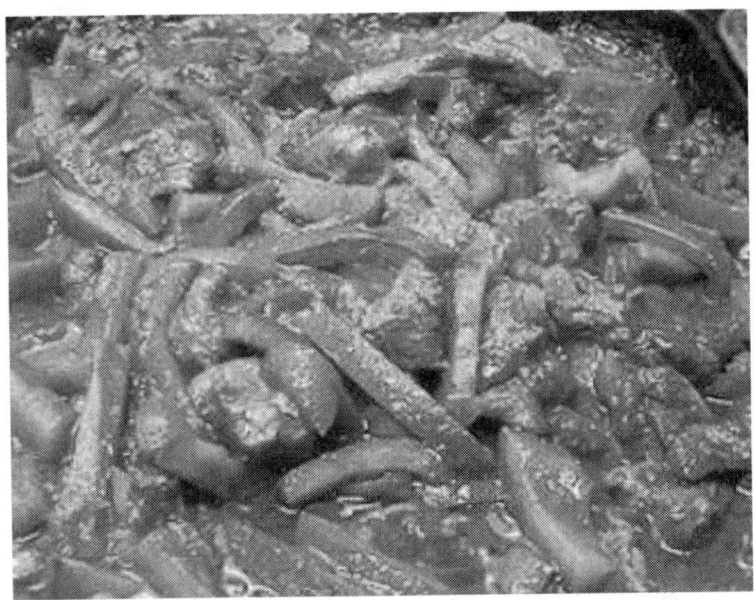

Pork, Mushrooms & Herbs Stew
Serves 8

Ingredients - Allergies: SF, GF, DF, EF, NF

- 2 cups chopped onions
- 2 tbsp. coconut oil
- Salt, ground black pepper according to taste
- 4 pounds pork shoulder
- 3 cups sliced mushrooms
- 1/2 cup each parsley, cilantro and dill
- 2 Tbsp. minced garlic.

Instructions

Put ingredients in the slow cooker. Cover, & cook on low for 8 hours.

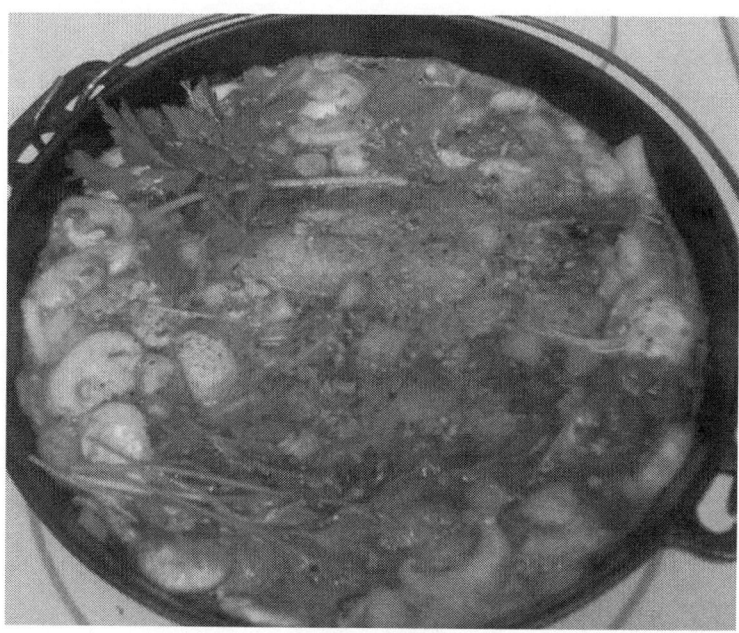

Chicken Green Curry
Serves 8

Ingredients - Allergies: SF, GF, DF, EF, NF

- 1 cup chopped onions
- 1 cup coconut milk
- 1 lime - juice & 1 cup chicken broth
- 1 cup chopped cilantro & 3 cloves garlic.
- 4 pounds chicken meat
- 2 cups sliced veggies (green beans and green peppers)
- 2 Tbsp. curry paste
- 4 Tbsp. fish sauce

Instructions

Blend lime, onions, curry paste, cilantro and spices. Put chicken and other ingredients in the slow cooker and pour blended ingredients over. Cover, & cook on low for 8 hours. Decorate with fresh basil leaves.

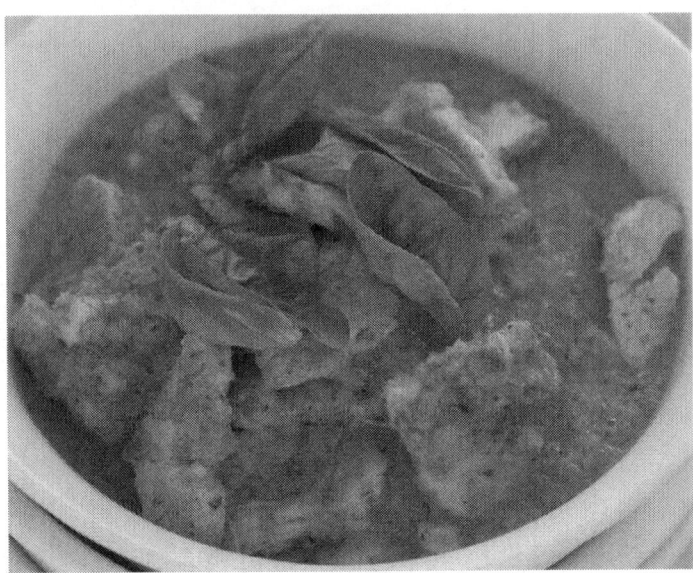

Two Beans Chili

Serves 8

Ingredients - Allergies: SF, GF, DF, EF, NF

- 2 tbsp. coconut oil
- 2 onions, chopped
- 3 cloves garlic, minced
- 1 pound ground beef
- 3/4 pound beef sirloin, cubed
- 2 cups diced tomatoes
- 1 cup strong brewed coffee
- 1 cup tomato paste
- 2 cups beef broth
- 1 tbsp. cumin seeds
- 1 tsp. dried oregano
- 1 tsp. ground cayenne pepper
- 1 tsp. ground coriander
- 1 tsp. salt
- 3 cups cooked kidney beans
- 3 cups cooked navy beans
- 4 fresh hot chili peppers, chopped

Instructions

Put ingredients in the slow cooker. Cover, & cook on low for 4 hours.

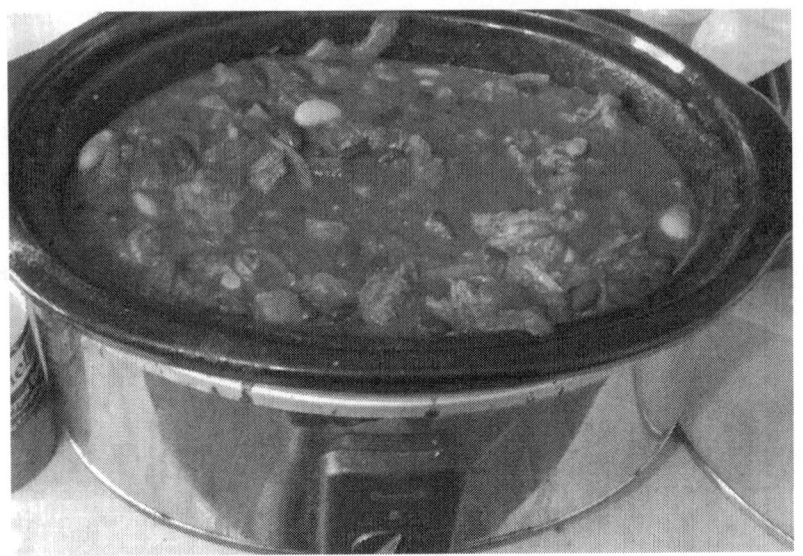

Chicken & Artichoke Hearts
Serves 8

Ingredients - Allergies: SF, GF, DF, EF, NF

- 2 cups chopped onions
- 2 tbsp. coconut oil
- Salt, ground black pepper according to taste
- 4 pounds chicken meat
- 2 cups chopped carrots.
- 8 Artichokes, tops sliced, trimmed
- 1 Tbsp. ground cumin.
- 1 cup chicken broth

Instructions

Put ingredients in the slow cooker. Cover, & cook on low for 8 hours.

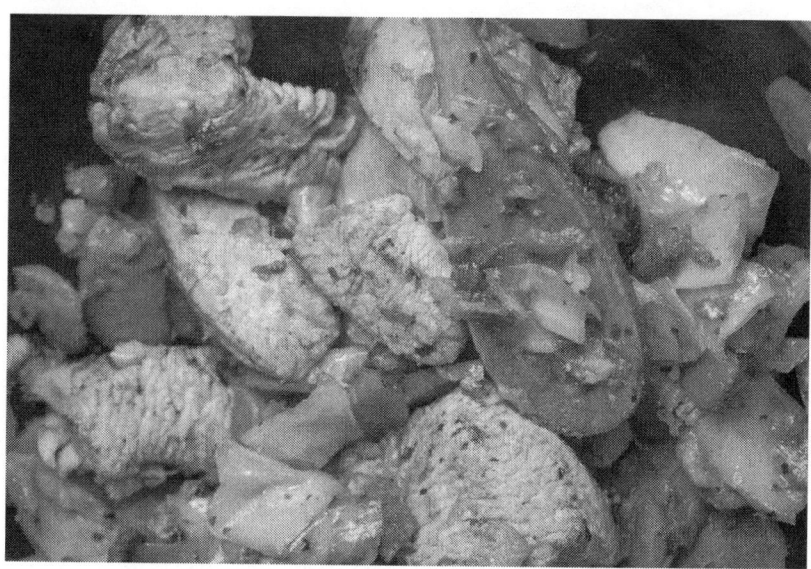

Green Peppers, Chicken and Green Onions

Serves 8

Ingredients - Allergies: SF, GF, DF, EF, NF

- 2 cups chopped green onions
- 2 tbsp. coconut oil
- Salt, ground black pepper according to taste
- 4 pounds chopped chicken meat
- 2 cups sliced green peppers
- 2 Tbsp. minced garlic.
- 1 Tbsp. ground cumin.

Instructions

Put ingredients in the slow cooker. Cover, & cook on low for 8 hours.

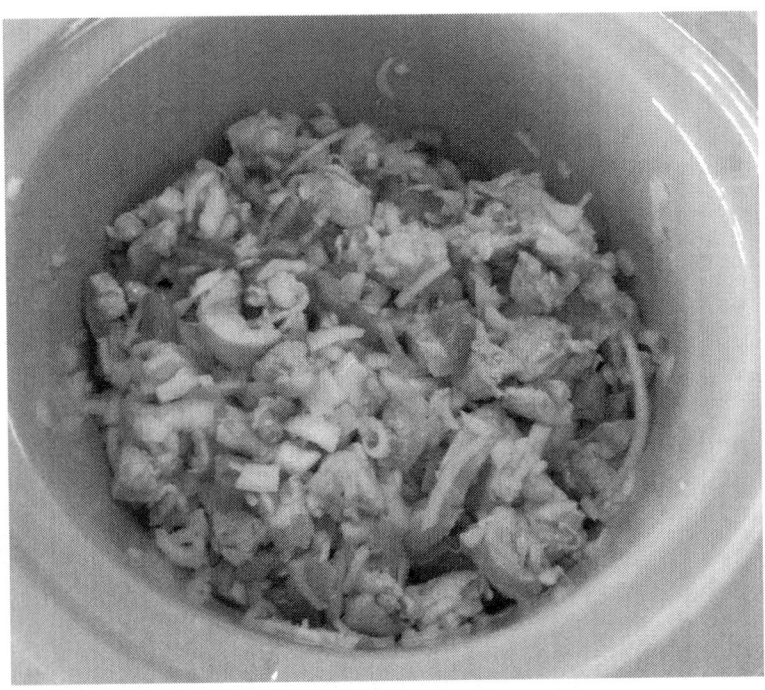

Black Bean Chicken Chili

Serves 8

Ingredients - Allergies: SF, GF, DF, EF, NF

- 2 tbsp. coconut oil
- 2 onions, chopped
- 3 cloves garlic, minced
- 2 pounds cubed chicken meat
- 2 cups diced red and yellow peppers
- 2 cups sliced celery
- 1 cup tomato paste
- 2 cups chicken broth
- 1 tbsp. cumin seeds
- 1 tsp. dried oregano
- 1 tsp. ground cayenne pepper
- 1 tsp. ground coriander
- 1 tsp. salt
- 2 cups black beans
- 4 fresh hot chili peppers, chopped

Instructions

Put ingredients in the slow cooker. Cover, & cook on low for 8 hours.

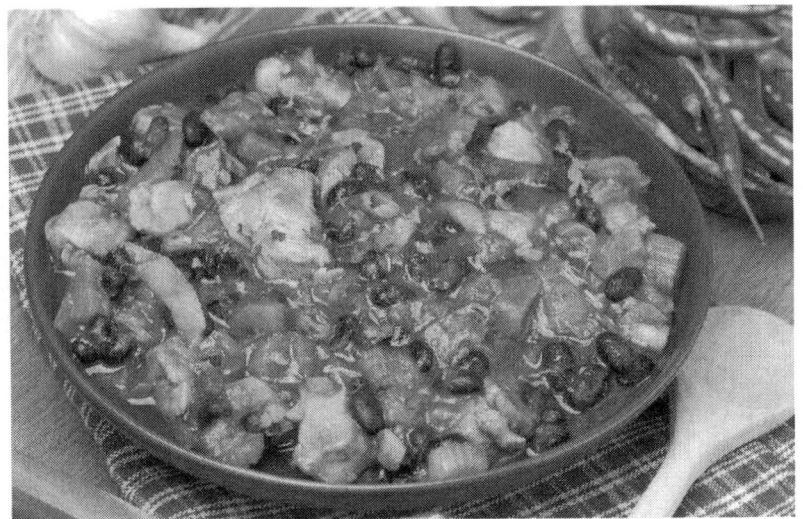

Haitian Spinach Shrimp Stew
Serves 8

Ingredients - Allergies: SF, GF, DF, EF, NF

- 2 cups chopped onions
- 2 tbsp. coconut oil
- Salt, ground black pepper to taste
- 4 pounds shrimp
- 3 cups spinach leaves
- 1 tsp. dried red pepper flakes (to taste).
- 4 whole cloves (discard after cooking)
- 2 cups fish broth
- 1 cup tomato paste.
- 1 lime – juice only & 1/8 ground cloves

Instructions

Put ingredients in the slow cooker. Cover, and cook on low for 8 hours.

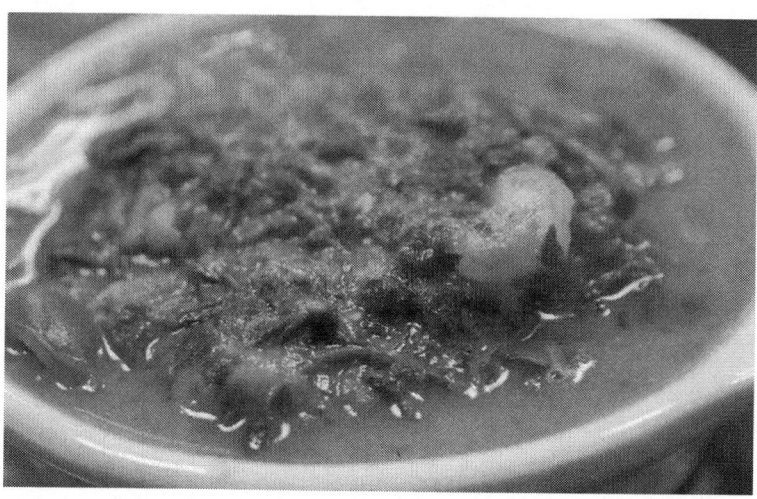

Duck Curry

Serves 8

Ingredients - Allergies: SF, GF, DF, EF, NF

- 2 cups chopped onions
- 1 cup chopped carrots
- 1 cup chopped zucchini
- 2 tbsp. coconut oil
- 4 cups duck meat
- Curry Paste, but go low on the heat
- 2 cups tomato paste
- 1/2 cup coconut milk or cream
- Cilantro for garnishing

Instructions

Make Curry Paste. Add the tomato paste, chicken, veggies and the cream. Stir to combine, add to crockpot and cook on low for 8 hours.

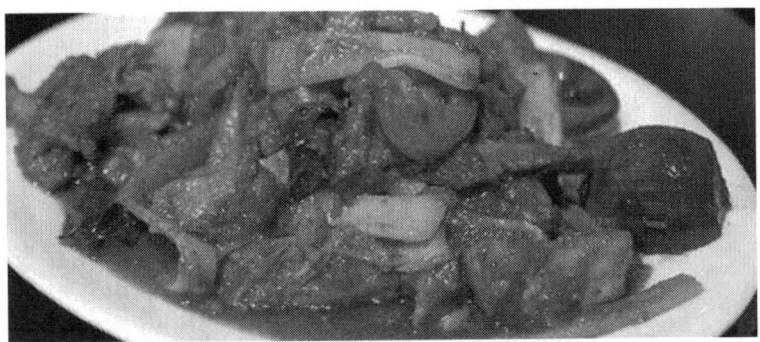

Eggplant Red Pepper Stew
Serves 8

Ingredients - Allergies: SF, GF, DF, EF, NF

- 2 cups chopped onions
- 4 tbsp. coconut oil
- Salt, ground black pepper to taste
- 4 pounds cubed eggplant
- 2 cups sliced red peppers
- 1 tsp. dried red pepper flakes (to taste).
- 1 cup tomato paste.

Instructions

Put ingredients in the slow cooker. Cover, and cook on low for 8 hours.

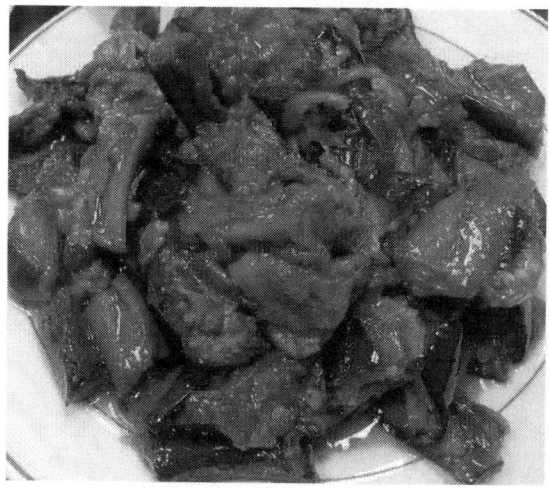

Irish Lamb Stew

Serves 8

Ingredients - Allergies: SF, GF, DF, EF, NF

- 2 cups chopped onions
- 2 tbsp. coconut oil
- Salt, ground black pepper to taste
- 4 pounds lamb neck meat
- 3 cups chopped sweet potato
- 1 cup chopped carrots
- 2 cups beef broth

Instructions

Put ingredients in the slow cooker. Cover, and cook on low for 8 hours.

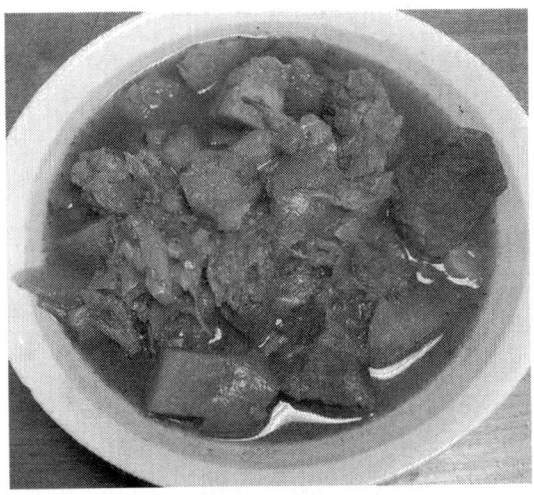

Shrimp, Onion & Cilantro Stew
Serves 8

Ingredients - Allergies: SF, GF, DF, EF, NF

- 4 cups quartered onions
- 2 tbsp. coconut oil
- Salt, ground black pepper to taste
- 4 pounds shrimp
- 1 tsp. dried red pepper flakes (to taste).
- 1 cup cilantro
- 2 cups fish broth
- 1 cup tomato paste.

Instructions

Put ingredients in the slow cooker. Cover, and cook on low for 8 hours.

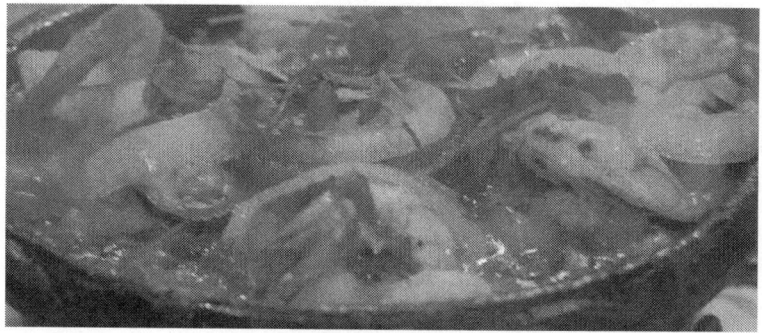

Venison Green Beans Onion Stew

Serves 8

Ingredients - Allergies: SF, GF, DF, EF, NF

- 4 cups quartered onions
- 2 tbsp. coconut oil
- Salt, ground black pepper to taste
- 4 pounds venison meat
- 1 tsp. dried red pepper flakes (to taste).
- 4 whole cloves (discard after cooking)
- 2 cups beef broth
- 2 cups green beans

Instructions

Put ingredients in the slow cooker. Cover, and cook on low for 8 hours.

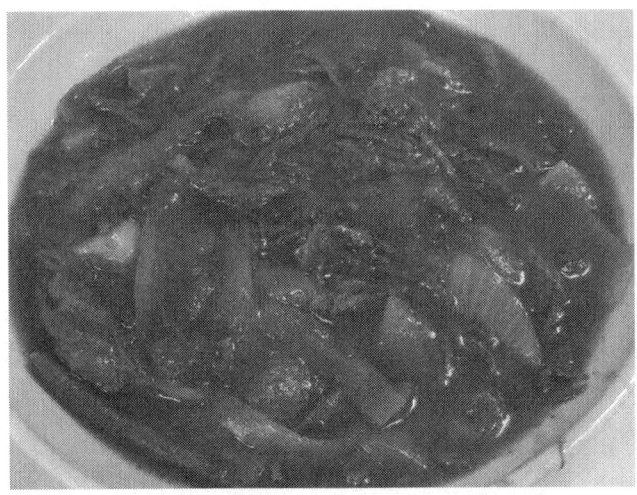

Pork Cauliflower Stew

Serves 8

Ingredients - Allergies: SF, GF, DF, EF, NF

- 2 cups chopped onions
- 2 tbsp. coconut oil
- Salt, ground black pepper to taste
- 4 pounds pork neck meat
- 1 cup sliced green onions
- 1 cup chopped carrots
- 2 cups beef broth
- 3 cups cauliflower
- 1 cup sliced tomatoes

Instructions

Put ingredients in the slow cooker. Cover, and cook on low for 8 hours. Sprinkle with sliced green onions.

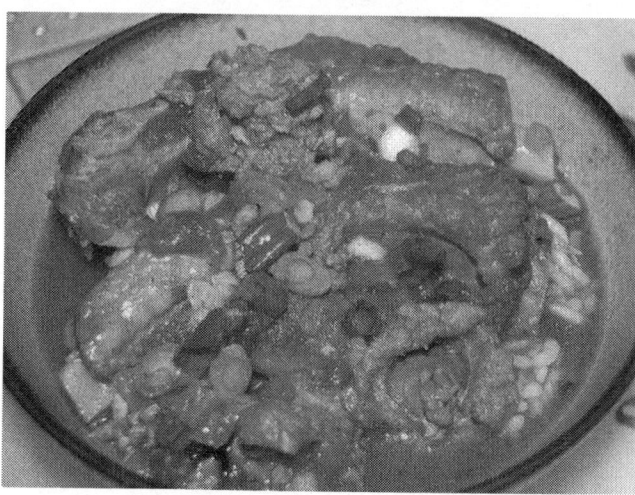

Sweet Potato Veal Stew

Serves 8

Ingredients - Allergies: SF, GF, DF, EF, NF

- 2 cups chopped onions
- 2 tbsp. coconut oil
- Salt, ground black pepper to taste
- 4 pounds veal neck meat
- 3 cups chopped sweet potato
- 2 cups beef broth

Instructions

Put ingredients in the slow cooker. Cover, and cook on low for 8 hours.

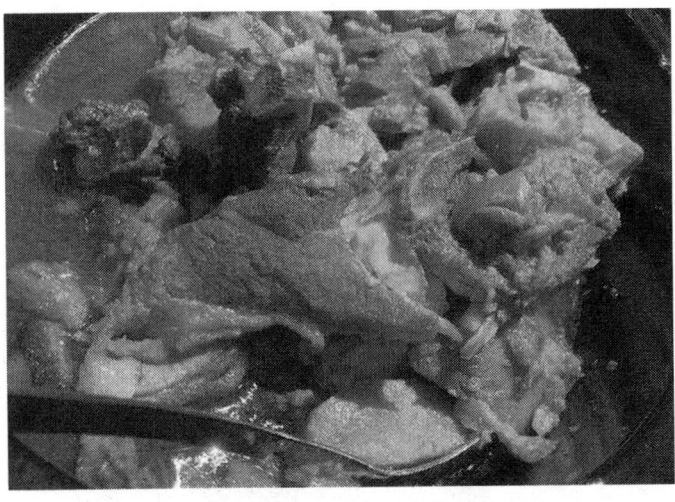

Pork Broccoli Carrot Stew

Serves 8

Ingredients - Allergies: SF, GF, DF, EF, NF

- 2 cups chopped onions
- 2 tbsp. coconut oil
- Salt, ground black pepper to taste
- 4 pounds cubed pork meat
- 3 cups broccoli
- 2 cups beef broth
- 2 cups sliced carrots

Instructions

Put ingredients in the slow cooker. Cover, and cook on low for 8 hours.

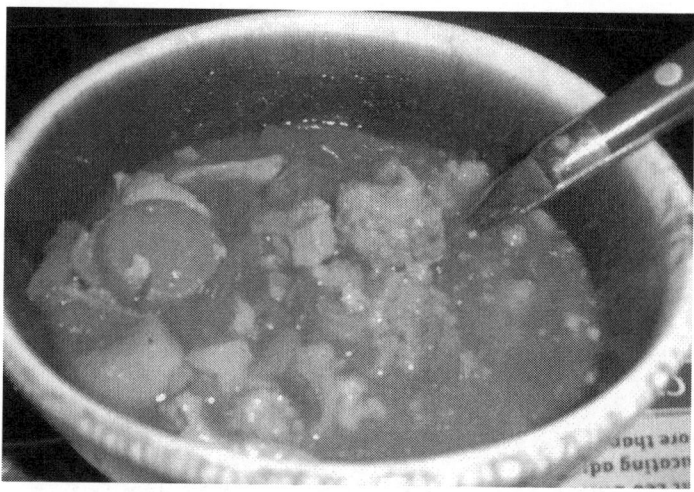

Moroccan Lamb & Mushrooms Stew

Serves 8

Ingredients - Allergies: SF, GF, DF, EF, NF

- 2 cups chopped onions
- 2 tbsp. coconut oil
- Salt, ground black pepper to taste
- 4 pounds lamb neck meat
- 1 tsp. each: cumin, coriander, fennel seeds
- 1 tsp. dried red pepper flakes (to taste).
- 1/2 cup dried apricots
- 1 cup beef broth
- 1 cup tomato paste.
- 2 cups whole mushrooms
- ½ cup cilantro

Instructions

Put ingredients in the slow cooker. Cover, and cook on low for 8 hours. Sprinkle with cilantro.

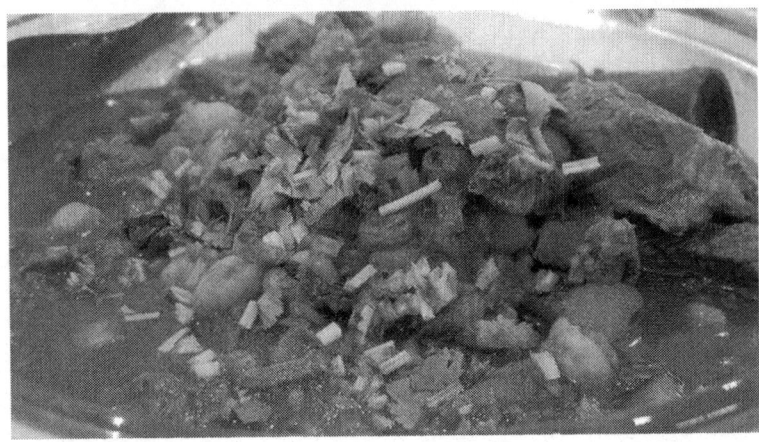

Shrimp Peppers Stew

Serves 8

Ingredients - Allergies: SF, GF, DF, EF, NF

- 2 cups chopped onions
- 2 tbsp. coconut oil
- Salt, ground black pepper to taste
- 4 pounds shrimp
- 1 tsp. dried red pepper flakes (to taste).
- 3 cups sliced red peppers
- 1 cup tomato paste.

Instructions

Put ingredients in the slow cooker. Cover, and cook on low for 8 hours.

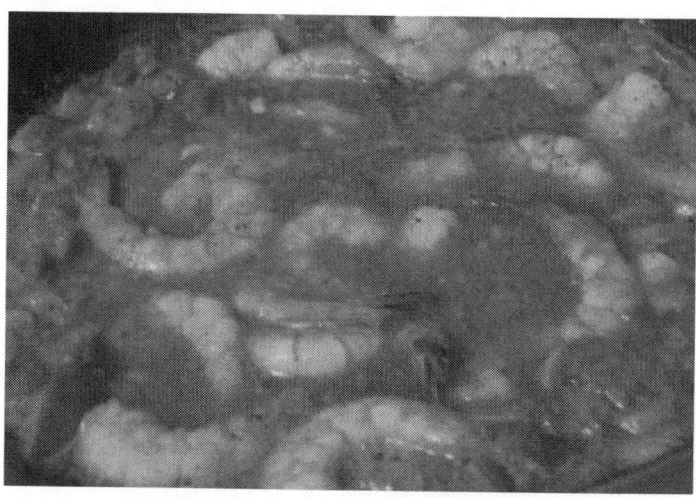

Afghan Stew

Serves 8

Ingredients - Allergies: SF, GF, DF, EF, NF

- 2 cups chopped onions & 2 minced garlic cloves
- 2 tbsp. coconut oil
- Salt, ground black pepper to taste
- 4 pounds chicken thighs
- 1 tsp. dried red pepper flakes (to taste).
- 1/2 tsp. cinnamon & 1 tsp. turmeric.
- 1/4 tsp. ground cardamom.
- 1 tbsp. parsley for decoration.
- 2 cups whole green peppers
- 1 cup beef broth & 2 cups tomato paste

Instructions

Put ingredients in the slow cooker. Cover, and cook on low for 8 hours. Decorate with parsley.

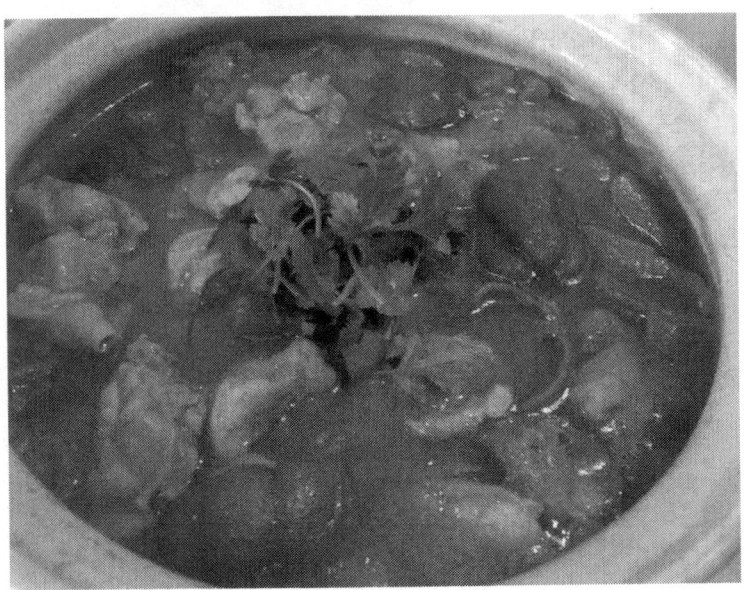

Chicken, Capers, Olives, Anchovy & Zucchini Stew

Serves 8

Ingredients - Allergies: SF, GF, DF, EF, NF

- 2 cups chopped onions
- 2 tbsp. coconut oil
- Salt, ground black pepper to taste
- 4 pounds cubed chicken
- 3/4 cup olives.
- 1/4 cup capers & 1/4 cup anchovy
- 3 cups sliced zucchini
- 1 cup tomato paste.

Instructions

Put ingredients in the slow cooker. Cover, and cook on low for 8 hours.

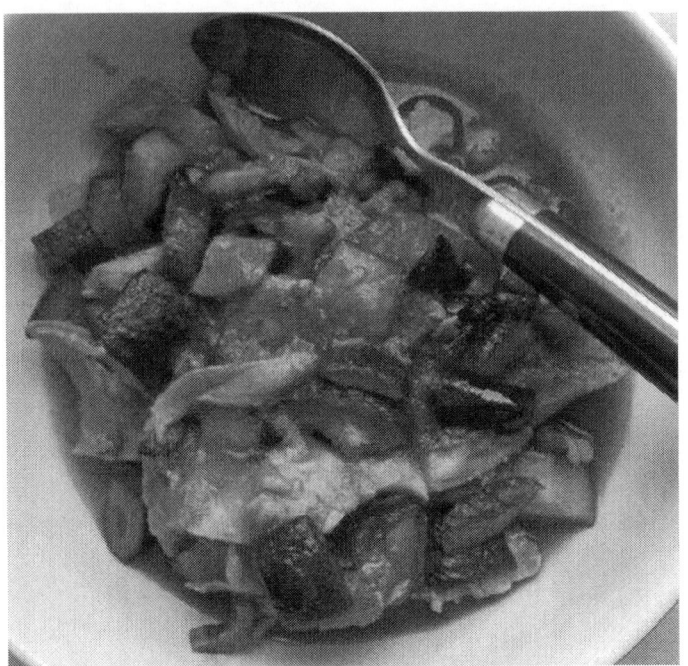

Hunter's Green Beans Chicken Stew

Serves 8

Ingredients - Allergies: SF, GF, DF, EF, NF

- 2 cups chopped onions & 2 minced garlic cloves
- 2 tbsp. coconut oil
- Salt, ground black pepper to taste
- 4 pounds chicken thighs
- 1 tsp. dried red pepper flakes (to taste).
- 1 cup mushrooms & 2 bay leaves
- 1 cup chopped tomatoes & 1 rosemary sprig
- 2 cups green beans cut in 2 inch pieces
- 2 cups chicken broth & 1 cup white wine

Instructions

Put ingredients in the slow cooker. Cover, and cook on low for 8 hours.

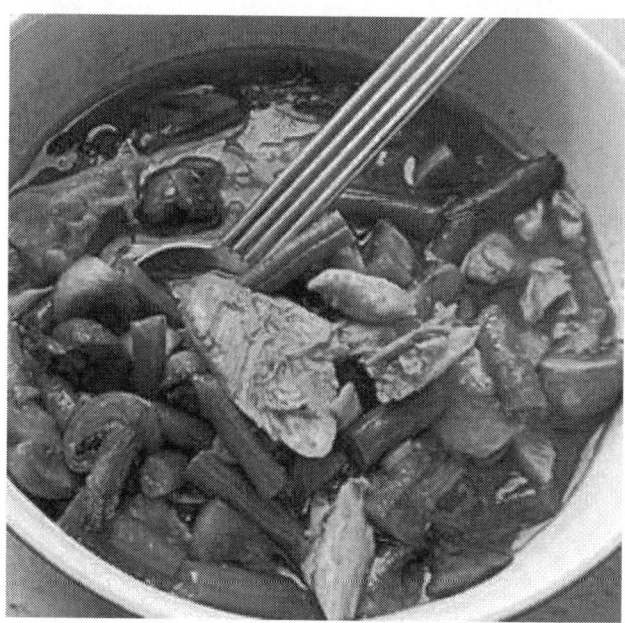

Kale Chicken Jambalaya

Serves 8

Ingredients - Allergies: SF, GF, DF, EF, NF

- 1 cup chopped onions & 2 minced garlic cloves
- 2 tbsp. coconut oil & 1 tsp. turmeric
- Salt, ground black pepper to taste
- 3 pounds cubed chicken & 1 pound shrimp
- 1 tsp. dried red pepper flakes (to taste).
- 3 cups kale & 1 cup mushrooms
- 1 cup tomato paste & 1 cup chicken broth
- 1 cup corn & 1 cup chopped carrot

Instructions

Put ingredients in the slow cooker. Cover, and cook on low for 8 hours.

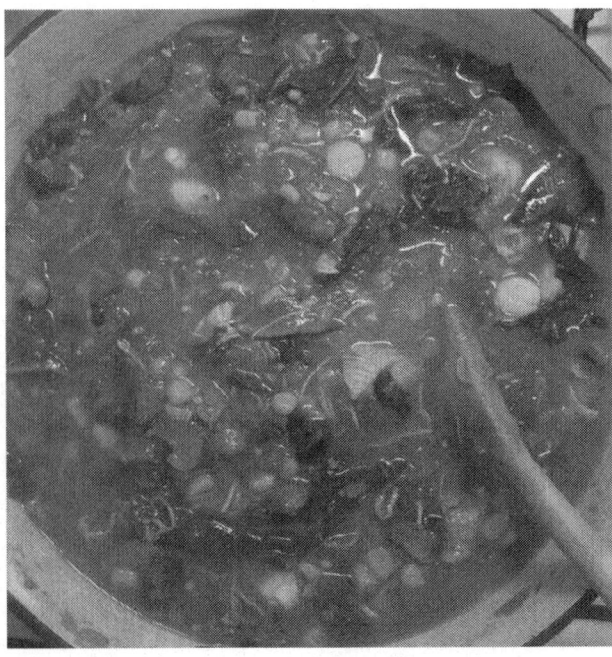

Minced Pork and Veal Stew
Serves 8

Ingredients - Allergies: SF, GF, DF, EF, NF

- 2 cups finely chopped onions
- 2 tbsp. coconut oil
- Salt, ground black pepper to taste
- 2 pounds minced pork and veal each
- 2 cloves garlic, minced
- 2 cups finely chopped celery
- 2 cups finely chopped carrot
- 1 cup beef broth

Instructions

Put ingredients in the slow cooker. Cover, and cook on low for 8 hours.

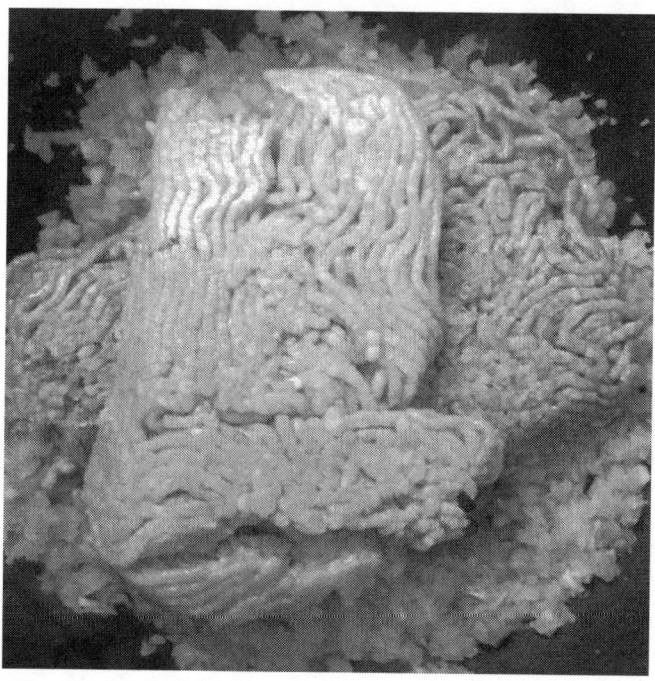

Olives & Chicken Stew

Serves 8

Ingredients - Allergies: SF, GF, DF, EF, NF

- 2 cups chopped onions
- 2 tbsp. coconut oil
- Salt, ground black pepper to taste
- 4 pounds chicken thigs
- 1 tsp. dried red pepper flakes (to taste).
- 2 cups sliced olives
- 3 cups tomato paste.

Instructions

Put ingredients in the slow cooker. Cover, and cook on low for 8 hours.

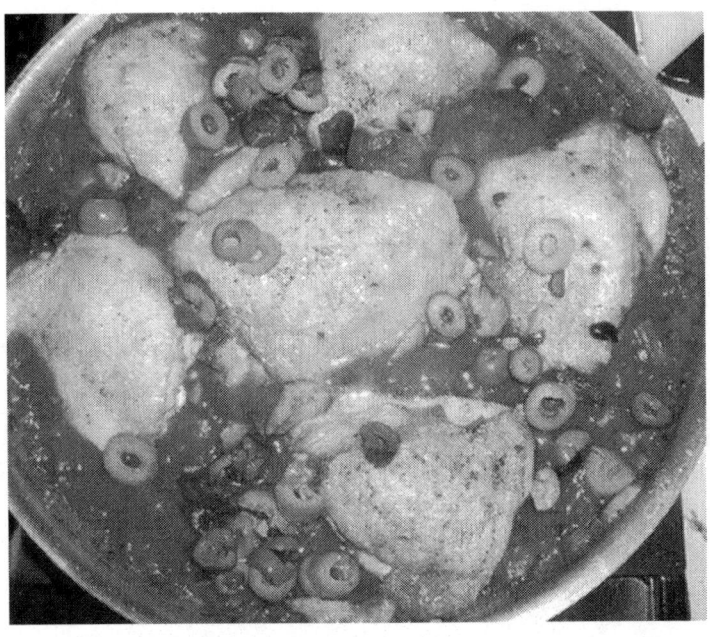

Pulled Pork

Serves 8

Ingredients - Allergies: SF, GF, DF, EF, NF

- 2 cups chopped onions & 2 minced garlic cloves
- 2 tbsp. coconut oil
- Salt, ground black pepper to taste
- 4 pounds pork shoulder
- 1 tsp. dried red pepper flakes (to taste).
- 1/2 cup chicken broth & 1/2 cup apple cider vinegar
- 1 cup tomato paste & 2 tsp. ground cumin
- 1 tbsp. mustard powder & 1 cup tomato paste

Instructions

Put ingredients in the slow cooker. Cover, and cook on low for 8 hours.

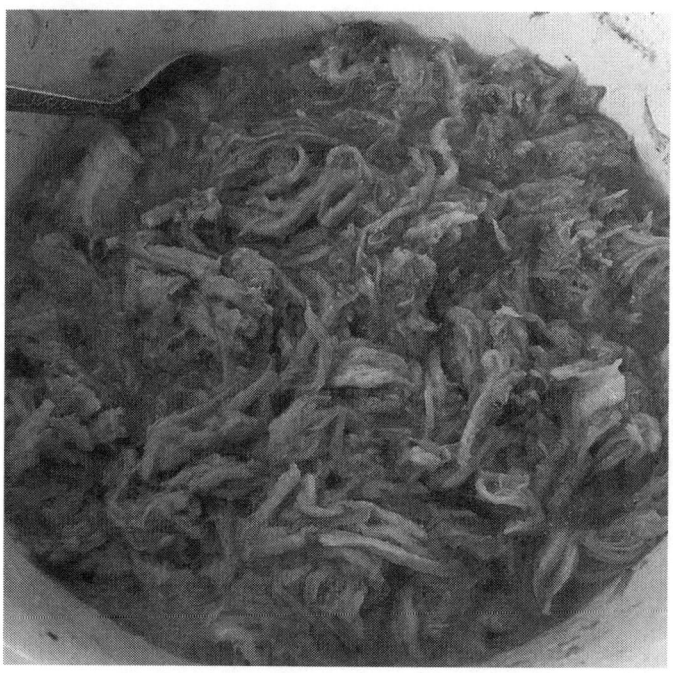

Chicken, Olives, Capers & Eggplant Stew

Serves 8

Ingredients - Allergies: SF, GF, DF, EF, NF

- 2 cups chopped onions
- 2 tbsp. coconut oil
- Salt, ground black pepper to taste
- 4 pounds cubed chicken
- 3/4 cup olives & 1/4 cup capers
- 1 cup cauliflower florets
- 3 cups sliced eggplant
- 1 cup tomato paste.

Instructions

Put ingredients in the slow cooker. Cover, and cook on low for 8 hours.

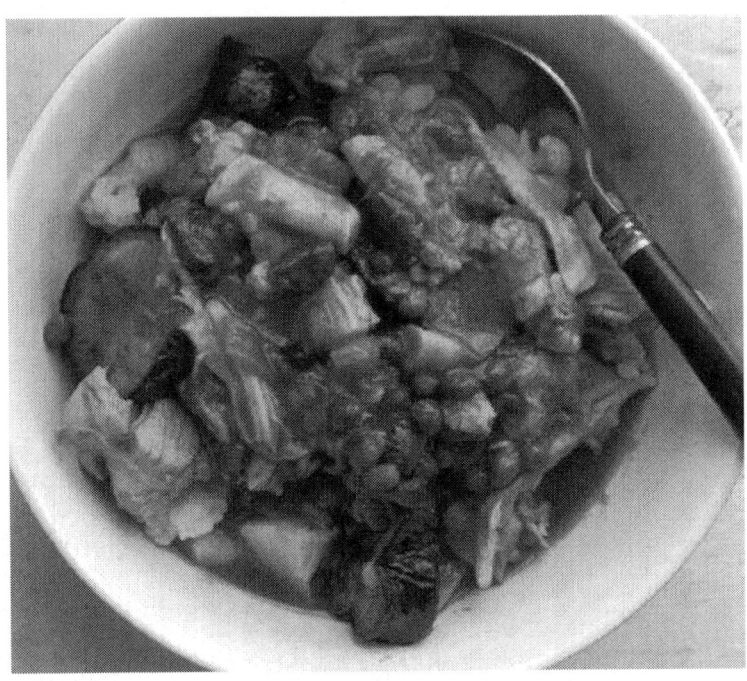

Turkish Chicken Stew
Serves 8

Ingredients - Allergies: SF, GF, DF, EF, NF

- 2 cups chopped onions & 2 minced garlic cloves
- 2 tbsp. coconut oil
- Salt, ground black pepper to taste
- 4 pounds chicken thighs
- 1 tsp. dried red pepper flakes (to taste).
- 2 cups sliced red peppers
- 2 cups sliced eggplant or zucchini
- 1 cup tomato paste. & 1/2 cups brown rice
- ½ tsp. ground cumin & 2 star anise (discard before serving)

Instructions

Put ingredients in the slow cooker. Cover, and cook on low for 8 hours.

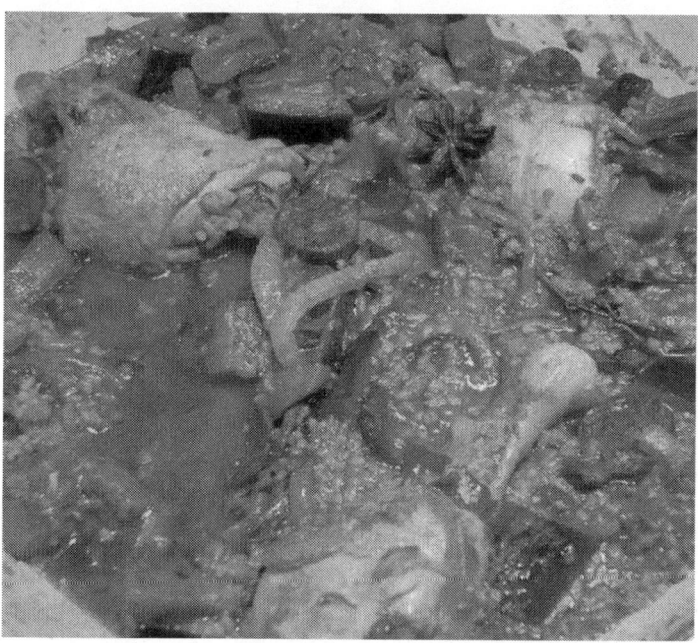

Veal & Red Peppers Stew

Serves 8

Ingredients - Allergies: SF, GF, DF, EF, NF

- 2 cups chopped onions & 2 minced garlic cloves
- 2 tbsp. coconut oil
- Salt, ground black pepper to taste
- 4 pounds cubed veal
- 1 tsp. dried red pepper flakes (to taste).
- 3 cups sliced red peppers
- 1 cup tomato paste.

Instructions

Put ingredients in the slow cooker. Cover, and cook on low for 8 hours.

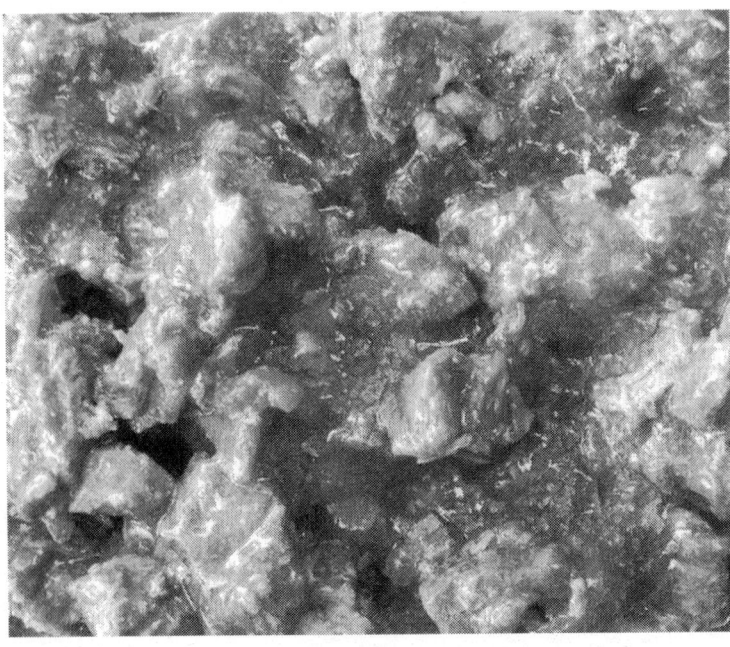

Chinese Eggplant, Chicken & Green Onions Stew
Serves 8

Ingredients - Allergies: SF, GF, DF, EF, NF

- 2 cups chopped onions
- 2 tbsp. coconut oil
- Salt, ground black pepper to taste
- 4 pounds cubed chicken
- 3/4 cup sliced green onions
- 2 cups chicken broth
- 3 cups halved Chinese eggplants
- 1 cup tomato paste.

Instructions

Put ingredients in the slow cooker. Cover, and cook on low for 8 hours.

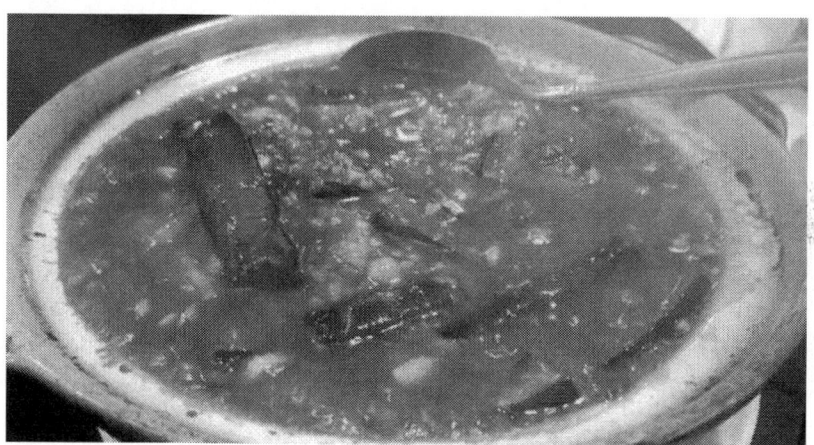

Pumpkin, Chicken, & Chinese Celery Stew

Serves 8

Ingredients - Allergies: SF, GF, DF, EF, NF

- 2 cups chopped onions
- 2 tbsp. coconut oil
- Salt, ground black pepper to taste
- 4 pounds dark chicken meat
- 3/4 cup Chinese Celery
- 1/2 cup green peas & 1/2 cup sliced carrots
- 3 cups sliced pumpkin
- 2 cups chicken broth

Instructions

Put ingredients in the slow cooker. Cover, and cook on low for 8 hours.

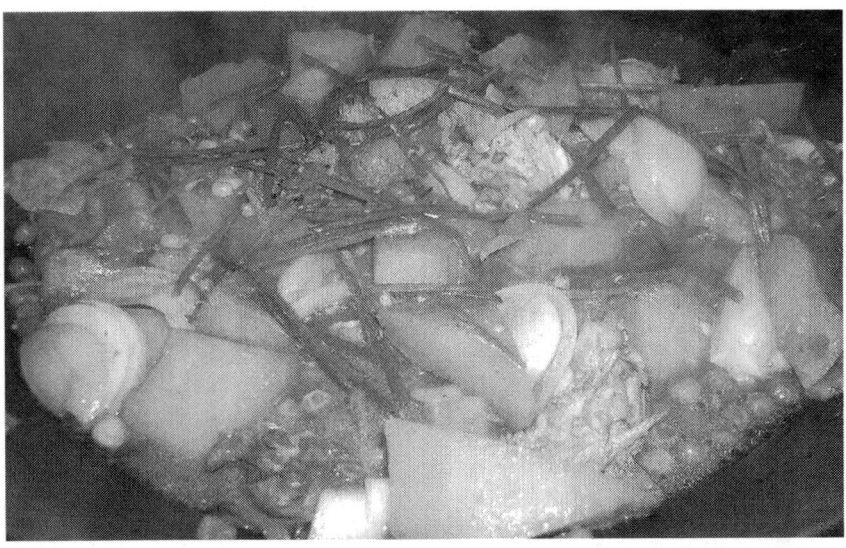

Spicy Shrimp & Eggplant Stew

Serves 8

Ingredients - Allergies: SF, GF, DF, EF, NF

- 2 cups chopped onions
- 2 tbsp. coconut oil
- Salt, ground black pepper to taste
- 4 pounds shrimp
- 3/4 cup sliced celery
- 1/4 cup chopped parsley
- 3 cups sliced eggplant
- 2 cups tomato paste

Instructions

Put ingredients in the slow cooker. Cover, and cook on low for 8 hours.

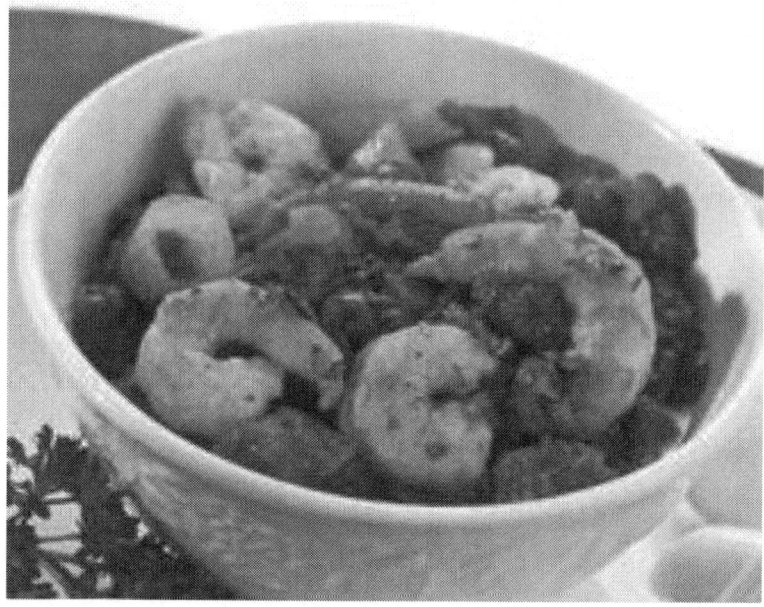

Veal, Tomato, Garlic, Corn & Zucchini Stew

Serves 8

Ingredients - Allergies: SF, GF, DF, EF, NF

- 2 cups chopped onions
- 2 tbsp. coconut oil
- Salt, ground black pepper to taste
- 4 pounds cubed veal
- 3/4 cup corn
- 12 cloves garlic
- 3 cups sliced zucchini
- 2 cups sliced tomatoes.

Instructions

Put ingredients in the slow cooker. Cover, and cook on low for 8 hours.

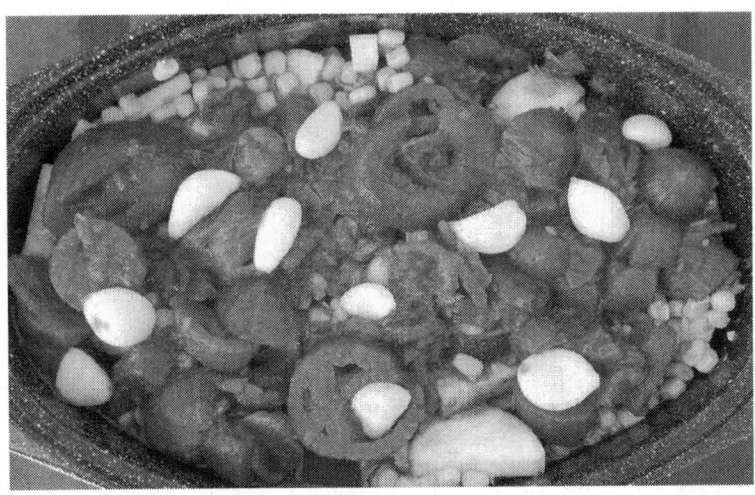

Chicken, Chickpeas, Tomato, Peppers & Eggplant Stew

Serves 8

Ingredients - Allergies: SF, GF, DF, EF, NF

- 2 cups chopped onions
- 2 tbsp. coconut oil
- Salt, ground black pepper to taste
- 4 pounds cubed chicken
- 1 cup chickpeas
- 1 cup sliced peppers
- 3 cups sliced eggplant
- 1 cup sliced tomatoes

Instructions

Put ingredients in the slow cooker. Cover, and cook on low for 8 hours.

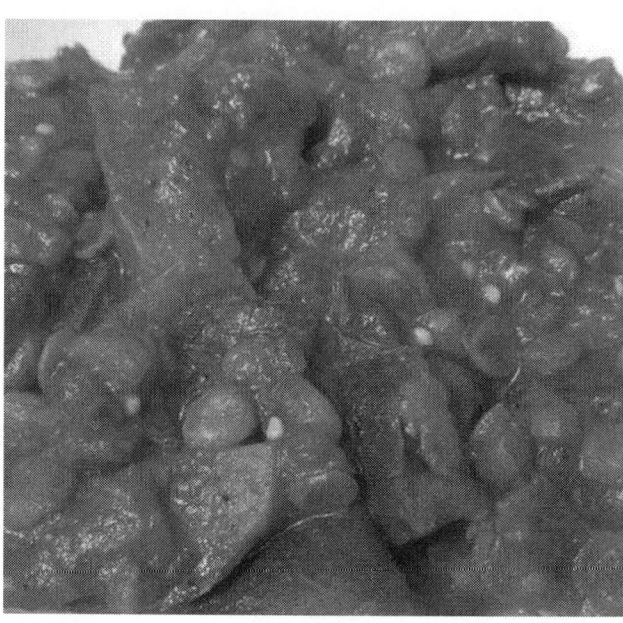

Pork, Chinese Celery & Mushrooms Stew

Serves 8

Ingredients - Allergies: SF, GF, DF, EF, NF

- 2 cups chopped onions
- 2 tbsp. coconut oil
- Salt, ground black pepper to taste
- 4 pounds cubed pork
- 3/4 cup olives.
- 1 cup Chinese celery
- 3 cups sliced mushrooms
- 1 cup beef broth

Instructions

Put ingredients in the slow cooker. Cover, and cook on low for 8 hours.

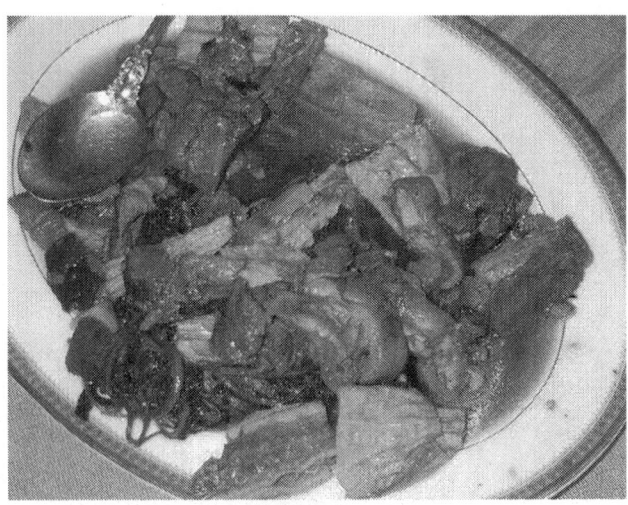

Shrimp, Yellow Peas & Green Onions Stew

Serves 8

Ingredients - Allergies: SF, GF, DF, EF, NF

- 2 cups chopped onions
- 2 tbsp. coconut oil
- Salt, ground black pepper to taste
- 4 pounds shrimp
- 2 cups yellow peas
- 1/4 cup sliced green onions
- 1 cup sliced carrot
- 4 cups vegetable broth

Instructions

Put ingredients in the slow cooker. Cover, and cook on low for 8 hours.

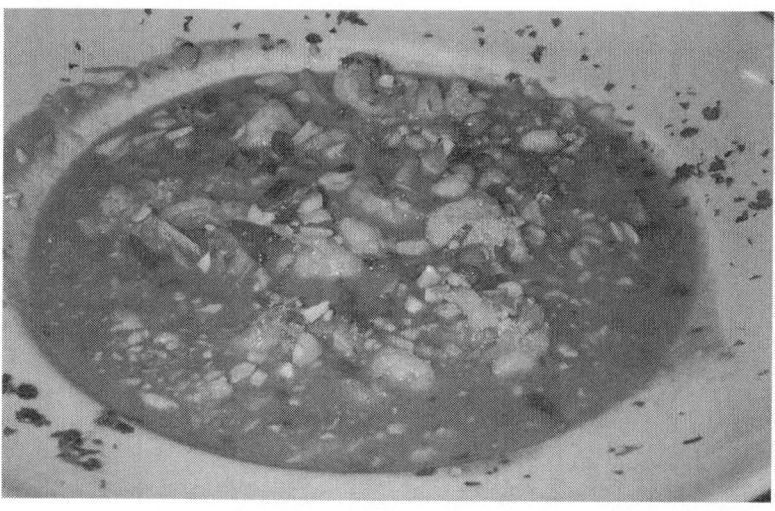

Pork & Bok Choy Stew

Serves 8

Ingredients - Allergies: SF, GF, DF, EF, NF

- 2 cups chopped onions
- 2 tbsp. coconut oil
- Salt, ground black pepper to taste
- 4 pounds pork roast
- 1 cup sliced carrots
- 1/4 cup sliced celery
- 3 cups bok choy
- 3 cups beef broth.

Instructions

Put ingredients in the slow cooker. Cover, and cook on low for 8 hours.

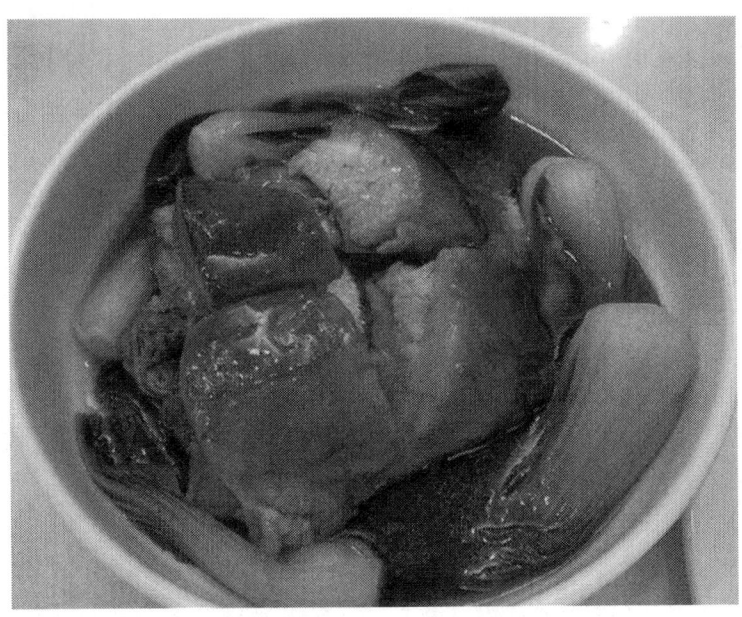

Shrimp & Red Peppers Stew

Serves 8

Ingredients - Allergies: SF, GF, DF, EF, NF

- 2 cups chopped onions
- 2 tbsp. coconut oil
- Salt, ground black pepper to taste
- 4 pounds shrimp
- 3 cups sliced red peppers
- 1 cup tomato paste.
- 2 cups fish broth

Instructions

Put ingredients in the slow cooker. Cover, and cook on low for 8 hours.

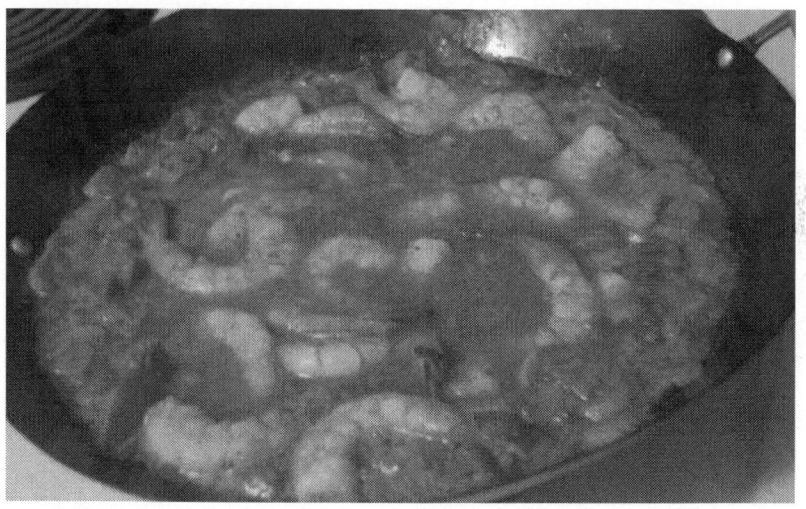

Pork, Mushrooms, Red Peppers & Zucchini Stew

Serves 8

Ingredients - Allergies: SF, GF, DF, EF, NF

- 2 cups chopped onions
- 2 tbsp. coconut oil
- Salt, ground black pepper to taste
- 4 pounds cubed pork
- 3/4 cup sliced carrots
- 2 cups sliced mushrooms
- 1 cup sliced zucchini
- 1 cup sliced red peppers
- 1 cup beef broth

Instructions

Put ingredients in the slow cooker. Cover, and cook on low for 8 hours.

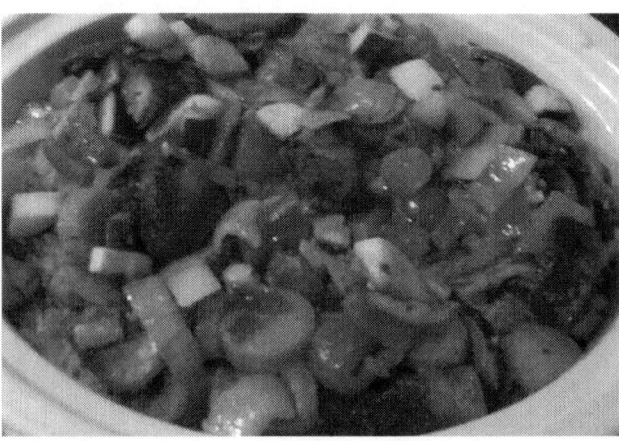

Beef, Leeks & Mushrooms Stew

Serves 8

Ingredients - Allergies: SF, GF, DF, EF, NF

- 2 cups chopped carrots
- 1 cup chopped onions
- 2 tbsp. coconut oil
- 1 cup chopped leeks
- Salt & ground black pepper to taste
- 1 cup sliced mushrooms
- 1 cup sliced tomatoes
- 4 pounds beef meat cut into stripes

Instructions

Put ingredients in the slow cooker. Cover, and cook on low for 7 to 9 hours.

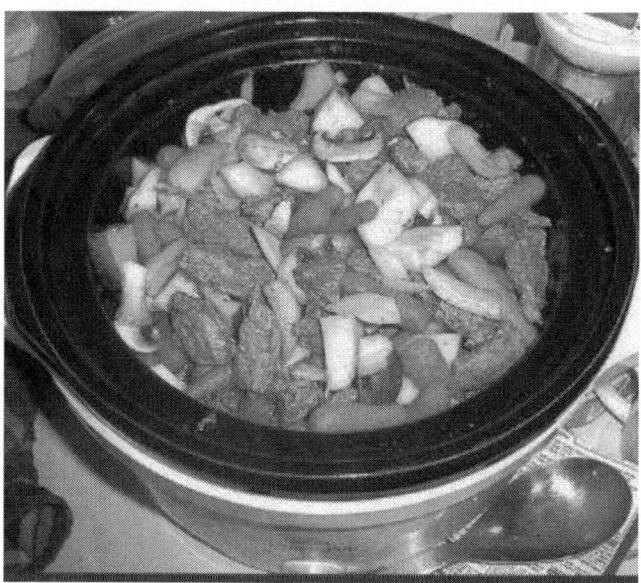

Chicken & Butternut Squash Stew

Serves 8

Ingredients - Allergies: SF, GF, DF, EF, NF

- 3 cups cubed uncooked butternut squash
- 1 cup chopped onions
- 2 tbsp. coconut oil
- 1 cup chopped red peppers
- Salt, ground black pepper to taste
- 1 cup chicken stock
- 4 pounds chicken dark, cubed

Instructions

Put ingredients in the slow cooker. Cover, and cook on low for 7 to 9 hours.

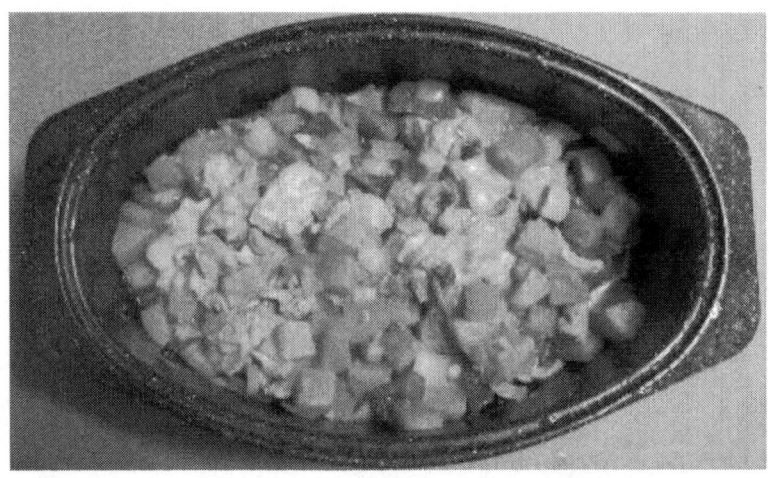

Chicken, Garlic & Tomato Stew

Serves 8

Ingredients - Allergies: SF, GF, DF, EF, NF

- 3 cups tomatoes
- 2 cups chopped onions
- 2 tbsp. coconut oil
- 1 garlic bulb, cut across
- Salt, ground black pepper and ground cumin to taste
- 1 Tbsp. minced garlic
- 4 pounds chicken breast meat cut into stripes

Instructions

Put ingredients in the slow cooker. Cover, and cook on low for 7 to 9 hours.

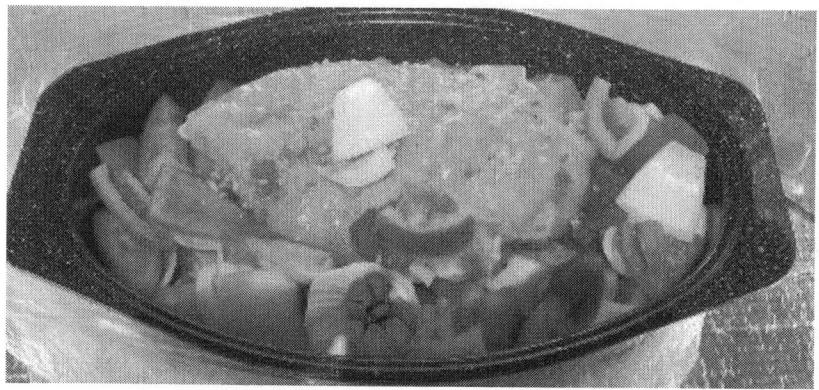

Minced Pork, Tomato & Red Peppers Stew

Serves 8

Ingredients - Allergies: SF, GF, DF, EF, NF

- 3 cups quartered tomatoes
- 1 cup chopped onions
- 2 tbsp. coconut oil
- 2 cups chopped red peppers
- Salt, ground black pepper and ground cumin to taste
- 1 cup shredded carrots
- 4 pounds minced pork meat

Instructions

Put ingredients in the slow cooker. Cover, and cook on low for 7 to 9 hours.

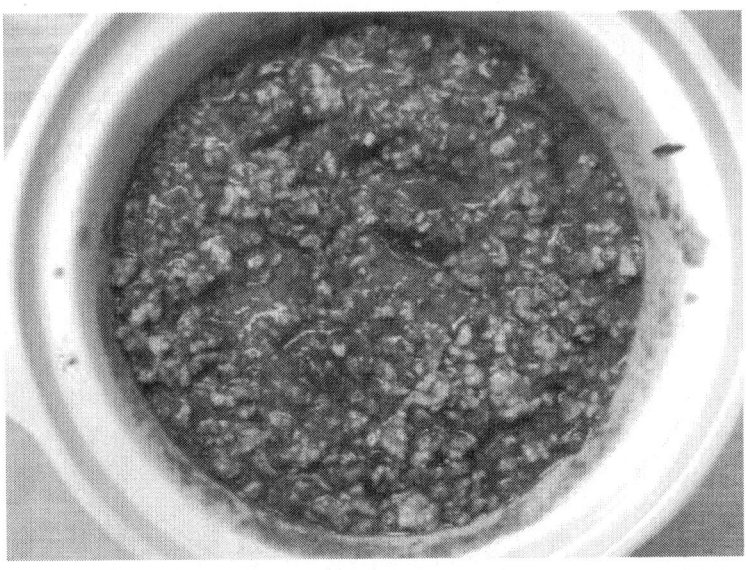

Beef, Eggplant, Celery & Peppers Stew
Serves 8

Ingredients - Allergies: SF, GF, DF, EF, NF

- 1 cup cubed eggplant
- 2 cups chopped onions
- 2 tbsp. coconut oil
- 1 cup sliced celery
- Salt, ground black pepper to taste
- 1 cup sliced red peppers
- 4 pounds beef meat cut into stripes

Instructions

Put ingredients in the slow cooker. Cover, and cook on low for 7 to 9 hours.

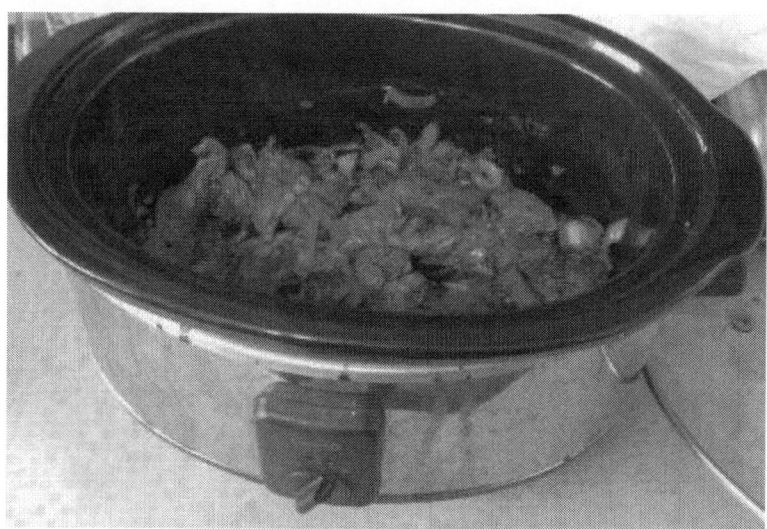

Chicken & Onion Stew

Serves 8

Ingredients - Allergies: SF, GF, DF, EF, NF

- 1 cup sliced mushrooms
- 6 large onions, quartered
- 2 tbsp. coconut oil
- Salt, ground black pepper to taste
- 2 cups chicken stock
- 4 pounds chicken drumsticks with skin on

Instructions

Put ingredients in the slow cooker. Cover, and cook on low for 7 to 9 hours.

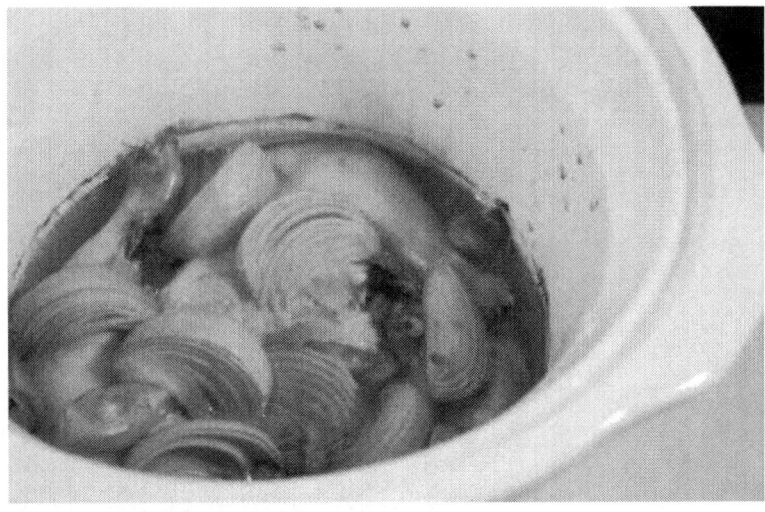

Pork & Black Eyed Peas Stew
Serves 8

Ingredients - Allergies: SF, GF, DF, EF, NF

- 1 cup chopped parsnips
- 2 cups chopped onions
- 2 tbsp. coconut oil
- 1 cup uncooked black eyed peas
- 1 cup chopped tomato
- 1 cup chopped celery
- Salt, ground black pepper and ground cumin to taste
- 2 cups beef stock
- 4 pounds cubed pork meat

Instructions

Put ingredients in the slow cooker. Cover, and cook on low for 7 to 9 hours.

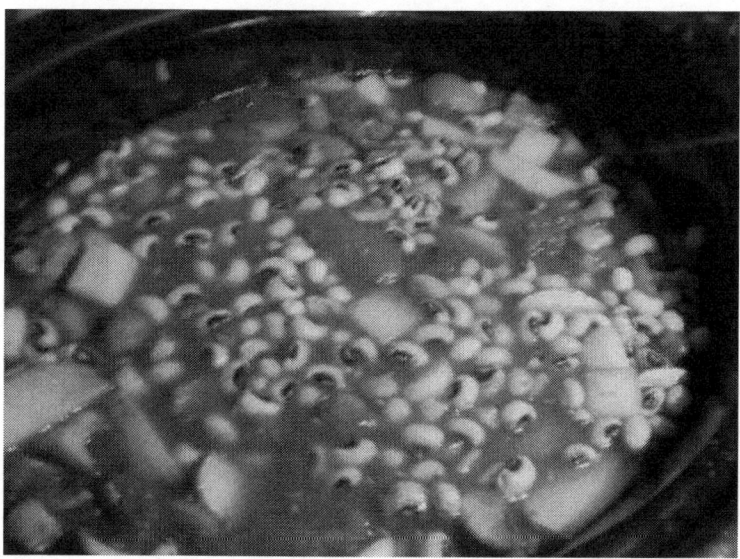

Zucchini Rolls

Serves 8

Ingredients - Allergies: SF, GF, DF, EF, NF

- 1 cup brown rice
- 2 cups chopped onions
- 2 tbsp. coconut oil
- 3-4 large zucchinis cut into thick stripes (see picture)
- Salt, ground black pepper and ground cumin to taste
- 2 cups beef stock
- 4 pounds minced beef meat

Instructions

Mix spices, meat, rice and onion, fill zucchini stripes with the mixture, make rolls and arrange them in the slow cooker. Add beef stock slowly by pouring by the sides. Cover, and cook on low for 7 to 9 hours.

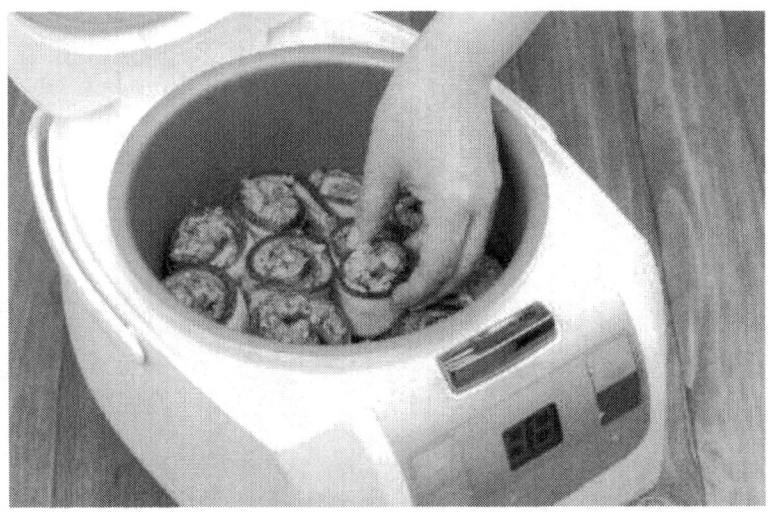

Beef Pot Roast with Broccoli

Serves 8

Ingredients - Allergies: SF, GF, DF, EF, NF

- 2 cups chopped onions
- 2 tbsp. coconut oil
- 3 cups broccoli
- Salt, ground black pepper & 2 bay leaves
- 2 cups beef stock
- 2 tsp. minced garlic
- 4 pounds beef pot roast

Instructions

Put ingredients in the slow cooker. Cover, and cook on low for 7 to 9 hours.

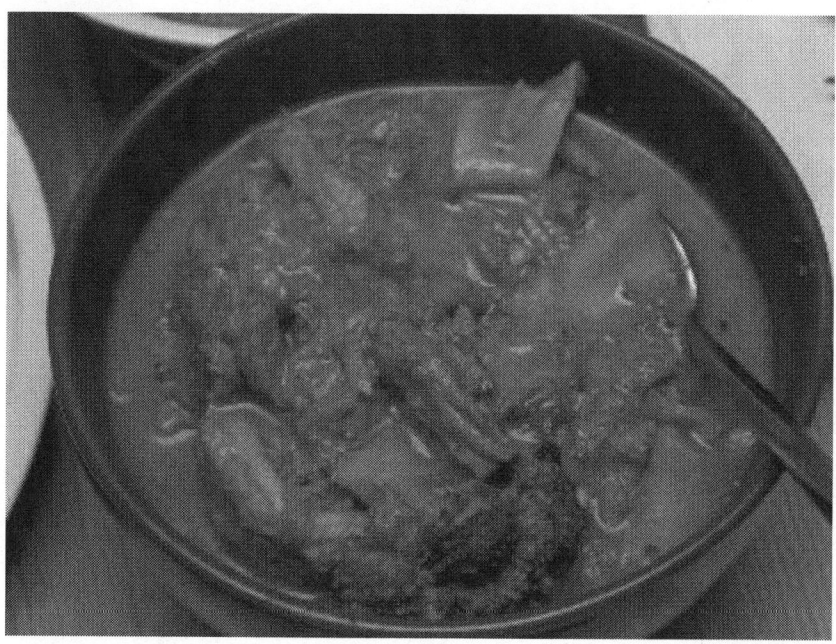

Mixed Seafood, Saffron & Sundried Tomatoes

Serves 8

Ingredients - Allergies: SF, GF, DF, EF, NF

- 1 cup sundried tomatoes
- 2 cups chopped onions
- 2 tbsp. coconut oil
- 1/4 cup olive oil mixed with 1 tsp. saffron
- Salt
- 2 cups white wine
- 4 pounds frozen mixed seafood

Instructions

Put ingredients in the slow cooker. Cover, and cook on high for 90 minutes.

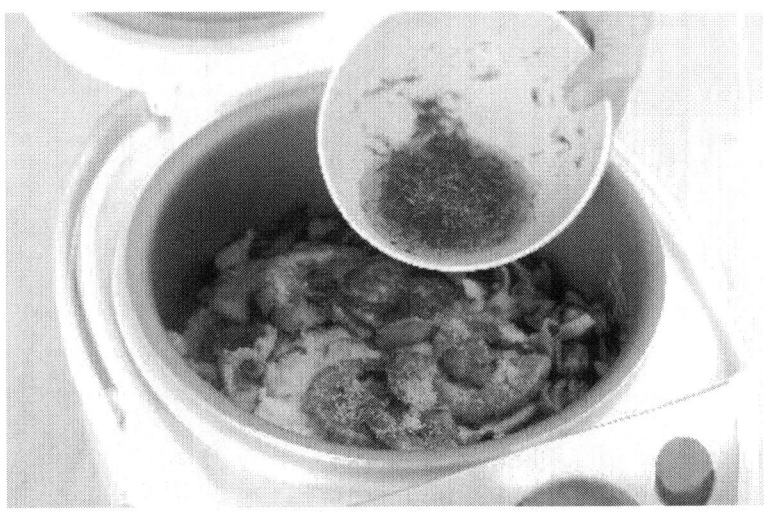

Chicken and Sweet Potato

Serves 8

Ingredients - Allergies: SF, GF, DF, EF, NF

- 2 cups cubed sweet potato
- 2 cups chopped onions
- 2 tbsp. coconut oil
- 3 red peppers, chopped
- Salt, ground black pepper and ground cumin to taste
- 2 cups chicken stock
- 4 pounds chicken meat

Instructions

Put ingredients in the slow cooker. Cover, and cook on low for 7 to 9 hours.

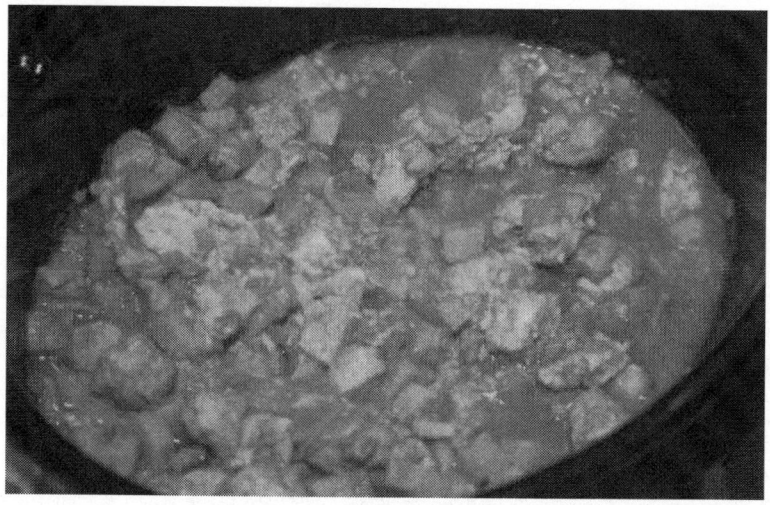

Black Bean Cuban Stew

Serves 8

Ingredients - Allergies: SF, GF, DF, EF, NF

- 1 cup sliced carrot
- 2 cups chopped onions
- 2 red peppers, chopped
- Salt, 1 Tsp. ground cayenne pepper and 1 Tbsp. cumin seeds
- 1 cup corn
- 3 cups dry black beans
- 1 cup tomato paste
- 2 cups beef broth
- 1 tsp. ground coriander
- 4 pounds pork neck meat, cubed

Instructions

Put ingredients in the slow cooker. Cover, and cook on low for 7 to 9 hours.

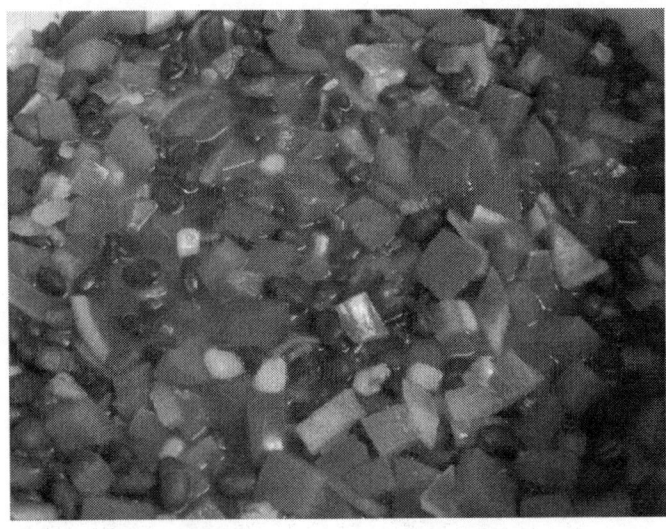

Chicken and Garbanzo Stew

Serves 8

Ingredients - Allergies: SF, GF, DF, EF, NF

- 2 cups dry garbanzo beans
- 2 cups chopped onions
- 2 tbsp. coconut oil
- 3 cups tomatoes, chopped
- 1 cup chopped carrot
- 1 cup sliced celery
- 2 garlic cloves, minced
- Salt, ground black pepper and ground cumin to taste
- 2 cups chicken stock
- 4 pounds chicken meat

Instructions

Put ingredients in the slow cooker. Cover, and cook on low for 7 to 9 hours.

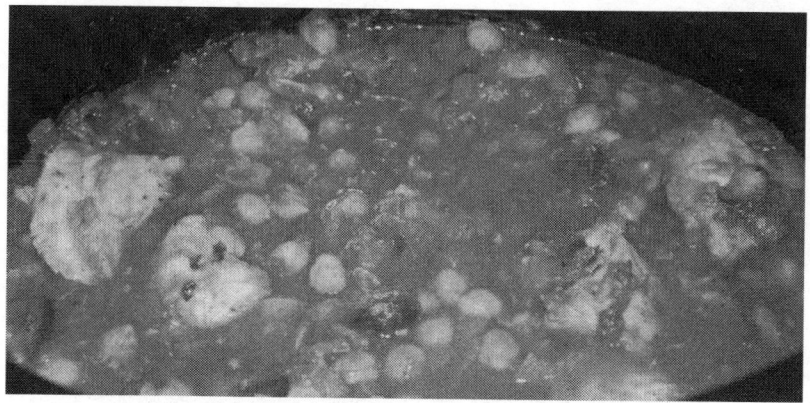

Spicy Beef Stew – Yukgaejang (Korean Recipe)

Serves 8

Ingredients - Allergies: SF, GF, DF, EF, NF

- 2 cups dried shiitake mushrooms
- 1 cup chopped onions
- 4 cloves minced garlic
- 1 Tbsp. minced ginger
- 2 cups green onions, cut in half
- 1 tbsp. sesame oil
- 2 cups sprouts
- 2 Tbsp. Fish sauce, hot pepper flakes to taste
- 2 cups chicken stock
- 4 pounds beef brisket

Instructions

Put ingredients in the slow cooker. Cover, and cook on low for 7 to 9 hours.

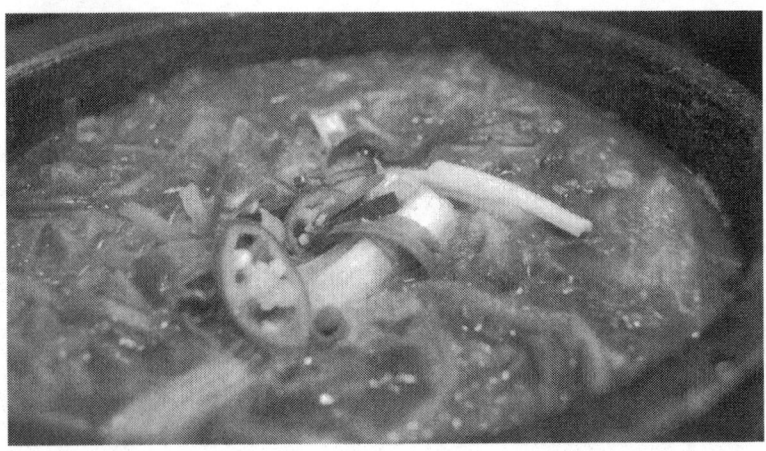

Kale, Quinoa and Beans Stew
Serves 8

Ingredients - Allergies: SF, GF, DF, EF, NF

- 2 cups raw kidney beans
- 2 cups chopped onions
- 2 cups chopped kale
- 1 cup sliced carrot
- 2 tbsp. coconut oil
- 2 cups tomatoes, chopped
- Salt, ground black pepper and ground cumin to taste
- 2 cups chicken or vegetable stock
- 1 cup quinoa

Instructions

Put ingredients in the slow cooker. Cover, and cook on low for 7 to 9 hours.

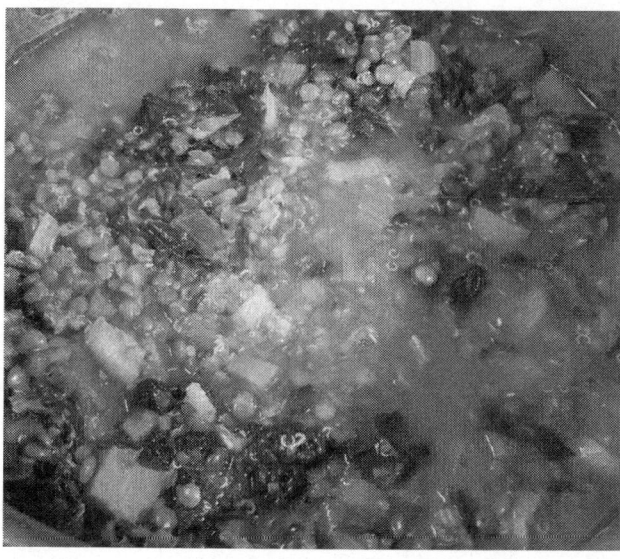

Veal & Sweet Potato Stew

Serves 8

Ingredients - Allergies: SF, GF, DF, EF, NF

- 2 cups cubed sweet potato
- 2 cups chopped onions
- 1 cup chopped carrots
- 1 cup chopped celery
- 2 tbsp. coconut oil
- 3 red peppers, chopped
- 1 cup tomato paste
- Salt, ground black pepper and ground cumin to taste
- 2 cups beef stock
- 4 pounds veal meat

Instructions

Put ingredients in the slow cooker. Cover, and cook on low for 7 to 9 hours.

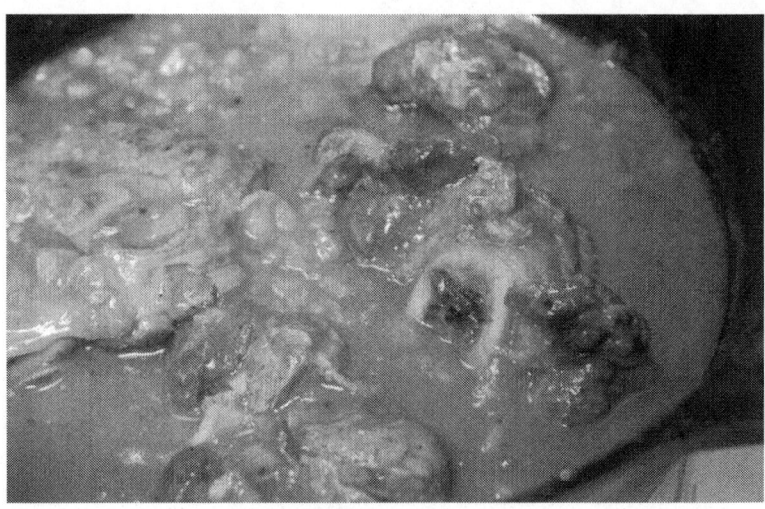

Teriyaki Chicken & Carrots
Serves 8

Ingredients - Allergies: SF, GF, DF, EF, NF

- 2 cups sliced carrots
- 1 Tbsp. minced ginger & 2 garlic cloves, minced
- 2 Tbsp. honey
- 1/4 cup rice or apple cider vinegar
- 2 tbsp. coconut oil
- 1 cup onions, chopped
- 3 Tbsp. fish sauce
- 1 cup chicken stock & 3 Tbsp. cornstarch (optional)
- 4 pounds chicken meat

Instructions

Put ingredients in the slow cooker. Cover, and cook on low for 7 to 9 hours.

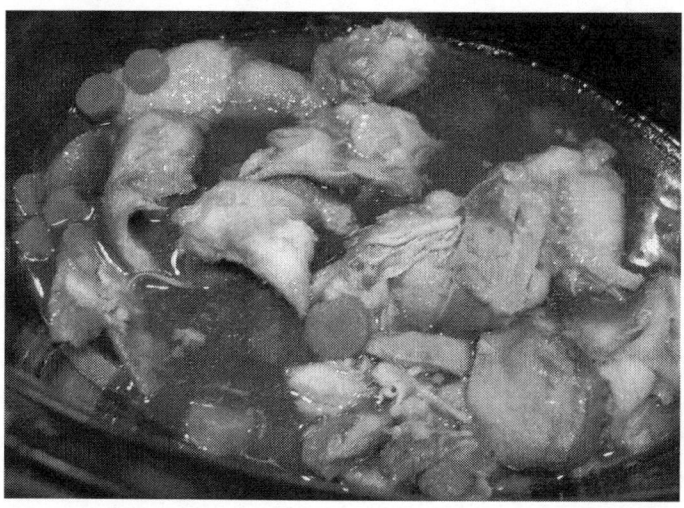

Spicy Garbanzo and Spinach Stew
Serves 8

Ingredients - Allergies: SF, GF, DF, EF, NF

- 2 cups dry garbanzo beans
- 2 cups chopped onions
- 2 cups spinach
- 2 tbsp. coconut oil
- 3 red peppers, chopped
- 2 cups tomato paste
- Salt, ground cayenne pepper and ground cumin to taste
- 2 cups chicken stock
- 4 pounds chicken meat

Instructions

Put ingredients in the slow cooker. Cover, and cook on low for 7 to 9 hours.

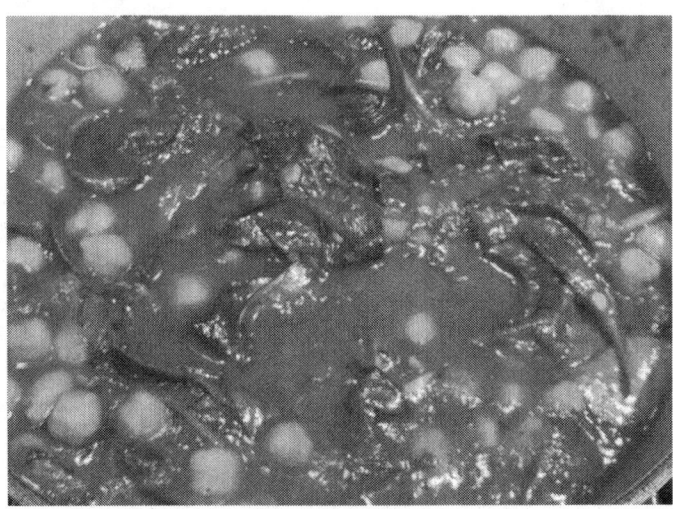

Cacciucco - Shrimp, Mussels, Fish & Scallops Stew
Serves 8

Ingredients - Allergies: SF, GF, DF, EF, NF

- 2 cups tomato paste
- 2 cups chopped onions
- 2 tbsp. coconut oil
- 1 cup cherry tomatoes
- Salt, 2 Tbsp. chopped dill
- 4 cups fish or vegetable stock
- 1 pound shrimp
- 1 pound mussels
- 1 pound scallops
- 1 pound local fish

Instructions

Put ingredients in the slow cooker. Cover, and cook on low for 7 to 9 hours.

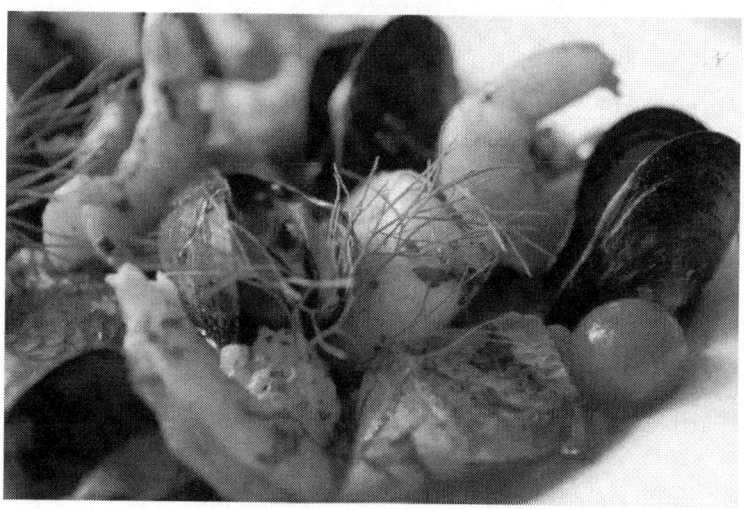

Lamb and Peppers Stew

Serves 8

Ingredients - Allergies: SF, GF, DF, EF, NF

- 2 cups chopped onions
- 2 tbsp. coconut oil
- 3 red peppers, chopped
- 3 yellow peppers, chopped
- Salt, ground black pepper and ground cumin to taste
- 2 cups beef stock
- 1 cup chopped parsley
- 4 pounds lamb, cubed

Instructions

Put ingredients in the slow cooker. Cover, and cook on low for 7 to 9 hours.

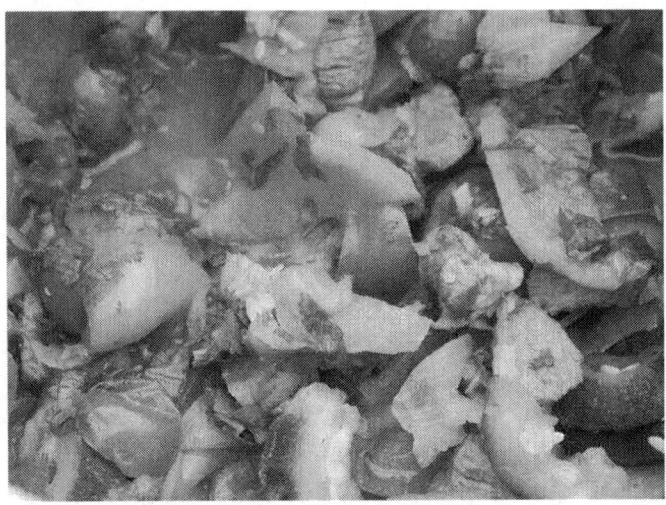

Plantain Chili

Serves 8

Ingredients - Allergies: SF, GF, DF, EF, NF

- 2 cups sliced plantain (1/2 inch thick)
- 1 cup sliced carrot
- 2 cups chopped onions
- Salt, 1 Tsp. ground cayenne pepper and 1 Tbsp. cumin seeds
- 1 cup corn
- 3 cups dry kidney beans
- 1 cup tomato paste
- 2 cups beef broth
- 1 tsp. ground coriander
- 1/2 cup chopped parsley
- 2 pounds pork neck meat, cubed

Instructions

Put ingredients in the slow cooker. Cover, and cook on low for 7 to 9 hours.

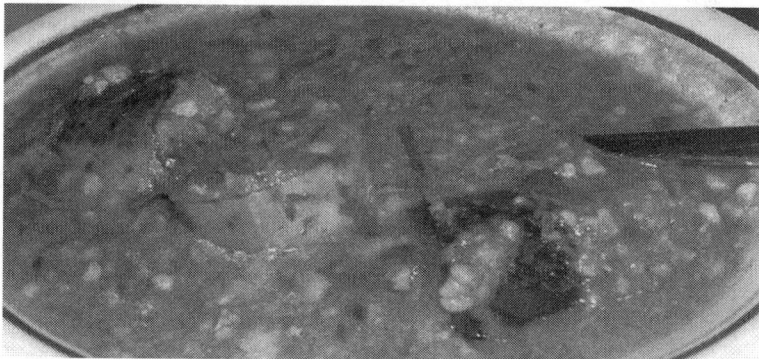

BBQ Pork
Serves 8

Ingredients - Allergies: SF, GF, DF, EF, NF

- 1-1/2 cups tomato paste
- 1/4 cup lemon juice
- 2 tbsp. mustard
- 1/2 tsp. salt
- 1/4 tsp. ground black pepper
- 1/2 tsp. minced garlic
- Salt, 1 Tsp. ground cayenne pepper and 1 Tbsp. cumin seeds
- 4 pounds pork neck meat

Instructions

Put ingredients in the slow cooker. Cover, and cook on low for 7 to 9 hours.

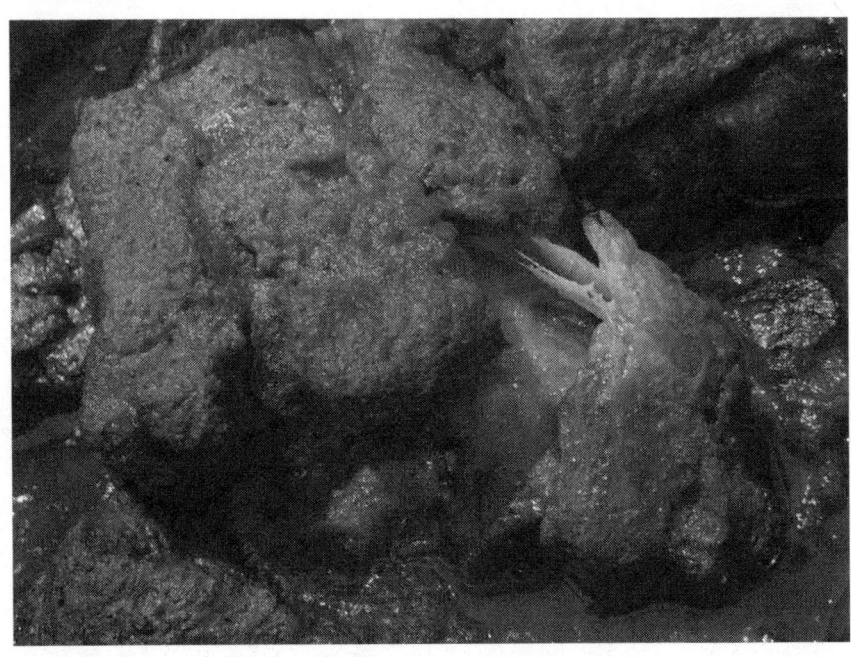

Penang Chicken Curry
Serves 8

Ingredients - Allergies: SF, GF, DF, EF, NF

- 4 pounds chicken meat
- Curry Paste, but go low on the heat
- 1 cup tomato paste
- 1 Tbsp. palm sugar (optional)
- 1/4 cup Thai basil leaves
- 1 cup coconut milk
- Cilantro or parsley for garnishing

Instructions

Put ingredients in the slow cooker. Cover, and cook on low for 7 to 9 hours.

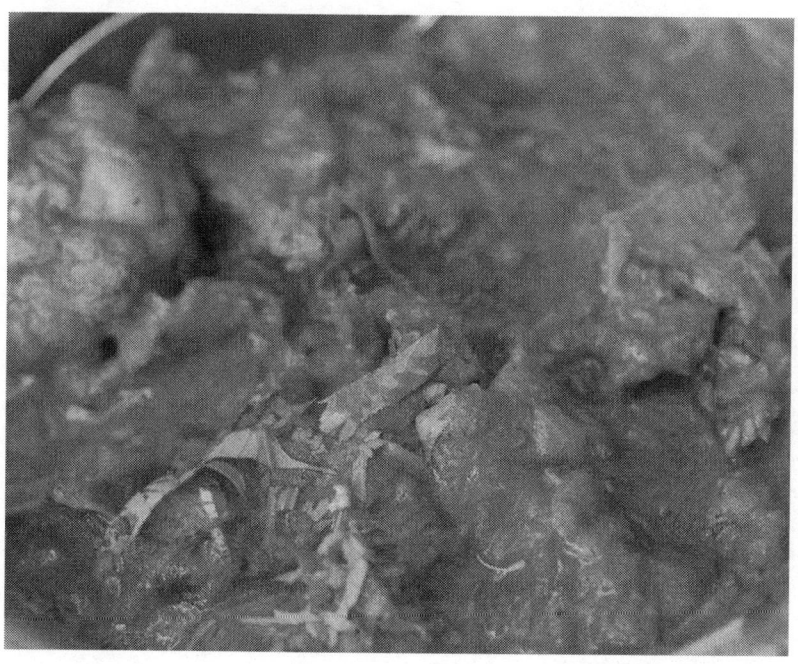

Chicken Fennel Stew
Serves 8

Ingredients - Allergies: SF, GF, DF, EF, NF

- 2 cups sliced fennel (bulb and tops)
- 1 cup sliced carrot
- 2 cups chopped onions
- Salt, 1 Tsp. ground pepper and 1 minced garlic clove
- 2 cups chicken broth
- 1/4 cup chopped parsley
- 2 pounds dark chicken meat

Instructions

Put ingredients in the slow cooker. Cover, and cook on low for 7 to 9 hours.

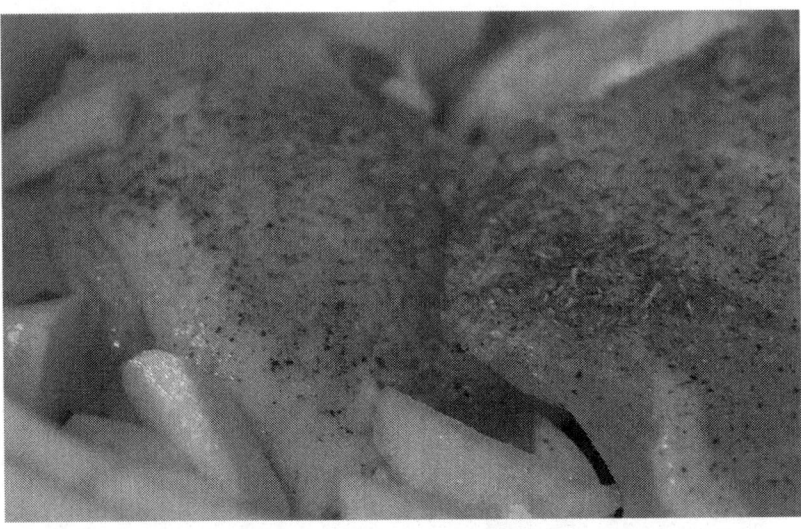

Garbanzo Kale Curry

Serves 8

Ingredients - Allergies: SF, GF, DF, EF, NF

- 4 cups dry garbanzo beans
- Curry Paste, but go low on the heat
- 1 cup sliced tomato
- 2 cups kale leaves
- 1/2 cup coconut milk

Instructions

Put ingredients in the slow cooker. Cover, and cook on low for 7 to 9 hours.

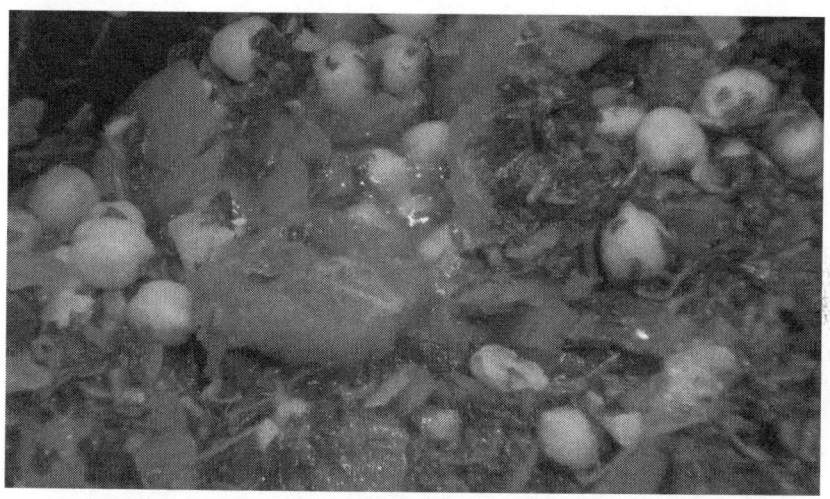

Mexican Veal

Serves 8

Ingredients - Allergies: SF, GF, DF, EF, NF

- 2 cups sliced carrot
- 2 cups chopped onions
- Salt, 1 Tsp. ground chili powder and 2 Tbsp. cumin seeds
- 1/2 cup tomato paste
- 2 cups beef broth
- 2 minced garlic cloves
- 2 tbsp. chili sauce
- 1/4 cup chopped mild green chiles
- 4 pounds veal, cubed

Instructions

Put ingredients in the slow cooker. Cover, and cook on low for 7 to 9 hours.

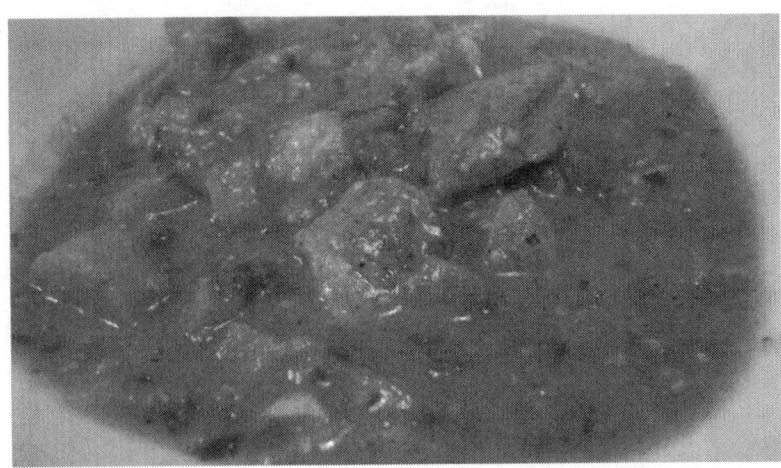

Okra Pork Spinach Stew

Serves 8

Ingredients - Allergies: SF, GF, DF, EF, NF

- 4 cups okra
- 1 cup sliced carrot
- 2 cups chopped onions
- Salt, 1 Tsp. ground pepper
- 1 cup sliced tomatoes
- 3 cups spinach
- 1 cup tomato paste
- 2 cups beef broth
- 1/2 cup chopped parsley
- 2 pounds pork neck meat, cubed

Instructions

Put ingredients in the slow cooker. Cover, and cook on low for 7 to 9 hours.

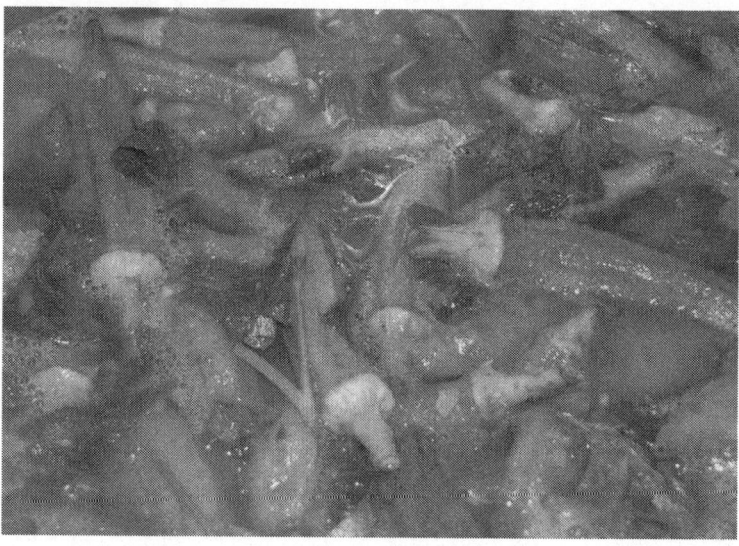

Red Curry

Serves 8

Ingredients - Allergies: SF, GF, DF, EF, NF

- 4 pounds chicken meat
- Curry Paste, but go low on the heat
- 1 cup tomato paste
- 1 Tbsp. palm sugar (optional)
- 1/4 cup Thai basil leaves
- 1 cup sliced tomato
- 1 cup coconut milk
- Cilantro or parsley for garnishing

Instructions

Put ingredients in the slow cooker. Cover, and cook on low for 7 to 9 hours.

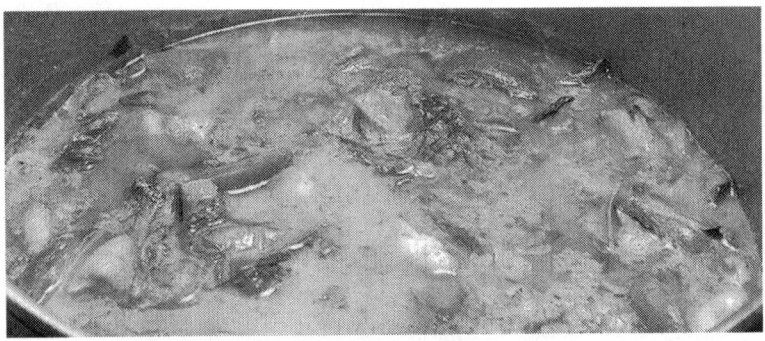

Shrimp & Green Peas
Serves 8

Ingredients - Allergies: SF, GF, DF, EF, NF

- 2 cups green peas
- 1 cup sliced carrot
- 2 cups chopped onions
- Salt & 1 Tsp. ground pepper to taste
- 1/2 cup tomato paste
- 1 cup fish broth
- 4 pounds shrimp

Instructions

Put ingredients in the slow cooker. Cover, and cook on low for 5 to 6 hours.

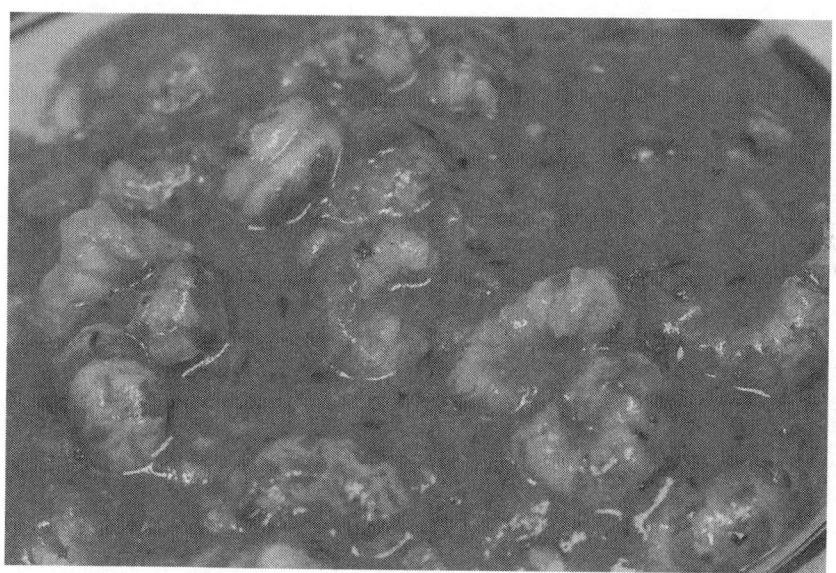

Shrimp & Peppers

Serves 8

Ingredients - Allergies: SF, GF, DF, EF, NF

- 2 cups sliced red peppers
- 1 cup sliced carrot
- 2 cups chopped onions
- Salt & 1 Tsp. ground pepper to taste
- 1 cup sliced green peppers
- 1/2 cup tomato paste
- 1 cup fish broth
- 4 pounds shrimp

Instructions

Put ingredients in the slow cooker. Cover, and cook on low for 5 to 6 hours.

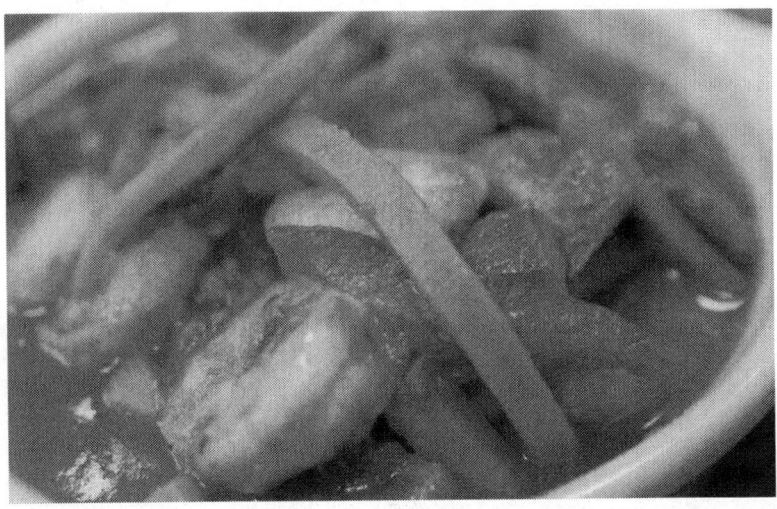

BBQ Pork Ribs

Serves 8

Ingredients - Allergies: SF, GF, DF, EF, NF

- 1-1/2 cups tomato paste
- 1/4 cup lemon juice
- 2 tbsp. mustard
- 1/2 tsp. salt
- 1/4 tsp. ground black pepper
- 1/2 tsp. minced garlic
- Salt, 1 Tsp. ground cayenne pepper and 1 Tbsp. cumin seeds
- 4 pounds pork ribs

Instructions

Put ingredients in the slow cooker. Cover, and cook on low for 7 to 9 hours. Serve with coleslaw.

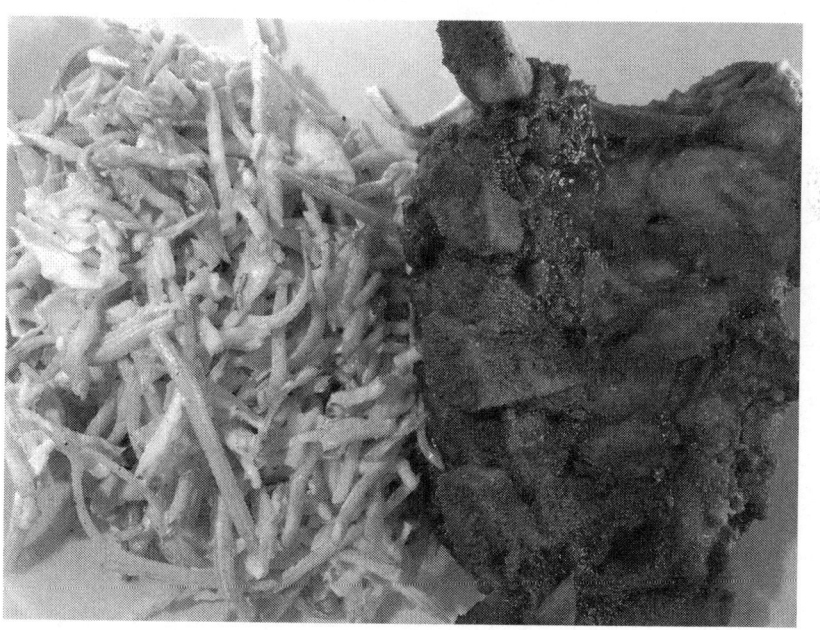

Pork Shoulder Stew

Serves 8

Ingredients - Allergies: SF, GF, DF, EF, NF

- 1 cup sliced red peppers
- 1 cup sliced carrot
- 2 cups sliced leeks
- Salt & 1 Tsp. ground pepper to taste
- 1 Tbsp. cumin seeds & 3 bay leaves
- 2 cups beef broth
- 3 garlic cloves, minced
- 1 cup beef broth
- 4 pounds pork shoulder

Instructions

Put ingredients in the slow cooker. Cover, and cook on low for 7 to 9 hours.

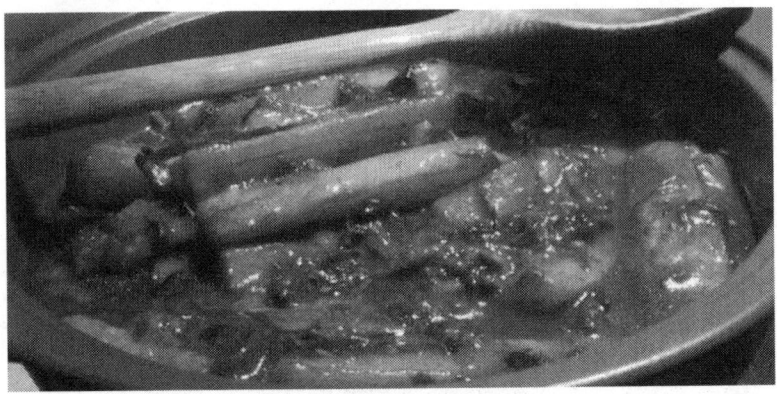

Fish, Onion & Fennel Stew

Serves 8

Ingredients - Allergies: SF, GF, DF, EF, NF

- 1 cup sliced yellow peppers
- 1 cup sliced carrot
- 2 cups chopped onions
- Salt & 1 Tsp. ground pepper to taste
- 2 cups sliced fennel bulb
- 1/2 cup tomato paste
- 1 cup fish broth
- 4 pounds local fish

Instructions

Put ingredients in the slow cooker. Cover, and cook on low for 6 hours.

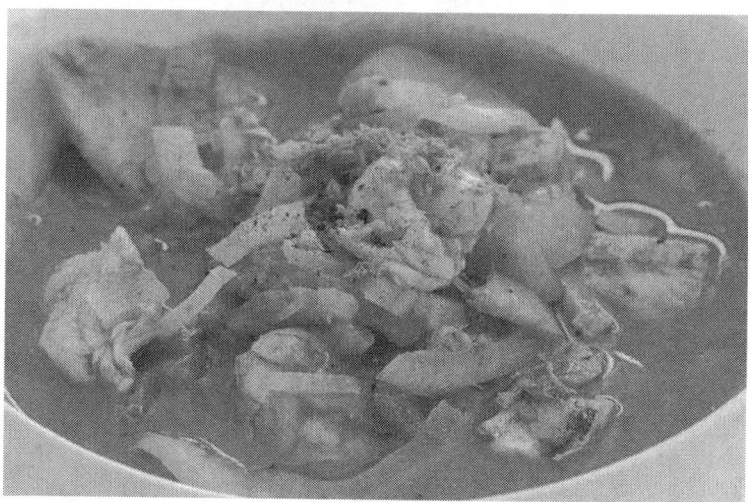

Kale & Shiitake Stew

Serves 8

Ingredients - Allergies: SF, GF, DF, EF, NF

- 3 garlic cloves, minced
- 2 cups chopped onions
- 1/2 cup olive oil
- Salt & 1 Tsp. ground pepper to taste
- 4 cups vegetable broth
- 2 pounds dry shiitake mushrooms

Instructions

Put ingredients in the slow cooker. Cover, and cook on low for 3 to 4 hours.

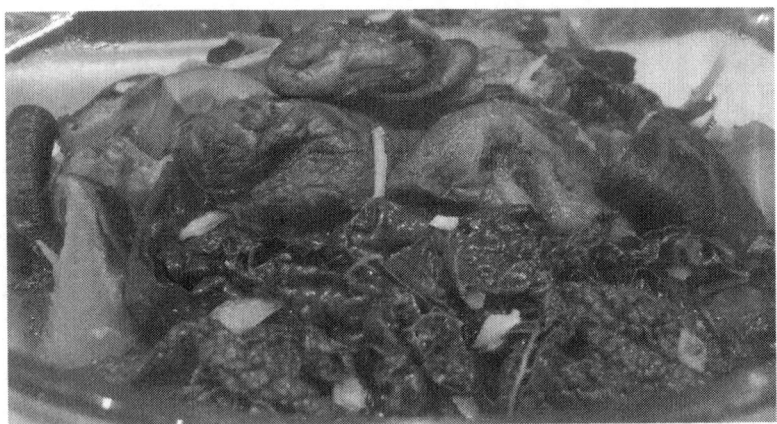

Kale & Chicken Stew

Serves 8

Ingredients - Allergies: SF, GF, DF, EF, NF

- 1 cup sliced leeks
- 1 sliced carrot
- 1 cup chopped onions
- Salt & 1 Tsp. ground pepper to taste
- 2 cups chicken broth
- 3 cups kale
- 4 pounds chicken

Instructions

Put ingredients in the slow cooker. Cover, and cook on low for 7 to 9 hours.

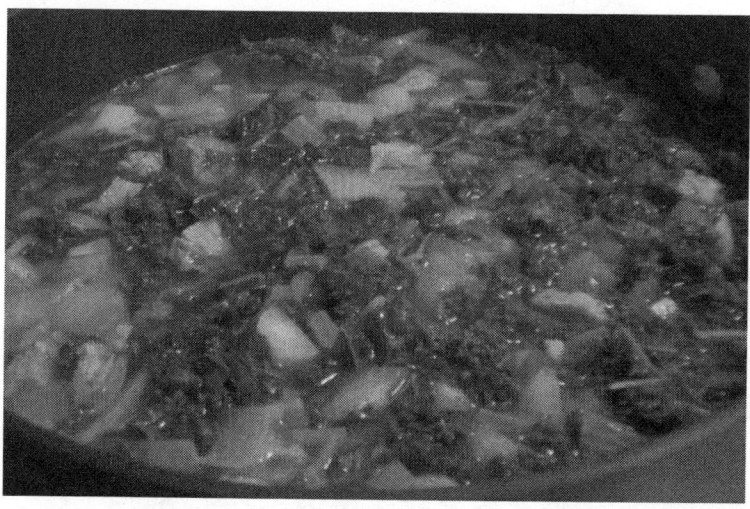

Mackerel & Bamboo Shoots Stew

Serves 8

Ingredients - Allergies: SF, GF, DF, EF, NF

- 2 cups sliced bamboo shoots
- 2 cup sliced carrot
- 1 cup chopped onions
- Salt & 1 Tsp. ground pepper to taste
- 1/2 cup tomato paste
- 2 cup fish broth
- 1/2 cup chopped green onions for sprinkling
- 4 pounds mackerel

Instructions

Put ingredients in the slow cooker. Cover, and cook on low for 5 to 6 hours.

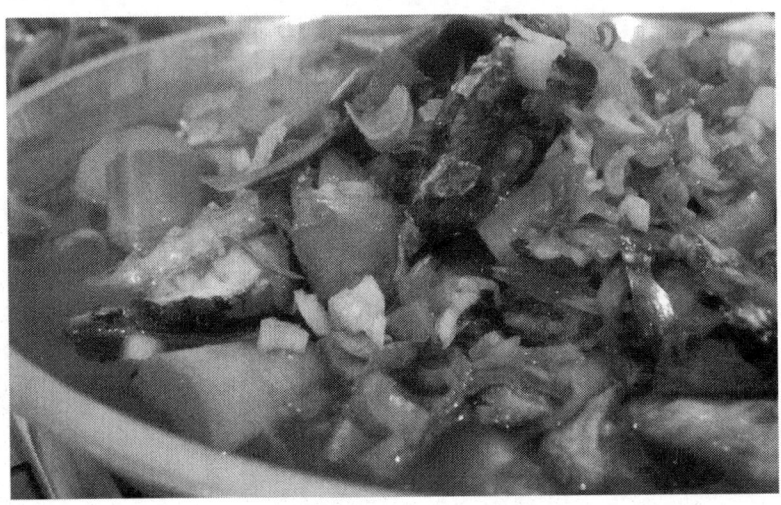

Korean Spicy Fish Soup – Mae Un Tang

Serves 8

Ingredients - Allergies: SF, GF, DF, EF, NF

- 2 cups sliced daikon (radish)
- 3 garlic cloves, minced
- 1 cup sliced green onions
- Salt & 1 Tsp. ground pepper to taste
- 1 Tbsp. chopped ginger
- 2 Tbsp. red pepper flakes (to taste)
- 1 cup tomato paste
- 6 cups water
- 4 pounds local fish (pieces)

Instructions

Put ingredients in the slow cooker. Cover, and cook on low for 5 to 6 hours.

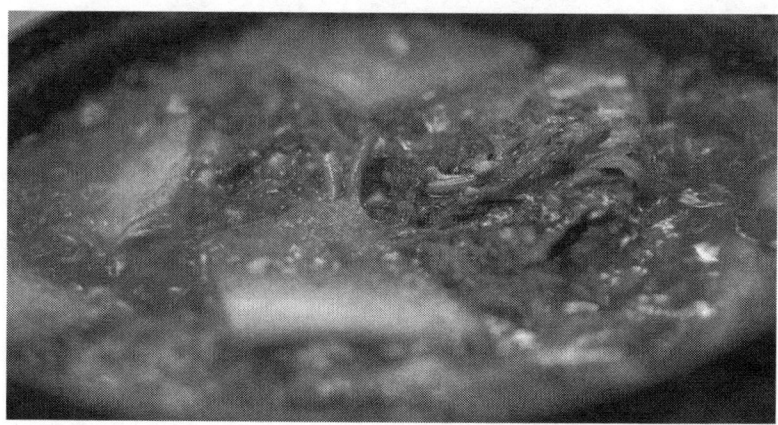

Mushrooms & Pork Ribs Stew

Serves 8

Ingredients - Allergies: SF, GF, DF, EF, NF

- 2 cups sliced bok choy
- 2 cups sliced mushrooms
- 2 cups chopped onions
- Salt & 1 Tsp. ground pepper to taste
- 2 cups beef broth
- 4 pounds pork ribs

Instructions

Put ingredients in the slow cooker. Cover, and cook on low for 7 to 9 hours.

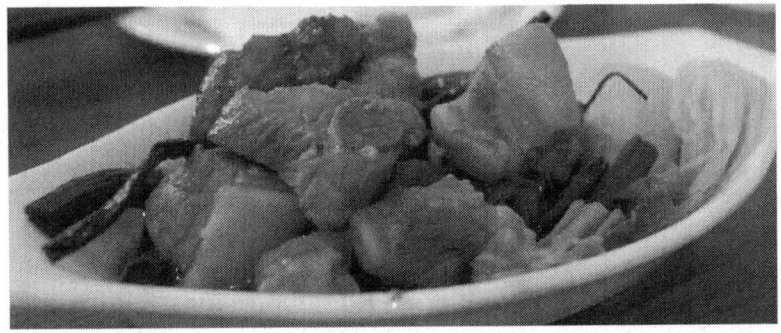

Olives Jambalaya

Serves 8

Ingredients - Allergies: SF, GF, DF, EF, NF

- 1 cup chopped onions & 2 minced garlic cloves
- 2 tbsp. coconut oil & 1 tsp. turmeric
- Salt, ground black pepper to taste
- 3 pounds cubed chicken & 1 pound shrimp
- 1 tsp. dried red pepper flakes (to taste).
- 3 cups kale & 1 cup mushrooms
- 1 cup tomato paste & 1 cup chicken broth
- 2 cups Kalamata olives & 1 cup chopped carrot

Instructions

Put ingredients in the slow cooker. Cover, and cook on low for 7 to 9 hours.

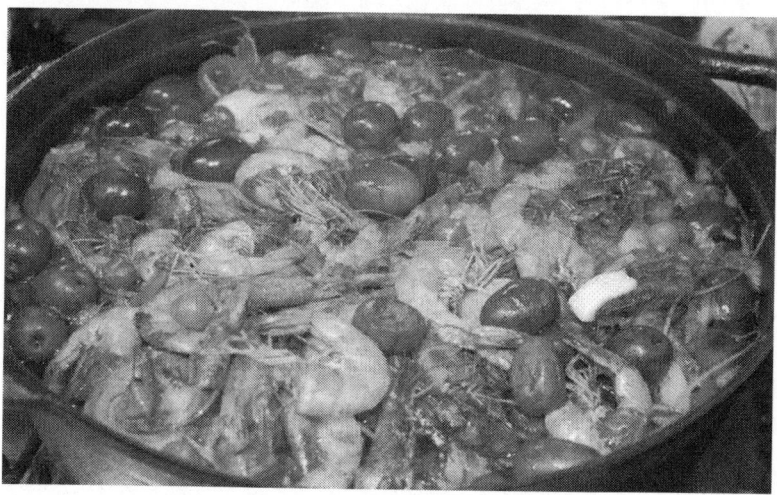

Pork & Cauliflower Stew

Serves 8

Ingredients - Allergies: SF, GF, DF, EF, NF

- 3 cups sliced cauliflower
- 1 cup sliced carrot
- 2 cups chopped onions
- Salt & 1 Tsp. ground pepper to taste
- 2 cups beef broth
- 4 pounds pork shoulder

Instructions

Put ingredients in the slow cooker. Cover, and cook on low for 7 to 9 hours.

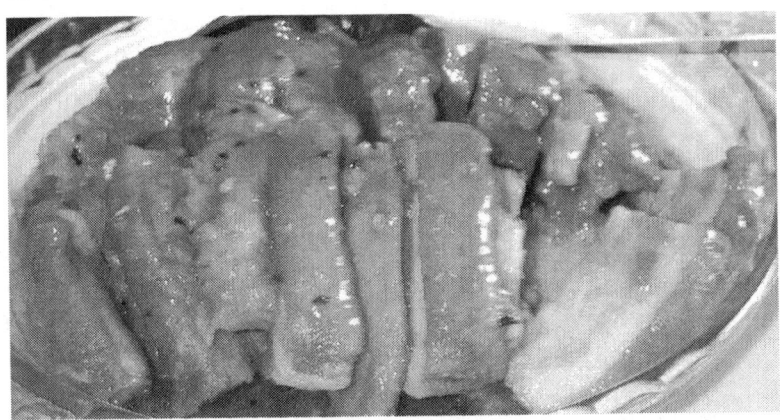

Shui Zhu Yu - Sichuan Fish Stew
Serves 8

Ingredients - Allergies: SF, GF, DF, EF, NF

- 2 cups dried shiitake
- 2 Tbsp. coconut oil
- 1 cup Chinese celery
- 1 Tsp. ground white pepper
- 12 dried chili red peppers (or more, to taste)
- Fish sauce or salt to taste & 1 Tsp. Sichuan peppercorns
- 1 cup sliced green onions
- 2 Tbsp. minced ginger & 5 garlic cloves, minced
- 6 cups water
- 4 pounds local fish

Instructions

Put ingredients in the slow cooker. Cover, and cook on low for 5 to 6 hours.

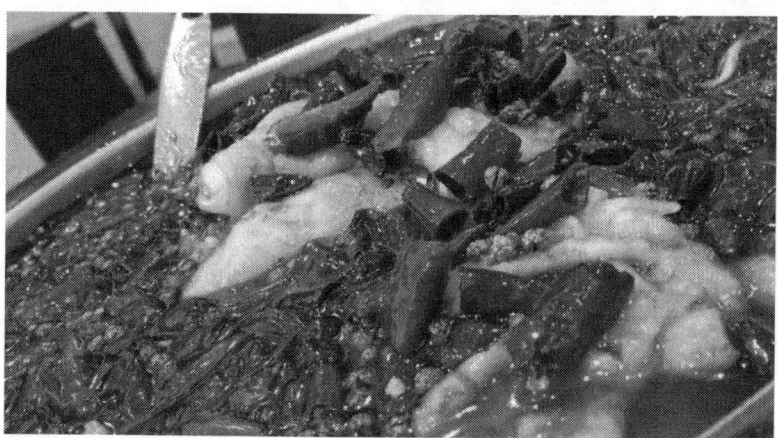

Haleem – Beef & Lentils Stew

Serves 8

Ingredients - Allergies: SF, GF, DF, EF, NF

- 3 cups dry brown lentils
- 2 cups chopped onions & 2 garlic cloves, minced
- Salt & 1 Tsp. ground pepper to taste
- 3 cups water
- 1/4 cup green chillies (to taste) & 1 Tbsp. minced ginger
- ¼ tsp. fenugreek seed, coriander, turmeric & cumin each
- 2 pounds cubed beef (or mutton)
- 1 Tbsp. cilantro leaves

Instructions

Put all ingredients except cilantro in the slow cooker. Cover, and cook on low for 7 to 9 hours. Sprinkle with cilantro and serve.

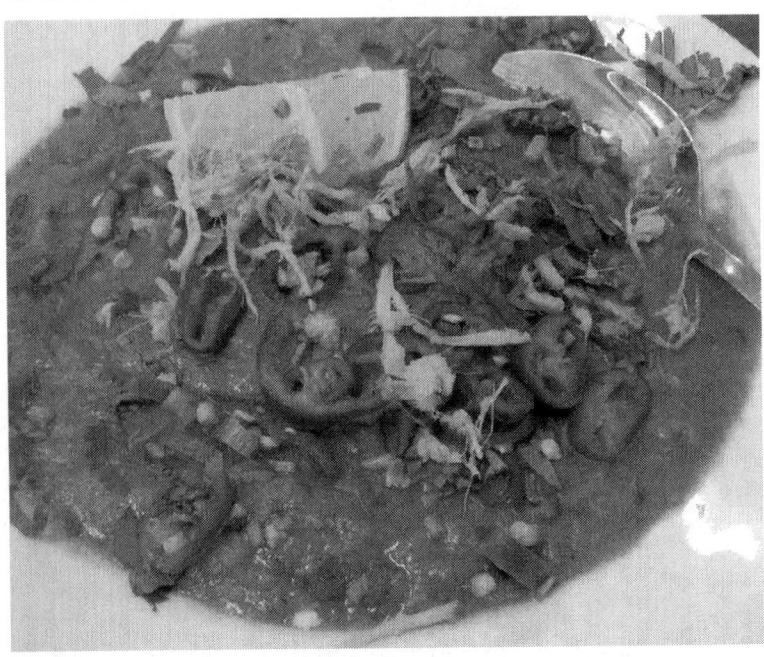

Hong Shao Rou Pork Stew

Serves 8

Ingredients - Allergies: SF, GF, DF, EF, NF

- 3 cups sliced leeks
- 1 cup sliced carrot
- 1 cup chopped green onion
- 1 Tbsp. minced ginger
- Salt & 1 Tsp. ground pepper to taste
- 1 cup beef broth
- 1 cup red cooking wine
- 2 Tbsp. fish sauce
- 4 pounds pork belly, cubed

Instructions

Put all ingredients except green onions in the slow cooker. Cover, and cook on low for 7 to 9 hours. Sprinkle with green onions.

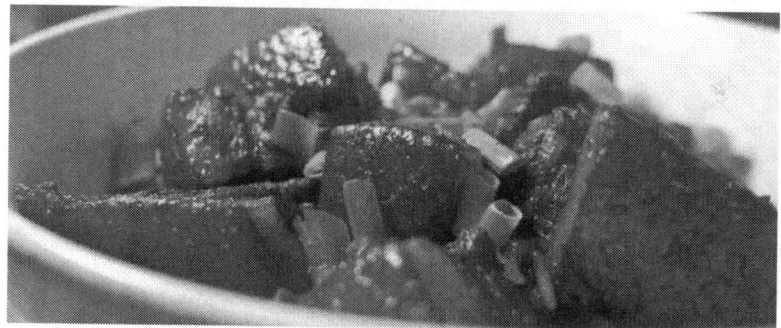

Pork Jambalaya

Serves 8

Ingredients - Allergies: SF, GF, DF, EF, NF

- 2 cups diced celery
- 1 cup sliced carrot
- 2 cups chopped onions & 2 cloves minced garlic
- 2 cup sliced mushrooms
- Salt & 1 Tsp. ground pepper to taste
- 2 cups beef broth & 1 cup tomato paste
- 1 Tsp. red pepper flakes &
- 4 pounds pork shoulder

Instructions

Put ingredients in the slow cooker. Cover, and cook on low for 7 to 9 hours.

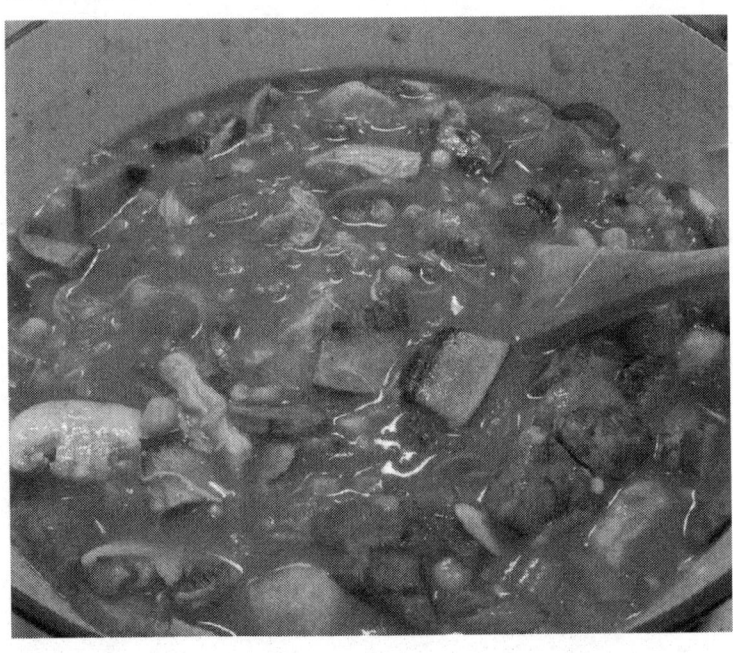

Khoresht – Green Peas Stew
Serves 8

Ingredients - Allergies: SF, GF, DF, EF, NF

- 2 cups green peas
- 1 sliced eggplant
- 1 tsp. turmeric, cumin, cardamom each
- 2 cups chopped onions
- Salt & 1 Tsp. ground pepper to taste
- 1 cup chicken broth & 1 cup tomato paste
- 3 pounds chicken breast meat

Instructions

Put ingredients in the slow cooker. Cover, and cook on low for 7 to 9 hours.

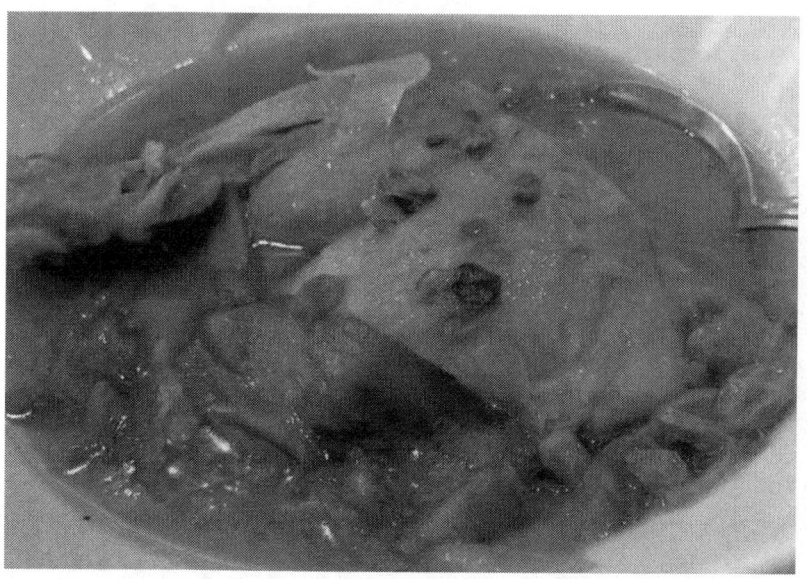

Kimchee Jjiagae – Kimchee Stew

Serves 8

Ingredients - Allergies: SF, GF, DF, EF, NF

- 3 cups kimchee
- 1/2 cup green peas
- 1/2 cup sliced green onions
- 1 cup chopped onions
- 1 Tbsp. dried kelp
- 1/2 cup sliced radish
- Salt & 1 Tsp. ground pepper to taste
- 1 cup beef broth & 1 cup Tomato paste
- 1 tsp. red pepper flakes (to taste)
- 3 pounds pork shoulder

Instructions

Put ingredients in the slow cooker. Cover, and cook on low for 7 to 9 hours.

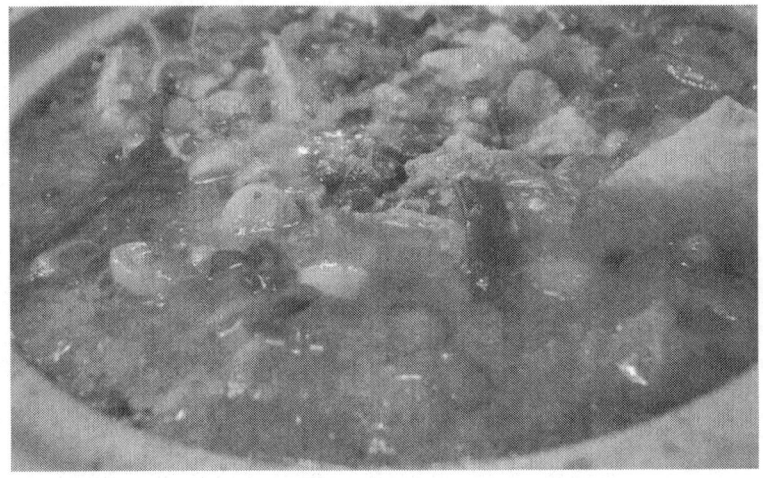

Locro Argentine Stew
Serves 8

Ingredients - Allergies: SF, GF, DF, EF, NF
- 1 cup dry, broken hominy
- 1 cup dry white beans
- 2 cups sliced red peppers
- 2 cups chopped onions & 2 garlic cloves, minced
- Salt & 1 Tsp. ground pepper to taste
- 2 cups beef broth
- 1 Tsp. cumin
- 2 pounds Osso buco, cubed

Instructions

Put ingredients in the slow cooker. Cover, and cook on low for 7 to 9 hours.

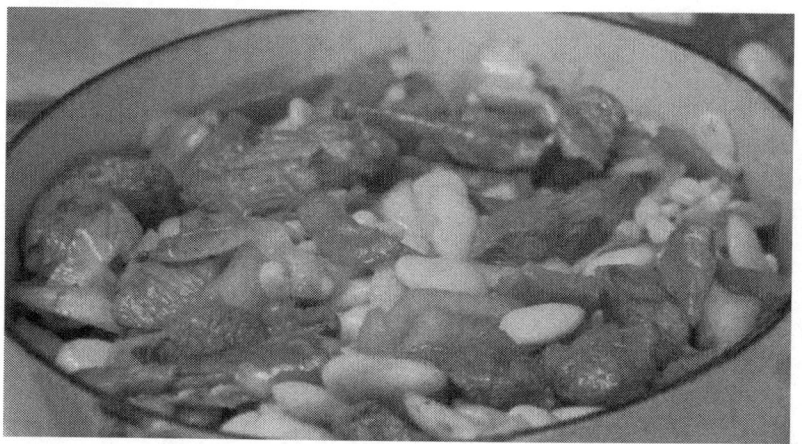

Mixed Fish Stew

Serves 8

Ingredients - Allergies: SF, GF, DF, EF, NF

- 2 cups sliced red peppers
- 1 cup sliced celery
- 1 cup shredded carrot
- 1/2 cup white wine (optional)
- 2 cups chopped leeks
- Salt & 1 Tsp. ground pepper to taste
- 3 cups fish broth
- 4 pounds fish steaks, mixed (e.g. salmon, cod etc.)

Instructions

Put ingredients in the slow cooker. Cover, and cook on low for 7 to 9 hours.

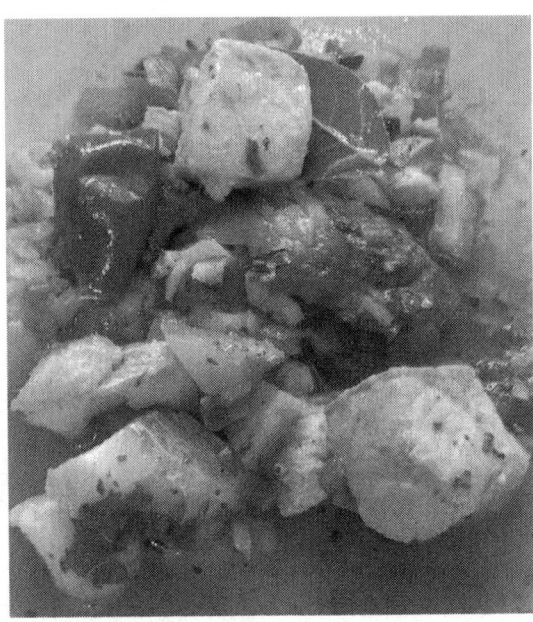

Onion, Leeks & Chicken Breast Stew
Serves 8

Ingredients - Allergies: SF, GF, DF, EF, NF

- 2 cups sliced leeks
- 1 cup shredded carrot
- 2 large onions, sliced in rings
- Salt & 1 Tsp. ground pepper to taste
- 2 cups chicken broth & ½ cup tomato paste
- 4 pounds chicken breast meat

Instructions

Put ingredients in the slow cooker. Cover, and cook on low for 7 to 9 hours.

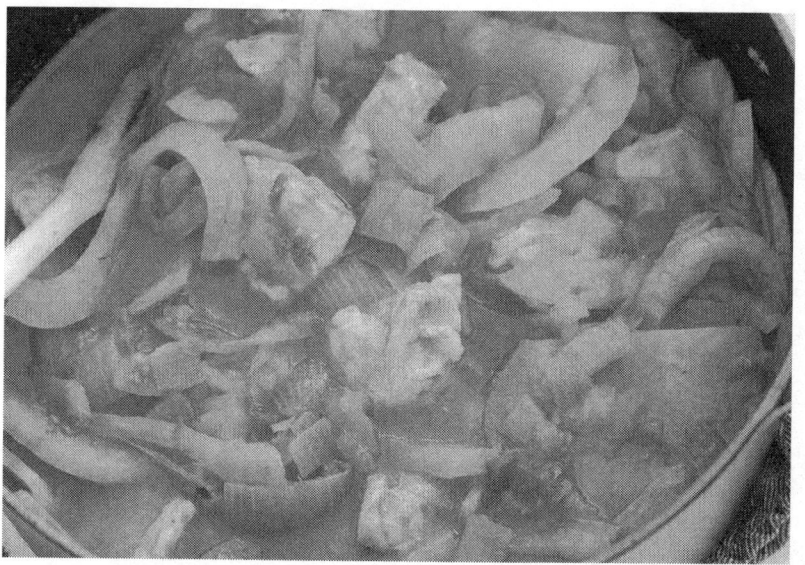

Pork & Onion Stew

Serves 8

Ingredients - Allergies: SF, GF, DF, EF, NF

- 2 cups sliced red onions
- 1 cup sliced carrot
- 2 cups chopped leeks
- Salt & 1 Tsp. ground pepper to taste
- 1 cup beef broth
- 4 pounds pork shoulder

Instructions

Put ingredients in the slow cooker. Cover, and cook on low for 7 to 9 hours.

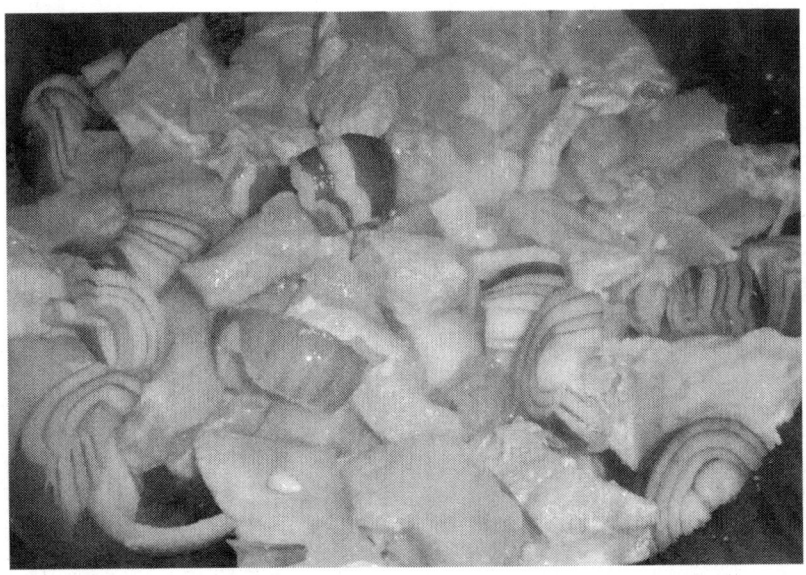

Shrimp Gumbo Stew
Serves 8

Ingredients - Allergies: SF, GF, DF, EF, NF

- 1 cup chopped celery
- 1 cup sliced red peppers
- 1 cup sliced carrot
- 2 cups chopped onions
- Salt & 1 Tsp. ground pepper to taste
- 2 cups fish broth & 1 cup tomato paste
- 1 pound cubed chicken
- 3 pounds shrimp

Instructions

Put ingredients in the slow cooker. Cover, and cook on low for 7 to 9 hours.

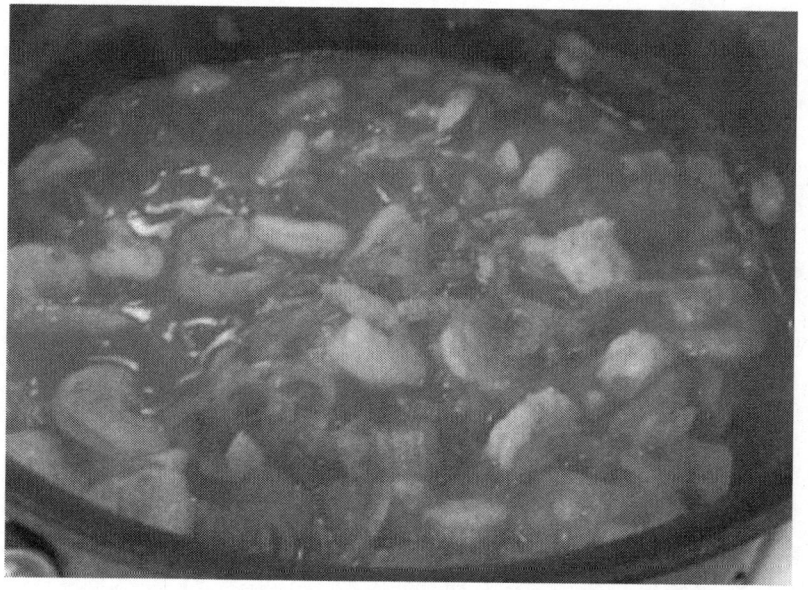

Cholent – Jewish Brisket & Beans Stew
Serves 8

Ingredients - Allergies: SF, GF, DF, EF, NF

- 2 cups diced celery
- 1 cup sliced carrot
- 2 cups chopped onions & 2 cloves minced garlic
- 1 cup dried butter beans
- 1 cup dried kidney beans
- Salt & 1 Tsp. ground pepper to taste
- 3 cups water or beef broth
- 1 Tsp. red pepper flakes (to taste)
- 3 pounds beef brisket, cubed

Instructions

Put ingredients in the slow cooker. Cover, and cook on low for 7 to 9 hours.

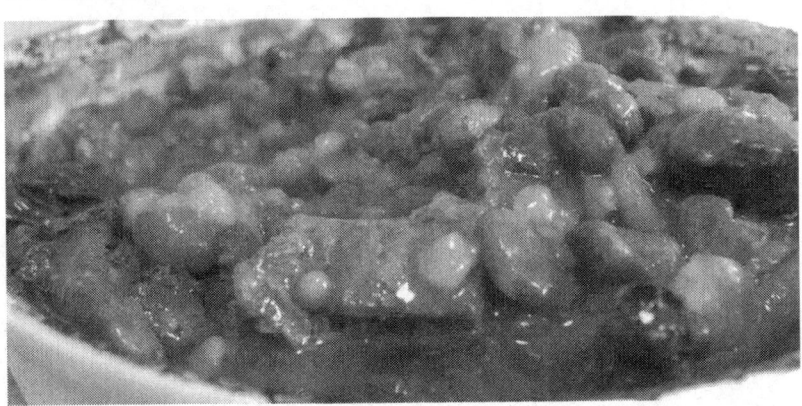

Beef Daube Stew

Serves 8

Ingredients - Allergies: SF, GF, DF, EF, NF

- 1 cup mushrooms & 1 rosemary spring
- 1 cup sliced carrot & 4 thyme sprigs
- 2 cups chopped onions & 2 cloves minced garlic
- Salt & 1 Tsp. ground pepper to taste
- 1 cup beef broth & 1 cup tomato paste
- 1 Tsp. red pepper flakes &
- 4 pounds beef chuck, cubed

Instructions

Put ingredients in the slow cooker. Cover, and cook on low for 7 to 9 hours.

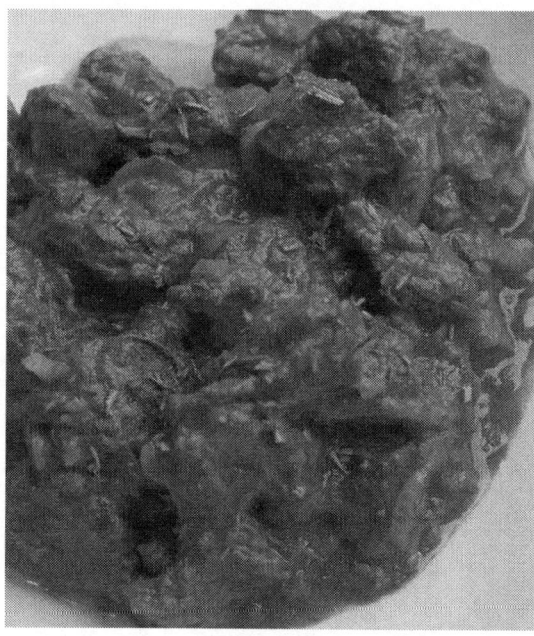

Dinuguan – Filipino Stew

Serves 8

Ingredients - Allergies: SF, GF, DF, EF, NF

- 1 cup sliced green peppers
- 1 cup sliced carrot
- 2 cups chopped onions & 2 cloves minced garlic
- ½ cup vinegar
- Salt & 1 Tsp. ground pepper to taste
- 2 cups beef broth or water
- 1 Tbsp. minced ginger
- 2 pounds pork shoulder, cubed
- 1 pound pork liver, cubed
- 1 pound pork kidney (optionally swap with liver or pork shoulder)

Instructions

Put ingredients in the slow cooker. Cover, and cook on low for 7 to 9 hours.

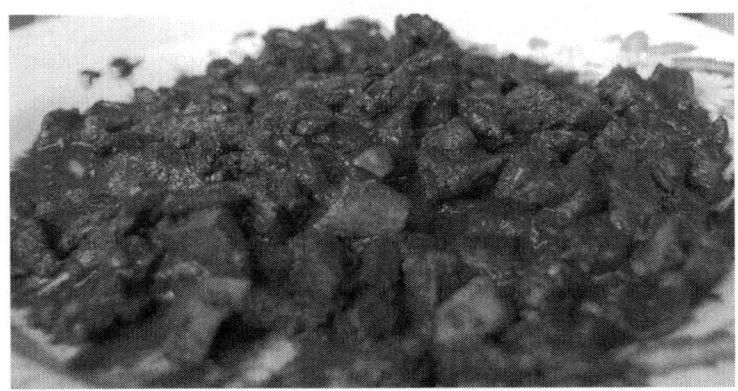

Fabada Asturiana – Spanish Pork Belly & Beans Stew

Serves 8

Ingredients - Allergies: SF, GF, DF, EF, NF

- 2 cups chopped onions & 2 cloves minced garlic
- 2 cup dried butter beans
- Salt & 1 Tsp. ground pepper to taste
- 2 cups beef broth
- 1 cup kale
- 1/2 Tsp. saffron
- 4 pounds pork belly, cubed

Instructions

Put ingredients in the slow cooker. Cover, and cook on low for 7 to 9 hours.

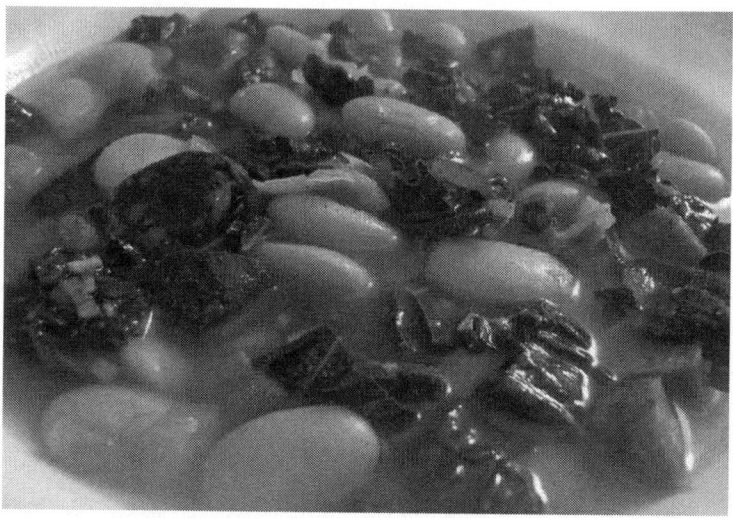

Ghormeh Sabzi – Persian Stew

Serves 8

Ingredients - Allergies: SF, GF, DF, EF, NF

- 2 cups spinach or kale
- 1 cup sliced green onions
- 1 cup chopped onions & 2 cloves minced garlic
- 1 tbsp. minced ginger
- Salt & 1 Tsp. ground pepper to taste
- 2 cups beef broth
- 1/2 cup lemon juice
- 1 Tsp. turmeric
- 1 cup cilantro
- 1 cup parsley
- 4 pounds lamb or beef stewing meat

Instructions

Put ingredients in the slow cooker. Cover, and cook on low for 7 to 9 hours.

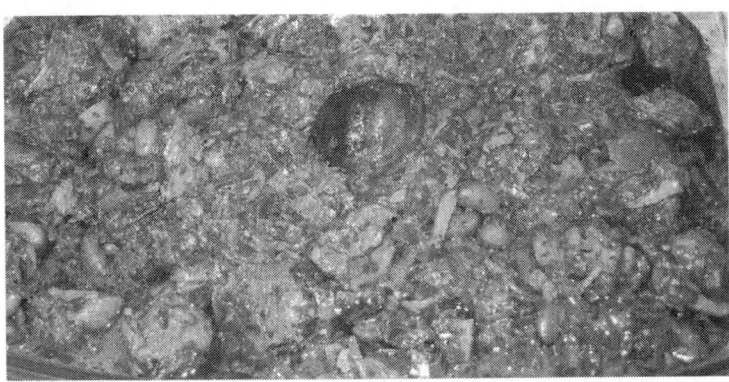

Goulash – Spicy Beef Stew
Serves 8

Ingredients - Allergies: SF, GF, DF, EF, NF

- 2 cups diced celery
- 1 cup shredded carrot
- 2 cups chopped onions & 2 cloves minced garlic
- 2 Tbsp. sweet paprika
- Salt & 1 Tsp. ground pepper to taste
- 2 cups beef broth & 1 cup tomato paste
- 1 Tsp. red pepper flakes
- 4 pounds beef stew meat
- 1 Tbsp. chopped parsley

Instructions

Put ingredients in the slow cooker. Cover, and cook on low for 7 to 9 hours. Sprinkle with parsley.

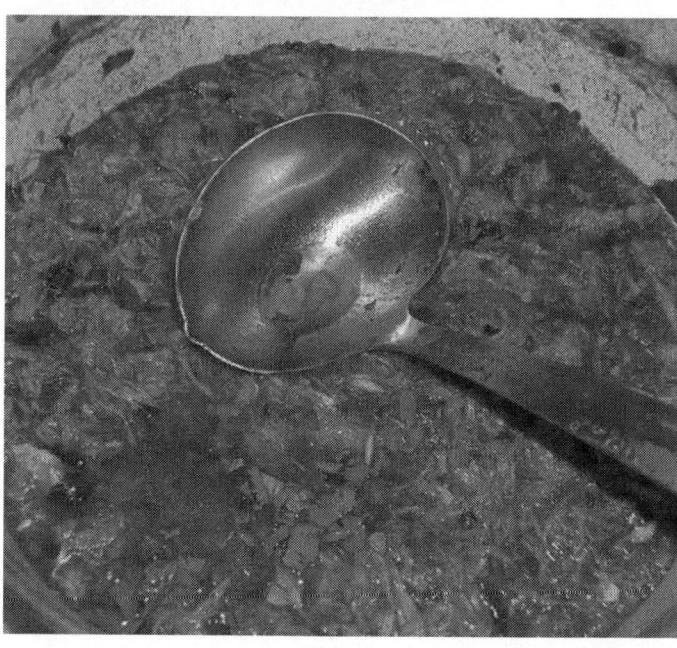

Letscho Chicken

Serves 8

Ingredients - Allergies: SF, GF, DF, EF, NF

- 2 cups sliced green peppers
- 2 cups chopped onions & 2 cloves minced garlic
- 2 cup sliced red peppers
- Salt & 1 Tsp. ground pepper to taste
- 3 tomatoes, sliced
- 1 Tsp. red pepper flakes
- 2 Tbsp. sweet paprika
- 1 cup green beans
- 4 pounds chicken meat, cubed

Instructions

Put ingredients in the slow cooker. Cover, and cook on low for 7 to 9 hours.

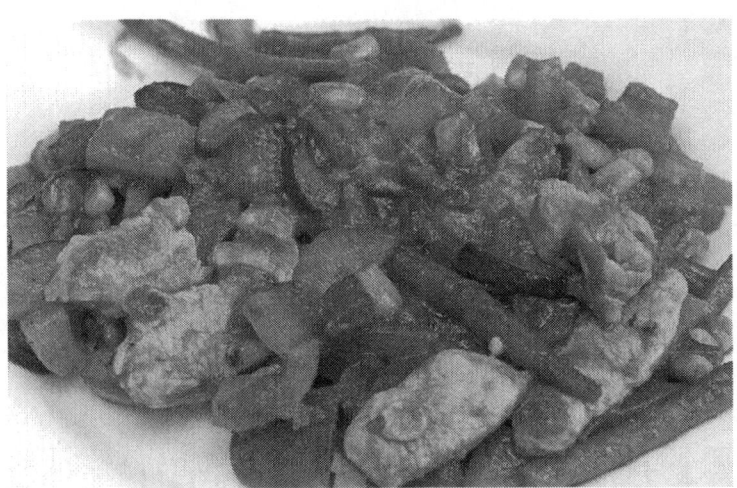

Narial Murgh Shorba Stew

Serves 8

Ingredients - Allergies: SF, GF, DF, EF, NF

- 1 cup diced celery
- 1 cup curry paste (see recipe at the beginning of the book)
- 2 cup chopped onions & 2 cloves minced garlic
- 2 cup sliced mushrooms
- Salt & 1 Tsp. ground pepper to taste
- 4 cups water
- 4 pounds chicken meat

Instructions

Put ingredients in the slow cooker. Cover, and cook on low for 7 to 9 hours.

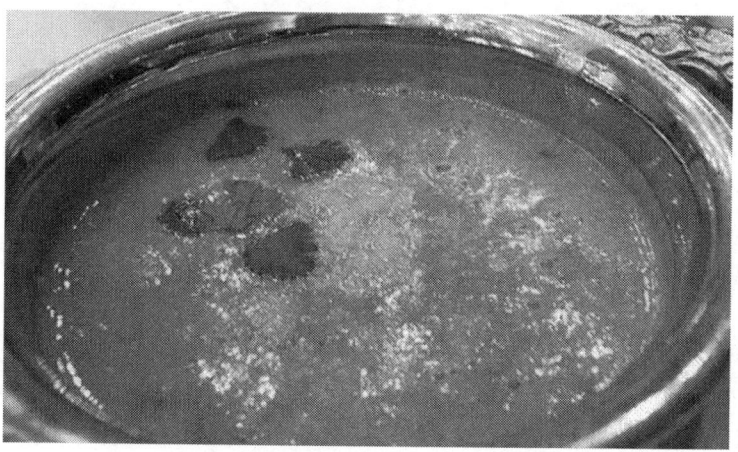

Stir Fries

Pork and Bok Choy / Celery Stir Fry

Serves 1 - Allergies: SF, GF, DF, EF, NF

5 oz. Lean Pork Tenderloin and Bok Choy / Celery stir fry. Use as much veggies as you want or replace Bok Choy with Kale. Season with fish sauce.

Nutrition Facts

Serving Size 574 g

Amount Per Serving

Calories 316 — Calories from Fat 39

	% Daily Value*
Total Fat 4.3g	**7%**
Saturated Fat 1.1g	**6%**
Trans Fat 0.0g	
Cholesterol 82mg	**27%**
Sodium 1156mg	**48%**
Potassium 1314mg	**38%**
Total Carbohydrates 34.6g	**12%**
Dietary Fiber 8.8g	**35%**
Sugars 8.8g	
Protein 34.5g	

Vitamin A 33%	•	Vitamin C 81%
Calcium 9%	•	Iron 30%

Nutrition Grade A

* Based on a 2000 calorie diet

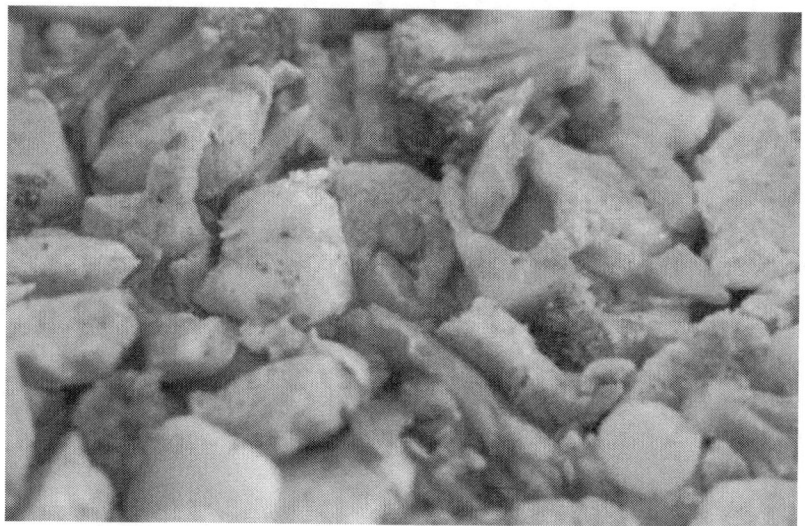

Lemon Chicken Stir Fry

Serves 3-4

Ingredients - Allergies: SF, GF, DF, EF, NF

- 1 lemon
- 1/2 cup chicken broth
- 3 tbsp. fish sauce
- 2 teaspoons arrowroot flour
- 1 tbsp. coconut oil
- 1 pound boneless, skinless cubed chicken breasts
- 10 ounces mushrooms, halved or quartered
- 2 cups snow peas, stems and strings removed
- 1 bunch scallions, cut into 1-inch pieces, white and green parts divided
- 1 tbsp. chopped garlic

Instructions

Grate 1 tsp. lemon zest. Juice the lemon and mix 3 tbsp. of the juice with broth, fish sauce and arrowroot flour in a small bowl.

Heat oil in a skillet over high heat. Add chicken and cook, stirring occasionally, until just cooked through. Transfer to a plate. Add mushrooms to the pan and cook until the mushrooms are tender. Add snow peas, garlic, scallion whites and the lemon zest. Cook, stirring, around 30 seconds. Add the broth to the pan and cook, stirring, 2 to 3 minutes. Add scallion greens and the chicken and any accumulated juices and stir.

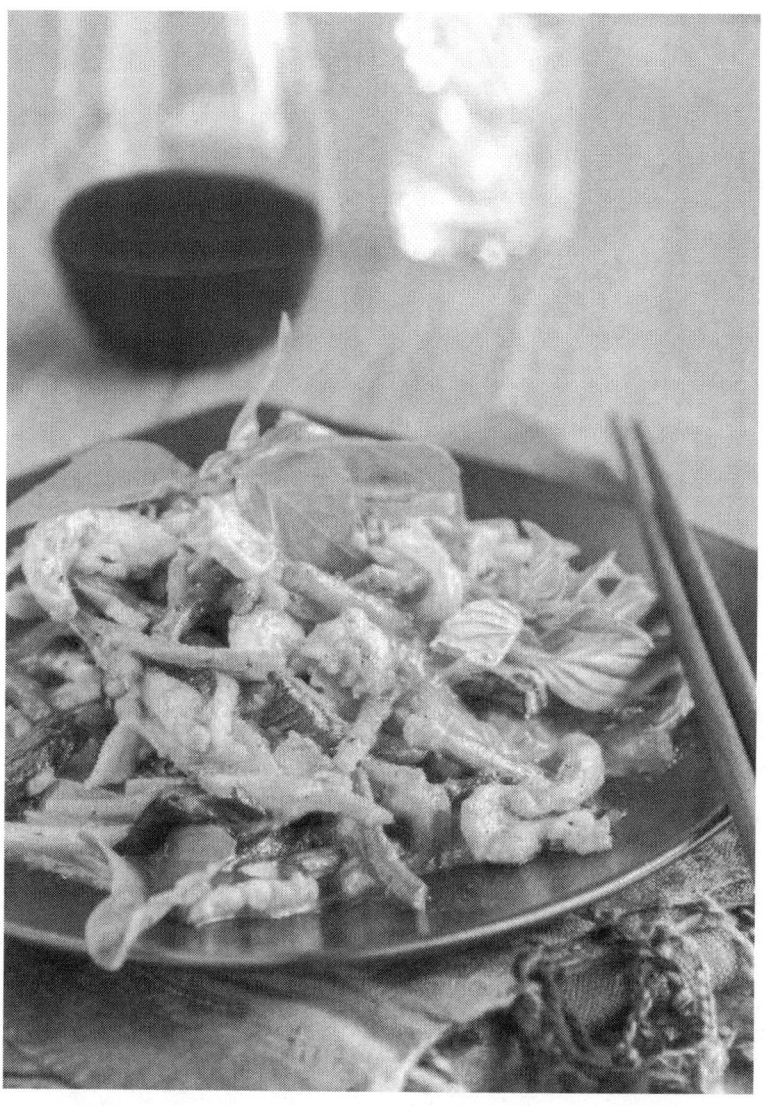

Pan seared Brussels sprouts

Serves 2

Ingredients - Allergies: SF, GF, DF, EF, NF

- 6 oz. cubed pork
- 2 tbsp. coconut oil
- 1 pound Brussels sprouts, halved
- 1/2 large onion, chopped
- Salt and ground black pepper

Instructions

Cook pork in a skillet over high heat. Remove to a plate and chop. In same pan with pork fat, add coconut oil over high heat. Add onions and Brussels sprouts and cook, stirring occasionally, until sprouts are golden brown. Season with salt and pepper, to taste, and put pork back into pan. Serve immediately.

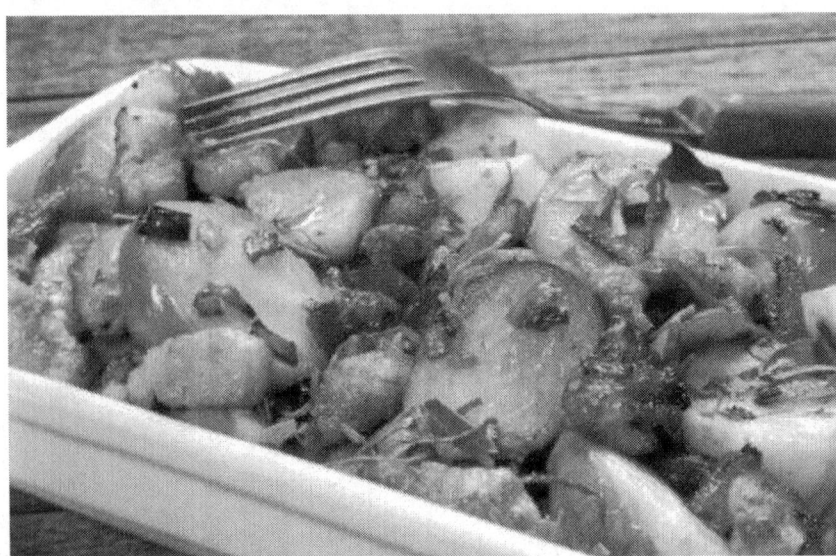

Beef and Broccoli Stir Fry

Serves 1 - Allergies: SF, GF, DF, EF, NF

- 5oz. of lean Beef and 1 cup broccoli stir fry. Use as much broccoli as you want or replace Broccoli with Kale.

Nutrition Facts

Serving Size 251 g

Amount Per Serving

Calories 342 — Calories from Fat 124

	% Daily Value*
Total Fat 13.8g	21%
Saturated Fat 4.0g	20%
Trans Fat 0.0g	
Cholesterol 127mg	42%
Sodium 1024mg	43%
Potassium 884mg	25%
Total Carbohydrates 7.0g	2%
Dietary Fiber 2.4g	10%
Sugars 1.7g	
Protein 46.5g	

Vitamin A 11% • Vitamin C 131%
Calcium 5% • Iron 154%

Nutrition Grade A-

* Based on a 2000 calorie diet

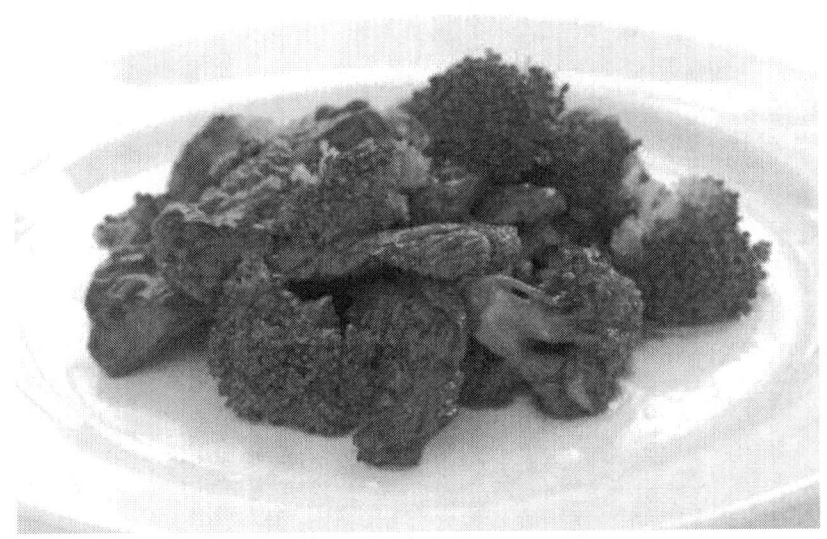

Garbanzo Stir Fry

Serves 2

Ingredients - Allergies: SF, GF, DF, EF, V, NF

- 2 tbsp. coconut oil
- 1 tbsp. oregano
- 1 tbsp. chopped basil
- 1 clove garlic, crushed
- ground black pepper according to taste
- 2 cups cooked garbanzo beans

- 1 large zucchini, halved and sliced
- 1/2 cup sliced mushrooms
- 1 tbsp. chopped cilantro
- 1 tomato, chopped

Heat oil in a skillet over medium heat. Stir in oregano, basil, garlic and pepper. Add the garbanzo beans and zucchini, stirring well to coat with oil and herbs. Cook for 10 minutes, stirring occasionally. Stir in mushrooms and cilantro; cook 10 minutes, stirring occasionally. Place the chopped tomato on top of the mixture to steam. Cover and cook 5 minutes more.

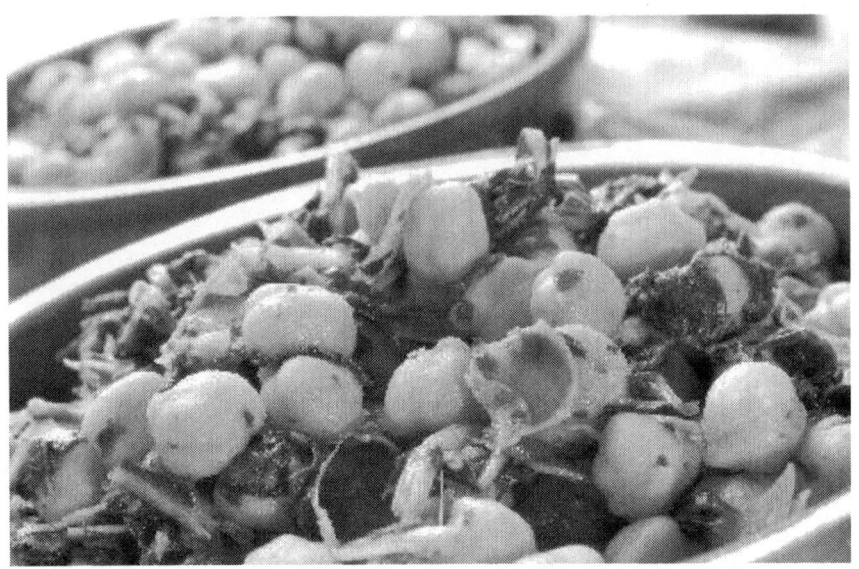

Thai Basil Chicken

Serves 1

Ingredients - Allergies: SF, GF, DF, NF

For the egg
- 1 egg
- 2 tbsp. of coconut oil for frying

Basil chicken
- 1 chicken breast (or any other cut of boneless chicken, about 200 grams)
- 5 cloves of garlic
- 4 Thai chilies
- 1 tbsp. coconut oil for frying
- Fish sauce
- 1 handful of Thai holy basil leaves

Instructions

First, fry the egg.

Basil chicken

Cut the chicken into small pieces. Peel the garlic and chilies, and chop them fine. Add basil leaves.

Add about 1 tbsp. of oil to the pan.

When the oil is hot, add the chilies and garlic. Stir fry for half a minute.

Toss in your chicken and keep stir frying. Add fish sauce.

Add basil into the pan, fold it into the chicken, and turn off the heat.

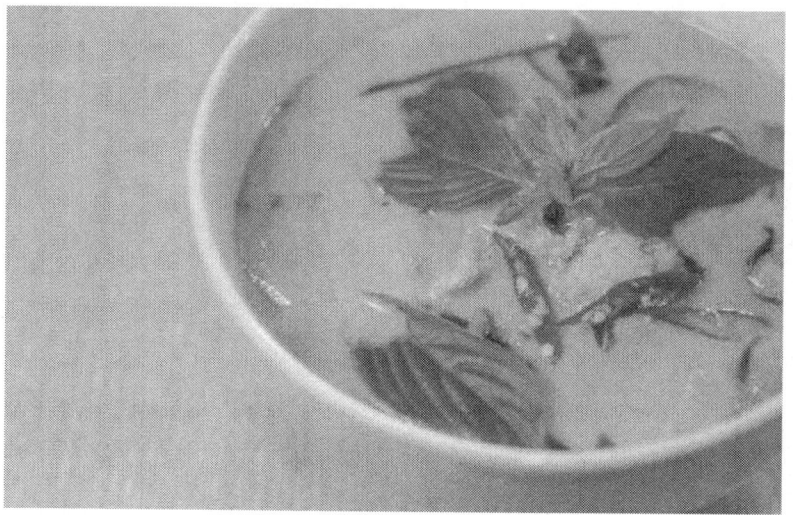

Shrimp with Snow Peas

Serves 4.

Ingredients - Allergies: SF, GF, DF, EF, NF

Marinade
- 2 teaspoons arrowroot flour
- 1 Tbsp wine
- 1/2 tsp. salt

Stir Fry
- 1 pound shrimp, peeled and deveined
- 2 Tbsp coconut oil
- 1 Tbsp minced ginger
- 3 garlic cloves, sliced thinly
- 1/2 pound snow peas, strings removed
- 2 teaspoons fish sauce
- 1/4 cup chicken broth
- 4 green onions, white and light green parts, sliced diagonally
- 2 teaspoons dark roasted sesame oil

Instructions

Mix all the ingredients for the marinade in a bowl and then add the shrimp. Mix to coat. Let it marinade 15 minutes while you prepare the peas, ginger, and garlic.

Add the coconut oil in the wok and let it get hot. Add the garlic and combine it with ginger. Stir-fry for about 30 seconds.

Add the marinade to the wok, add the snow peas, fish sauce and chicken broth. Stir-fry until the shrimp turns pink. Add the green onions and stir-fry for one more minute. Turn off the heat and add the sesame oil. Toss once more and serve with steamed brown rice or soba gluten free noodles.

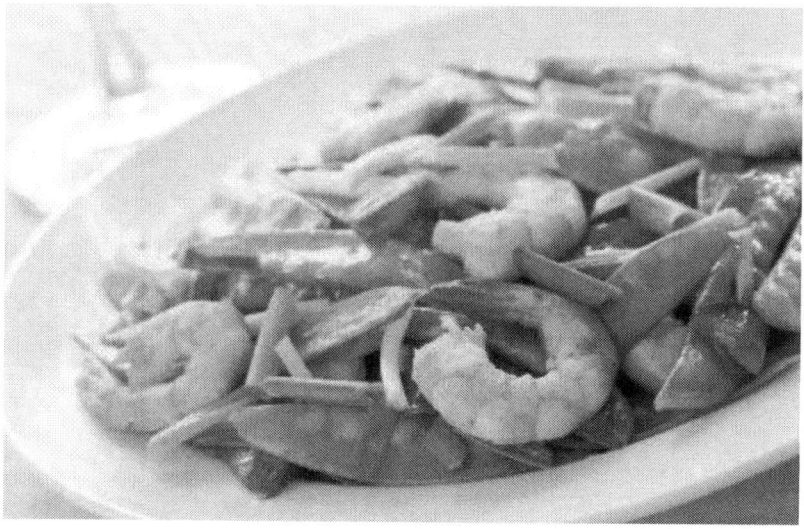

Pork and Green Beans Stir Fry

Serves 1 - Allergies: SF, GF, DF, EF, NF

- 6oz. of lean Pork
- 1 cup of Green Beans, snapped in half. Use as much veggies as you want or replace Green beans with Kale.
- 1 garlic clove, chopped
- 1/2 inch of peeled and chopped ginger
- Season with fish sauce.

Nutrition Facts

Serving Size 285 g

Amount Per Serving

Calories 317	Calories from Fat 97

	% Daily Value*
Total Fat 10.8g	17%
Saturated Fat 2.7g	14%
Trans Fat 0.1g	
Cholesterol 124mg	41%
Sodium 104mg	4%
Potassium 946mg	27%
Total Carbohydrates 7.8g	3%
Dietary Fiber 3.7g	15%
Sugars 1.5g	
Protein 46.5g	

Vitamin A 15%	•	Vitamin C 30%
Calcium 5%	•	Iron 17%

Nutrition Grade A
* Based on a 2000 calorie diet

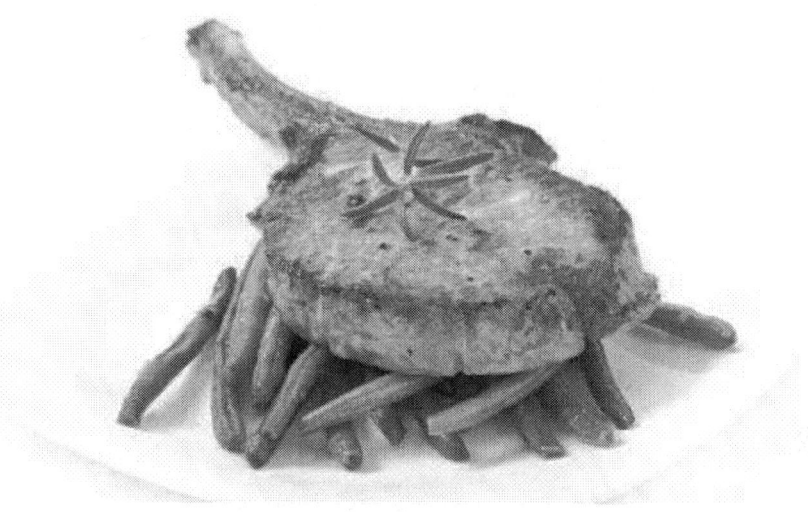

Cashew chicken

Serves 4

Ingredients - Allergies: SF, GF, DF, EF, NF

- 1 bunch scallions
- 1 pound skinless boneless chicken thighs
- 1/2 tsp. salt
- 1/4 tsp. black pepper
- 3 tbsp. coconut oil
- 1 red bell pepper and 1 stalk of celery, chopped
- 4 garlic cloves, finely chopped
- 1 1/2 tbsp. finely chopped peeled fresh ginger
- 1/4 tsp. dried hot red-pepper flakes
- 3/4 cup chicken broth
- 1 1/2 tbsp. fish sauce
- 1 1/2 teaspoons arrowroot flour
- 1/2 cup salted roasted whole cashews

Instructions

Chop scallions and separate green and white parts. Pat chicken dry and cut into 3/4-inch pieces and season with salt and pepper. Heat a wok or a skillet over high heat. Add oil and then stir-fry chicken until cooked through, 3 to 4 minutes. Transfer to a plate. Add garlic, bell pepper, celery, ginger, red-pepper flakes, and scallion whites to wok and stir-fry until peppers are just tender, 4 to 5 minutes.

Mix together broth, fish sauce and arrowroot flour, then stir into vegetables in wok. Reduce heat and simmer, stirring occasionally, until thickened. Stir in cashews, scallion greens, and chicken along with any juices.

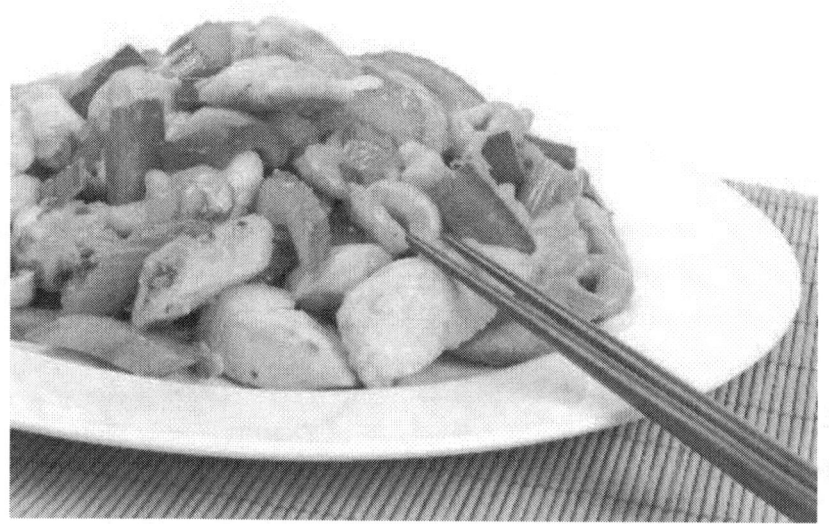

Chinese Celery, Mushrooms & Fish Stir Fry

Serves 2

Ingredients - Allergies: SF, GF, DF, EF

- 1/2 pound fish fillets
- 1 cup Chinese Celery
- 1 cup Mushrooms sliced in half
- 1/2 cup peppers sliced diagonally
- 1 Tsp. oil

Instructions

Marinade fish in a Superfoods marinade. Stir fry drained fish in coconut oil for few minutes, add all vegetables and stir fry for 2 more minutes. Add the rest of the marinade and stir fry for a minute. Serve with brown rice or quinoa.

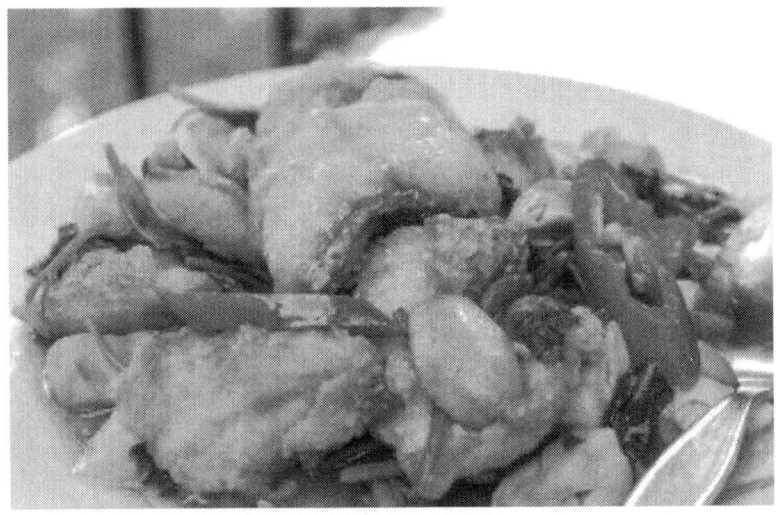

Pork, Green Pepper and Tomato Stir Fry
Serves 2

Ingredients - Allergies: SF, GF, DF, EF
- 1/2 pound cubed pork
- 1 cup Green Peppers
- 1/2 cup sliced Tomatoes
- 1 tsp. ground black pepper
- 1 Tsp. oil

Instructions
Marinade pork in a Superfoods marinade. Stir fry drained pork in coconut oil for few minutes, add all vegetables and stir fry for 2 more minutes. Add the rest of the marinade and stir fry for a minute. Serve with brown rice or quinoa.

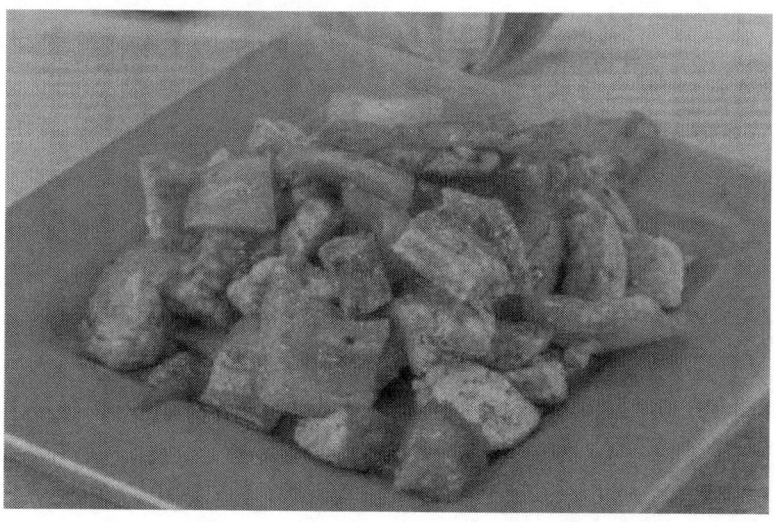

Pork, Red & Green Peppers, Onion & Carrots Stir Fry

Serves 2

Ingredients - Allergies: SF, GF, DF, EF

- 1/2 pound pork
- 1/2 cup chopped Red Peppers
- 1/2 cup chopped Green Peppers
- 1/2 cup sliced onion
- 1/2 cup sliced carrots
- 1 Tsp. oil

Instructions

Marinade pork in a Superfoods marinade. Stir fry drained pork in coconut oil for few minutes, add all vegetables and stir fry for 2 more minutes. Add the rest of the marinade and stir fry for a minute. Serve with brown rice or quinoa.

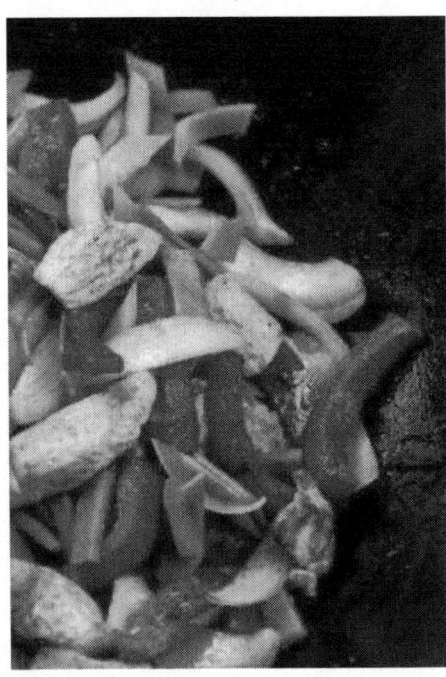

Chicken, Carrots & Snow Peas Stir Fry
Serves 2

Ingredients - Allergies: SF, GF, DF, EF
- 1/2 pound chicken
- 1 cup Carrots
- 1 cup Snow Peas
- 1 Tsp. oil

Instructions

Marinade chicken in a Superfoods marinade. Stir fry drained chicken in coconut oil for few minutes, add all vegetables and stir fry for 2 more minutes. Add the rest of the marinade and stir fry for a minute. Serve with brown rice or quinoa.

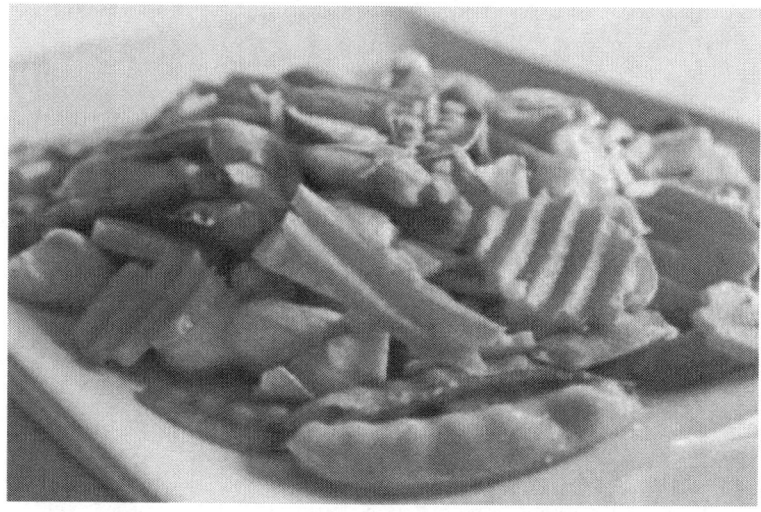

Beef, Green beans, Broccoli & Carrot Stir Fry

Serves 2

Ingredients - Allergies: SF, GF, DF, EF

- 1/2 pound beef
- 1/2 cup chopped Broccoli
- 1/2 cup chopped Green beans
- 1/2 cup sliced carrots
- 1/2 cup Baby Corn
- 1 Tsp. oil

Instructions

Marinade beef in a Superfoods marinade. Stir fry drained beef in coconut oil for few minutes, add all vegetables and stir fry for 2 more minutes. Add the rest of the marinade and stir fry for a minute. Serve with brown rice or quinoa.

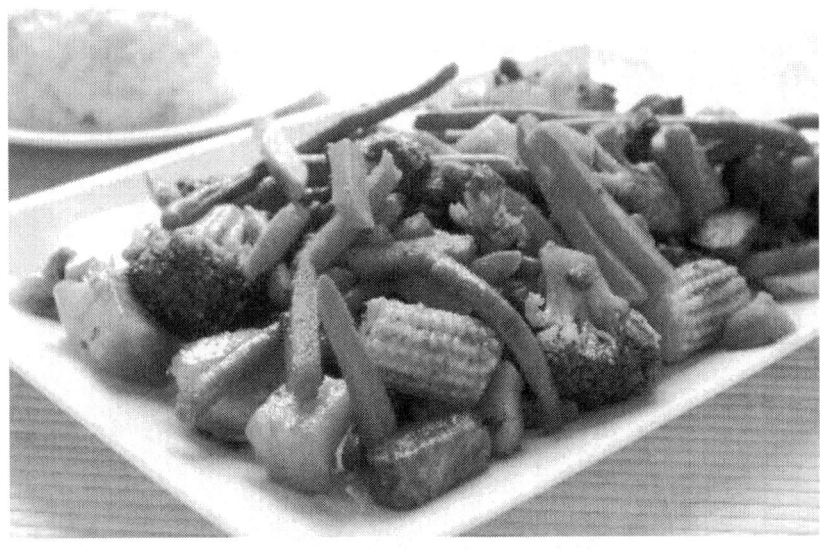

Pork, Onion & Bok Choy Stir Fry
Serves 2

Ingredients - Allergies: SF, GF, DF, EF

- 1/2 pound pork
- 1/2 cup sliced onions
- 1 cup sliced Bok Choy
- 1/2 cup sliced Chinese Celery
- 1 Tsp. oil

Instructions
Marinade pork in a Superfoods marinade. Stir fry drained pork in coconut oil for few minutes, add all vegetables and stir fry for 2 more minutes. Add the rest of the marinade and stir fry for a minute. Serve with brown rice or quinoa.

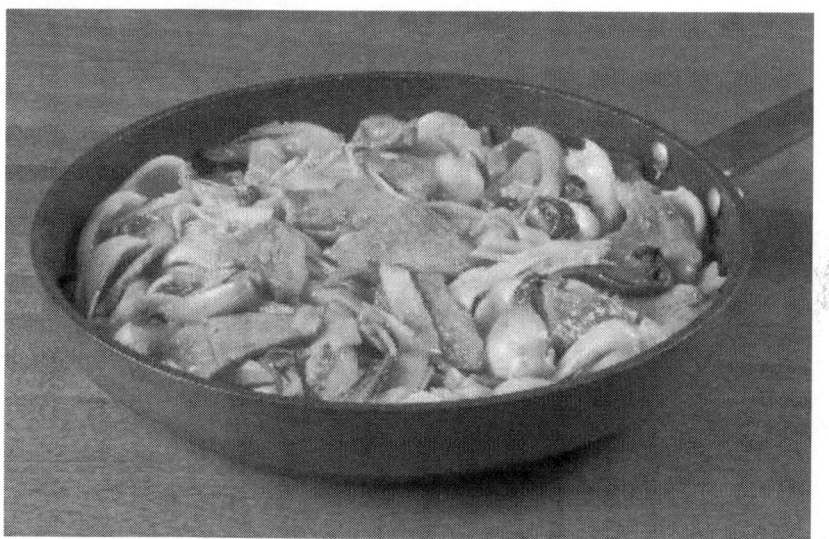

Chicken, Red Peppers & Bok Choy Stir Fry

Serves 2

Ingredients - Allergies: SF, GF, DF, EF

- 1/2 pound chicken
- 1/2 cup sliced onions
- 1 cup sliced Bok Choy
- 1/2 cup sliced Red Peppers
- 1 Tsp. oil

Instructions

Marinade chicken in a Superfoods marinade. Stir fry drained chicken in coconut oil for few minutes, add all vegetables and stir fry for 2 more minutes. Add the rest of the marinade and stir fry for a minute. Serve with brown rice or quinoa.

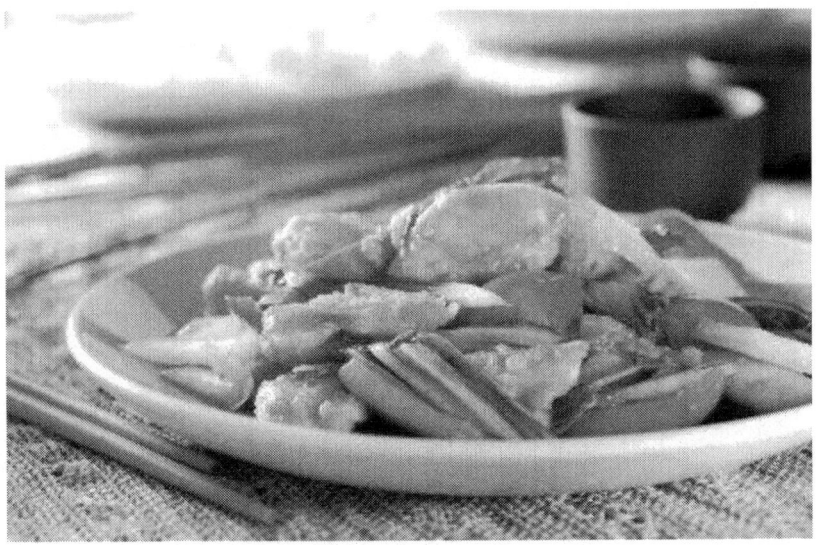

Cauliflower & Shiitake Stir Fry
Serves 2

Ingredients - Allergies: SF, GF, DF, EF

- 2 cups Cauliflower
- 1 cup sliced Shiitake mushrooms
- 1/2 cup sliced Green beans
- 1/2 cup sliced Broccoli
- 1/2 cup sliced carrot
- 1 Tsp. Coconut oil

Instructions

Stir fry cauliflower and broccoli in coconut oil for few minutes, add carrots and green beans and stir fry for 2 more minutes. Add the mushrooms and stir fry for 3 minutes more. Serve with brown rice or quinoa.

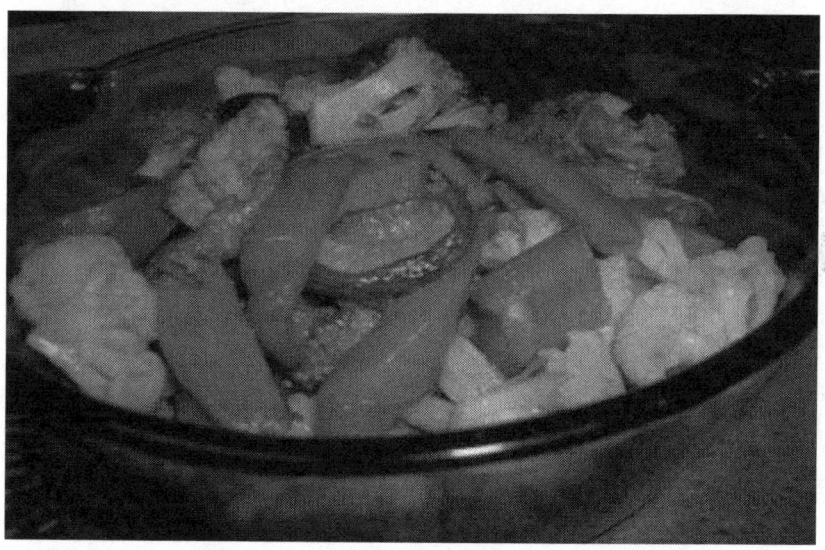

Pork, Cabbage & Bok Choy Stir Fry

Serves 2

Ingredients - Allergies: SF, GF, DF, EF

- 1/2 pound cubed pork
- 1 cup sliced Chinese cabbage
- 1/2 cup sliced bok choy
- 1/2 cup sliced red peppers
- 1 Tsp. oil

Instructions

Marinade pork in a Superfoods marinade. Stir fry drained pork in coconut oil for few minutes, add all vegetables and stir fry for 2 more minutes. Add the rest of the marinade and stir fry for a minute. Serve with brown rice or quinoa.

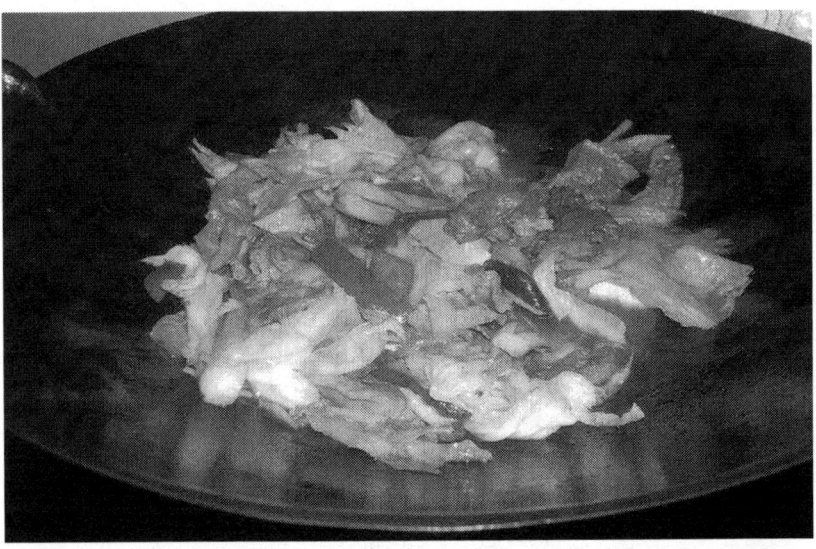

Chicken & Chinese Celery Stir Fry
Serves 2

Ingredients - Allergies: SF, GF, DF, EF

- 1/2 pound chicken
- 2 cups sliced Chinese Celery
- 1 Tsp. oil

Instructions

Marinade chicken in a Superfoods marinade. Stir fry drained chicken in coconut oil for few minutes, add Chinese celery and stir fry for 2 more minutes. Add the rest of the marinade and stir fry for a minute. Serve with brown rice or quinoa.

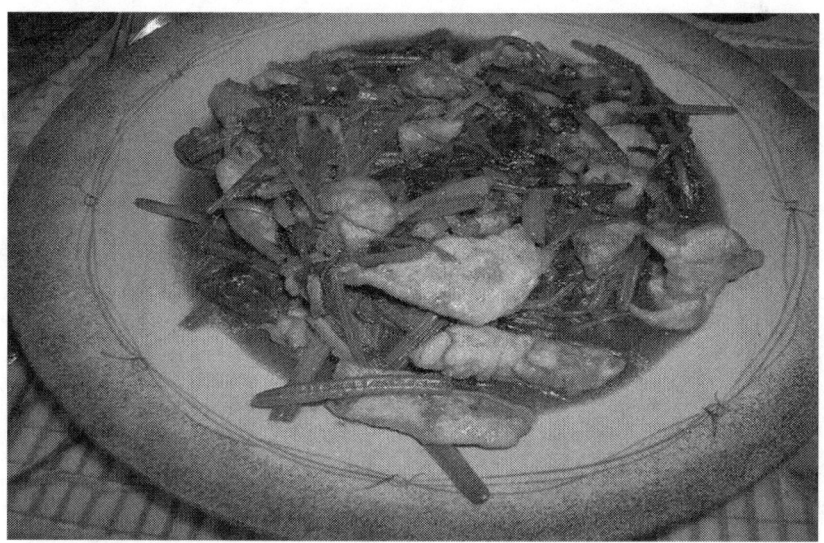

Meats

Baked Chicken Breast with Fresh Basil
Serves 10

Ingredients - Allergies: SF, GF, EF, NF

- 10 boneless skinless chicken breast
- 3/4 cup low-fat yogurt
- 1/2 cup chopped basil
- 2 tsp. arrowroot flour
- 1 cup oatmeal coarsely ground

Instructions

Arrange chicken in a baking dish. Combine basil, yogurt and arrowroot flour; mix well and spread over chicken.

Mix oatmeal with salt and pepper to taste & sprinkle over chicken.

Bake chicken in 375 degrees in the oven for half an hour. Makes 10 servings.

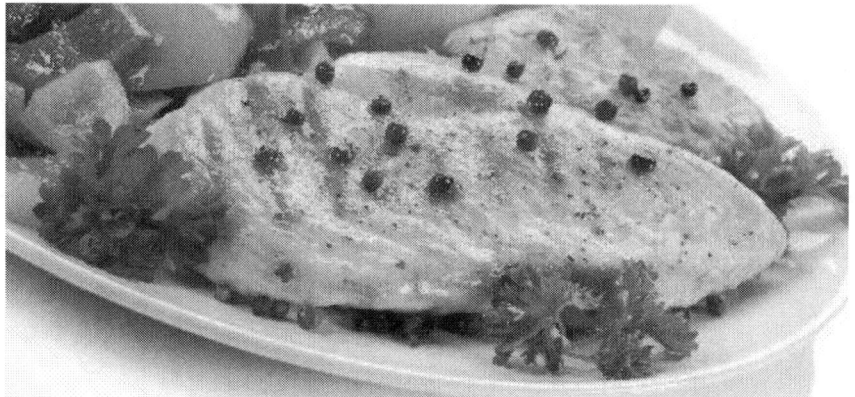

Roast Chicken with Rosemary

Serves 6-8

- 1 (3 pound) whole chicken, rinsed, skinned
- salt and pepper to taste
- 1 onion, quartered
- 1/4 cup chopped rosemary

Instructions - Allergies: SF, GF, DF, EF, NF

Heat the oven to 350F. Sprinkle salt and pepper on meat. Stuff with the onion and rosemary. Place in a baking dish and bake in the preheated oven until chicken is cooked through. Depending on the size of the bird, cooking time will vary.

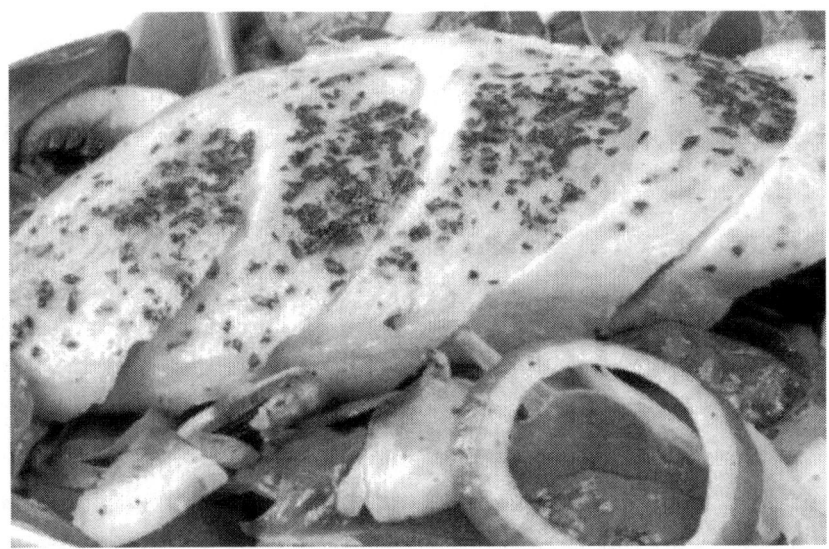

Carne Asada

Serves 4-6 - Allergies: SF, GF, DF, EF, NF

Marinade:

Mix together the garlic, jalapeno, cilantro, salt, and pepper to make a paste. Put the paste in a container. Add the oil, lime juice and orange juice. Shake it up to combine. Use as a marinade for beef or as a table condiment.

Instructions

Put the flank steak in a baking dish and pour the marinade over it. Refrigerate up to 8 hours.
Take the steak out of the marinade and season it on both sides with salt and pepper. Grill (or broil) the steak for 7 to 10 minutes per side, turning once, until medium-rare. Put the steak on a cutting board and allow the juices to settle (5 minutes). Thinly slice the steak across the grain.

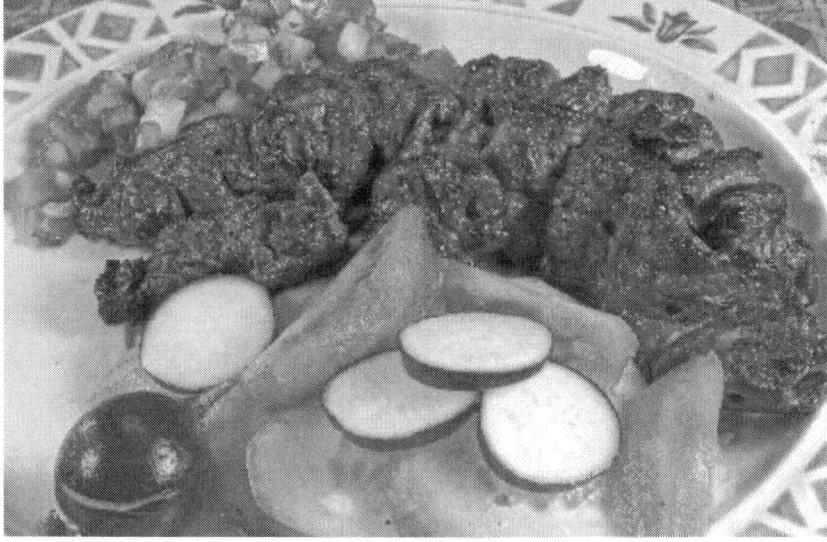

Meatballs

Baked Beef Meatballs

This amount is for 4 servings. Adjust for 2 if you want, eat one serving, freeze one or prepare it as is for 4 servings and then freeze 3/4 for some tasty casserole recipes like "Beef Meatballs Casserole with Green Beans" or with "Beef Meatballs Casserole with Broccoli".

Allergies: SF, GF, NF

- 1 pound lean ground beef
- 2 tbsp. minced onion
- 1/2 tsp. minced garlic
- 1 tsp. parmesan cheese
- 2 eggs
- 1/2 tsp. salt
- 1/4 tsp. pepper

Mix all of the ingredients in a large bowl using your fingers. Mix until the meat no long feels slimy from the eggs. Shape in small egg size meatballs. Place on a baking sheet. Bake at 375F for 20-25 minutes until the meatballs are cooked through. Serve with large Fiber Loaded salad with Italian Dressing.

Nutrition Facts

Serving Size 149 g

Amount Per Serving

Calories 268	Calories from Fat 97
	% Daily Value*
Total Fat 10.8g	17%
Saturated Fat 4.3g	22%
Trans Fat 0.0g	
Cholesterol 188mg	63%
Sodium 461mg	19%
Potassium 497mg	14%
Total Carbohydrates 1.1g	0%
Protein 39.5g	
Vitamin A 3%	Vitamin C 1%
Calcium 8%	Iron 121%

Nutrition Grade B
* Based on a 2000 calorie diet

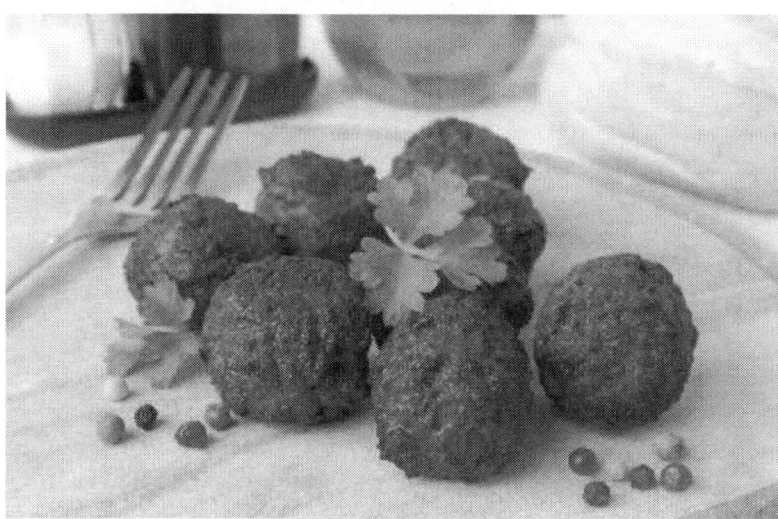

Middle Eastern Meatballs

Makes about 20 meatballs - Allergies: SF, GF, DF, EF, NF

Ingredients

- Ground lamb or beef, or a mixture of the two -- 2 pounds
- Onion, minced -- 1
- Fresh parsley or mint, finely chopped -- 1/2 bunch
- Ground cumin -- 1 tbsp.
- Cinnamon -- 2 teaspoons
- Allspice (optional) -- 1 tsp.
- Salt and pepper -- to season
- coconut oil -- 1/4 cup

Instructions

Place the ground beef or lamb, onion, herbs, spices, salt and pepper in a bowl and knead well. Chill for 1-2 hours and let the flavors mingle. Form the meat into patties or balls the size of a small egg.

Bake in the oven on 350F. Serve with brown rice with tzatziki sauce.

Variations

Experiment with different seasonings--coriander, cayenne, sesame seeds.

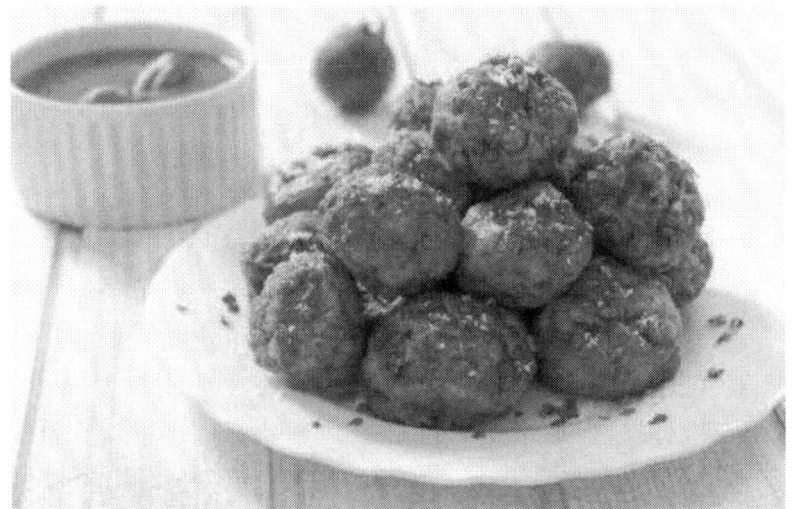

Casseroles

Some recipes are for 1 person, adjust for 2 or more

Broccoli Chicken Casserole

Serves 1

Ingredients - Allergies: SF, GF, NF

- 1 cup broccoli florets
- 6 oz. skinless, boneless chicken (or turkey) pieces (breast or dark meat)
- 1 tsp of flax seeds meal
- Salt, pepper
- 1 egg - beaten
- Half a cup of Yogurt Dressing (or coconut milk, if you don't like the sourish tang)
- 1/4 cup of chicken broth
- 2 tbsp of grated low-fat cheddar cheese

Heat the oven to 400°. Cook broccoli around 5 minutes. Take broccoli out and add chicken (or turkey) and simmer for 15 minutes. Cut chicken (or turkey) into cubes and add it to the broccoli.

Combine broth, flax, salt and pepper in a pan and mix. Bring to a boil over high heat and cook 1 minute, stirring constantly. Remove from heat. Add yogurt dressing, beaten egg and then half of the cheese, stirring until well combined. Add sauce to broccoli mixture; and stir gently until combined.

Put mixture in a small casserole dish oiled with some coconut oil. Put remaining cheese on top, sprinkle. Bake at 400° for 50 minutes or until mixture bubbles at the edges and cheese begins to brown. Remove from oven and let cool for 5 minutes.

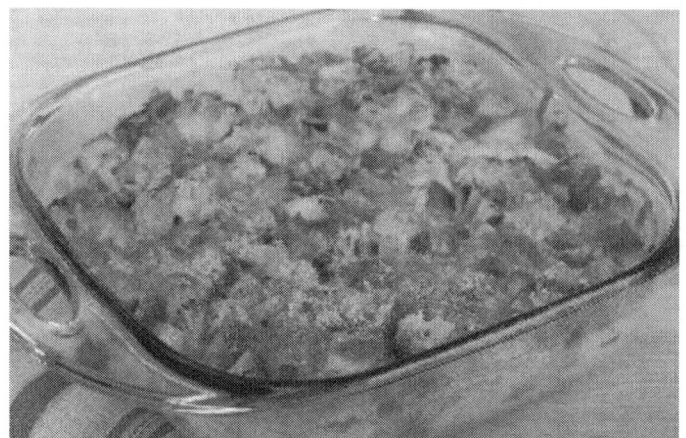

Beef Meatballs Broccoli Casserole

Serves 1

Ingredients - Allergies: SF, GF

- 1 cup broccoli florets
- 4 oz. beef meatballs (see separate recipe)
- 1 tsp of <u>almond</u> flour
- Salt, pepper
- 1 egg - beaten
- Half a cup of Yogurt Dressing
- 1/4 cup of chicken broth
- 2 tbsp of grated low-fat cheddar cheese

Instructions

Heat oven to 400F. Cook broccoli around 5 minutes. Prepare beef meatballs as in the recipe above. Combine broth, flour, salt and pepper in a saucepan, stirring with a whisk until smooth. Bring to a boil over medium-high heat; cook 1 minute, stirring constantly. Remove from heat. Add yogurt dressing, beaten egg and then half of the cheese, stirring until well combined. Add sauce to broccoli mixture; and stir gently until combined.

Put mixture in a small casserole dish oiled with some coconut oil. Sprinkle with remaining cheese. Bake at 400° for 50 minutes or until mixture bubbles at the edges and cheese begins to brown. Remove from oven and let cool for 5 minutes. Serve with large Fiber Loaded Salad with Italian Dressing.

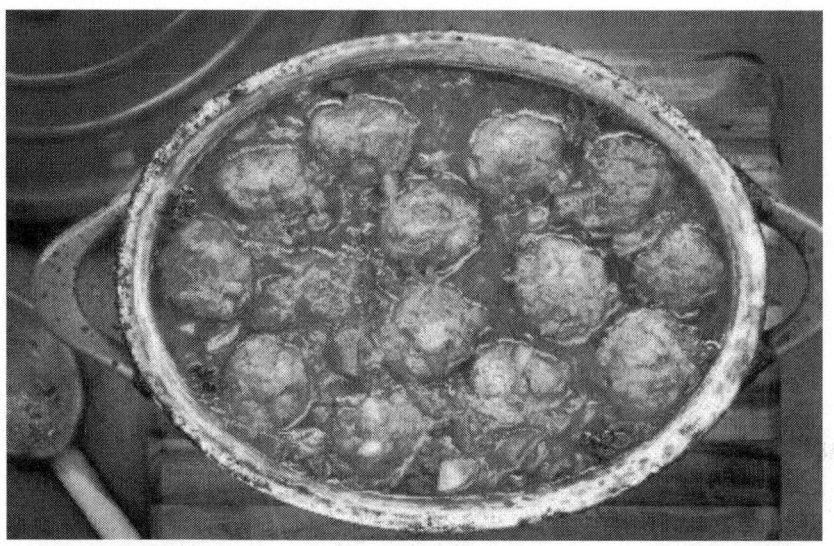

Nutrition Facts

Serving Size 352 g

Amount Per Serving

Calories 409   Calories from Fat 147

	% Daily Value*
Total Fat 16.3g	**25%**
Saturated Fat 6.5g	**32%**
Trans Fat 0.0g	
Cholesterol 277mg	**92%**
Sodium 745mg	**31%**
Potassium 958mg	**27%**
Total Carbohydrates 11.2g	**4%**
Dietary Fiber 2.2g	**9%**
Sugars 6.2g	
Protein 52.0g	

Vitamin A 29% • Vitamin C 104%
Calcium 30%   • Iron 128%

Nutrition Grade A-
* Based on a 2000 calorie diet

Beef Meatballs Cauliflower Casserole

Serves 1

Ingredients - Allergies: SF, GF

- 1 cup cauliflower florets
- 4 oz. beef meatballs (see separate recipe)
- 1 tsp of <u>almond</u> flour
- Salt, pepper
- 1 egg - beaten
- Half a cup of Yogurt Dressing
- 1/4 cup of chicken broth
- 2 tbsp of grated low-fat cheddar cheese

Instructions

Heat oven to 400°.

Cook cauliflower around 5 minutes. Prepare beef meatballs as in the recipe above. Combine soup, flour, salt and pepper in a saucepan, stirring with a whisk until smooth. Bring to a boil over medium-high heat; cook 1 minute, stirring constantly. Remove from heat. Add yogurt dressing, beaten egg and then half of the cheese, stirring until well combined. Add sauce to cauliflower mixture; and stir gently until combined.

Put mixture in a small casserole dish oiled with some coconut oil. Sprinkle with remaining cheese. Bake at 400° for 50 minutes or until mixture bubbles at the edges and cheese begins to brown. Remove from oven and let cool for 5 minutes. Serve with large Fiber Loaded

Nutrition Facts

Serving Size 361 g

Amount Per Serving

Calories 405	Calories from Fat 145
	% Daily Value*
Total Fat 16.1g	**25%**
Saturated Fat 6.5g	**32%**
Trans Fat 0.0g	
Cholesterol 277mg	**92%**
Sodium 745mg	**31%**
Potassium 976mg	**28%**
Total Carbohydrates 10.8g	**4%**
Dietary Fiber 2.3g	**9%**
Sugars 6.9g	
Protein 51.6g	
Vitamin A 21% •	Vitamin C 64%
Calcium 28% •	Iron 127%

Nutrition Grade A-

* Based on a 2000 calorie diet

Salad with Italian Dressing.

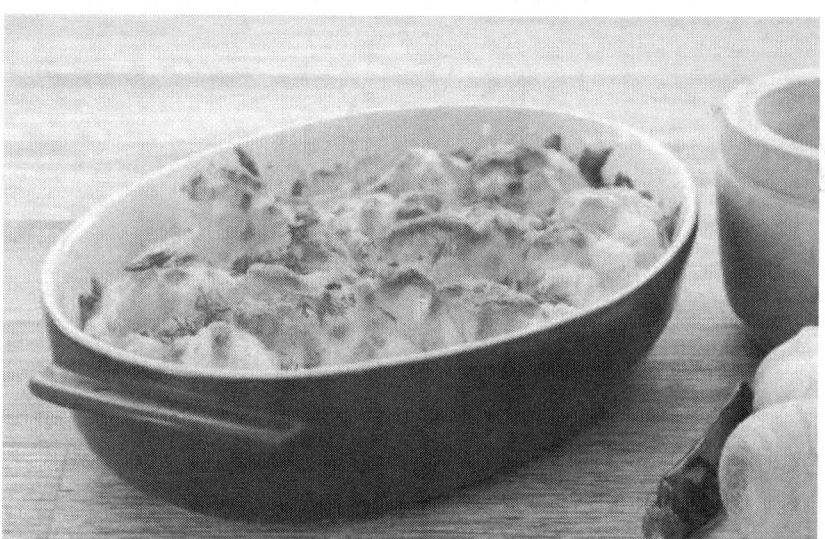

Cabbage Roll Casserole

Serves 8

Ingredients - Allergies: SF, GF, DF, EF, NF

2 pounds ground beef
1 cup chopped onion
1 liter tomato sauce
3 1/2 pounds cabbage or sauerkraut leaves
1 cup uncooked brown rice
1 tsp. salt
2 cups beef broth

Instructions

Heat oven to 350F.
Brown beef in coconut oil in a skillet over medium/high heat until through. In a large mixing bowl combine the onion, rice and salt. Add meat and mix all together. Roll mixture into cabbage leaves and arrange them in a casserole dish. Pour broth and tomato sauce over rolls and bake in the preheated oven, covered, for 1 hour.

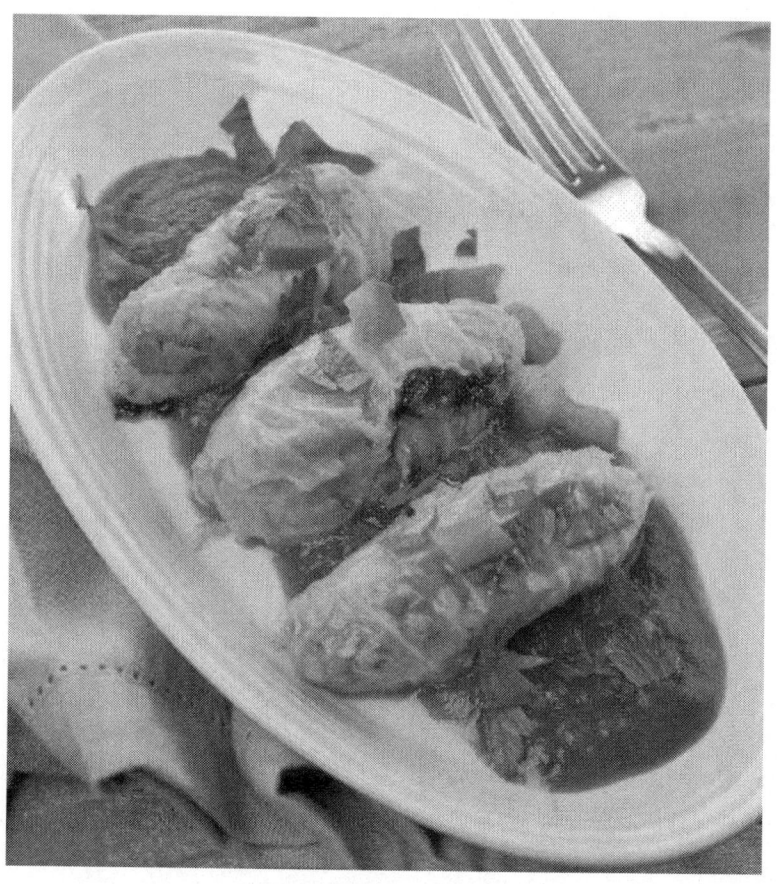

Pork Chop Casserole
Serves 6

Ingredients - Allergies: SF, GF, DF, EF, NF

- 3 cups vegetable broth
- 1 cup brown rice
- 5 ounce mushrooms
- salt and pepper to taste
- 6 (3/4 inch) thick pork chops

Instructions

Heat oven to 350F. Pour broth into a baking dish. Add rice and mushrooms and mix. Salt and pepper to taste. Add pork chops in a single layer on that mixture and push them down into mixture and make sure they are covered with it.
Cover baking dish with aluminum foil and bake for 1 hour.

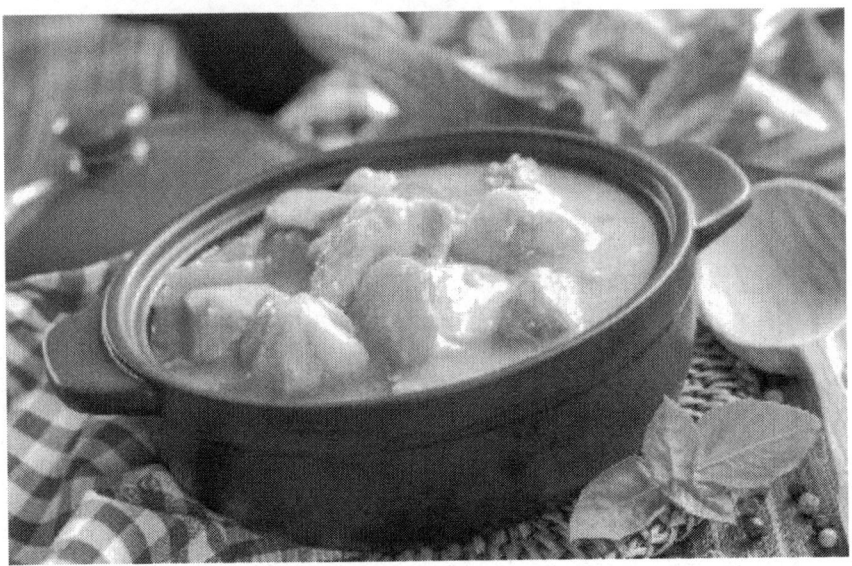

Chicken & Mushrooms Casserole

Serves 2

Ingredients - Allergies: SF, GF, DF, EF, NF

- 1 large onion, chopped
- 3 cups sliced mushrooms
- 2 tbsp. coconut oil
- 1/2 tsp. salt
- 1/4 tsp. ground black pepper
- 1/2 tsp. minced garlic
- 2 large chicken breast pieces with skin on

Instructions

Oil casserole dish with oil, put chicken pieces in. Mix onion, salt, pepper, mushrooms and garlic and put over chicken. Cover and bake for 1 ½ hours on 400F.

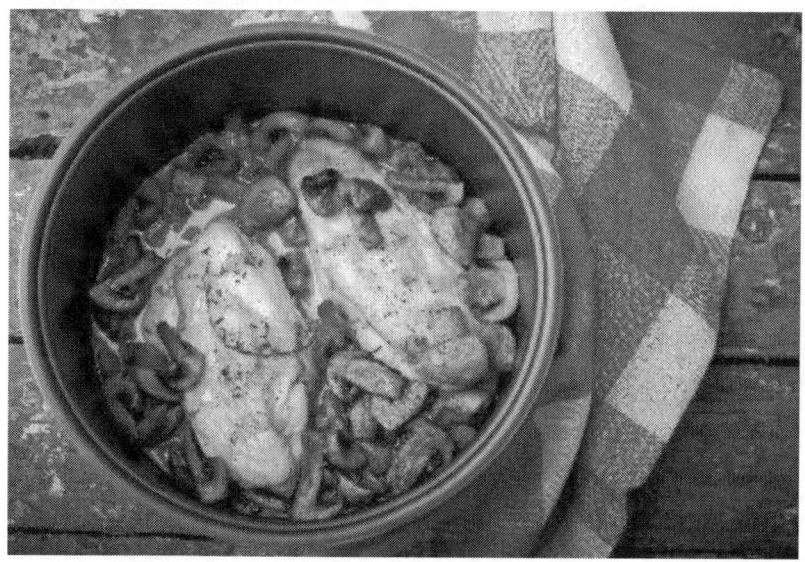

Pork & Red Peppers Casserole

Serves 8

Ingredients - Allergies: SF, GF, NF

- 1 cup chopped onions
- 2 cups sliced Red Peppers
- 4 pounds cubed pork
- 1 cup "healthy casserole sauce"

Instructions

Put all recipe ingredients in the casserole dish, pour sauce on top, cover and bake for 2 hours on 400F. Garnish with parsley.

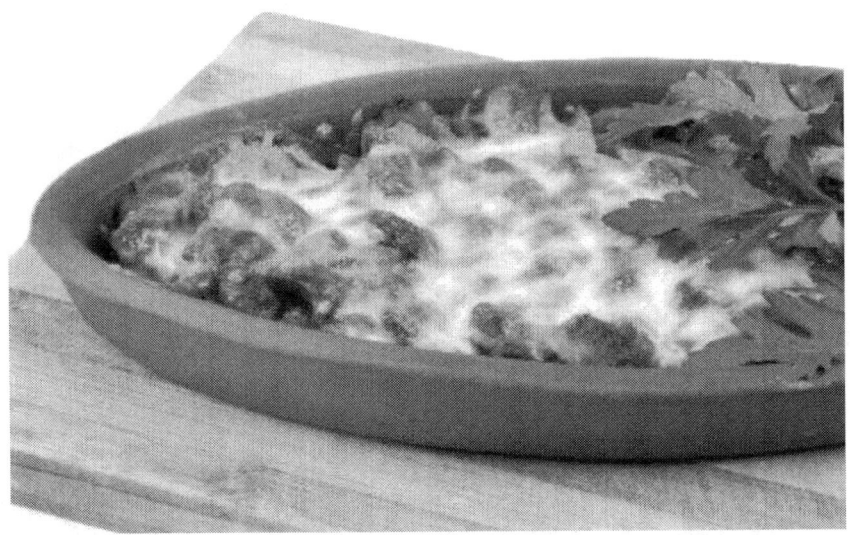

Chicken, Carrot and Cherry Tomatoes Casserole

Serves 8

Ingredients - Allergies: SF, GF, DF, EF, NF

- 1-1/2 cups chopped carrots
- 1 cup chopped onions
- 2 tbsp. coconut oil
- 1-1/2 cups yellow peppers
- 1/2 tsp. salt
- 1/4 tsp. ground black pepper
- 1/2 tsp. minced garlic
- 4 pounds cubed chicken
- 1/2 cups chopped parsley

Instructions

Put all recipe ingredients in the casserole dish, cover and bake for 2 hours on 400F.

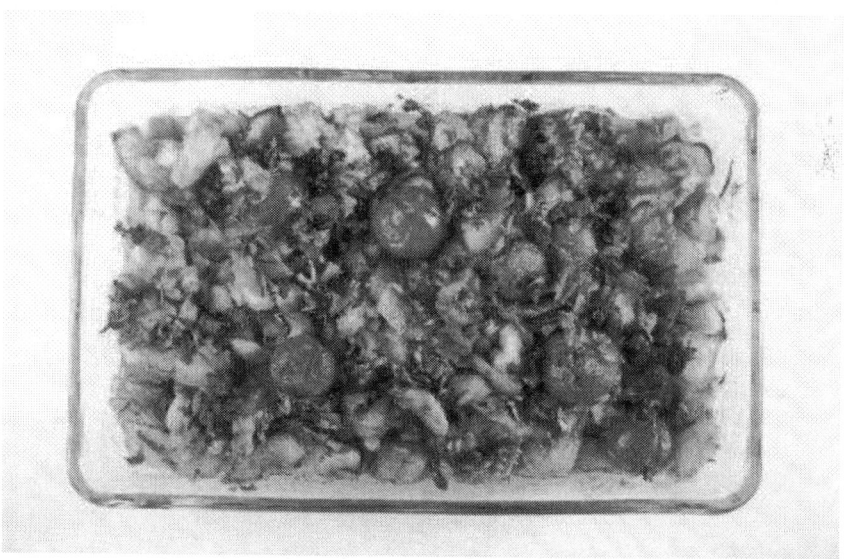

Chicken, Carrot and Onions Italian Casserole

Serves 6

Ingredients - Allergies: SF, GF, DF, EF, NF

- 1-1/2 cups chopped carrots
- 1 cup chopped onions
- 2 tbsp. coconut oil
- 1 cup sliced mushrooms
- 1/2 tsp. salt
- 1/4 tsp. ground black pepper
- 1/2 tsp. minced garlic
- 1 tsp. fresh rosemary
- 4 pounds chicken with skin on

Instructions

Put all recipe ingredients in the casserole dish, cover and bake for 2 hours on 400F.

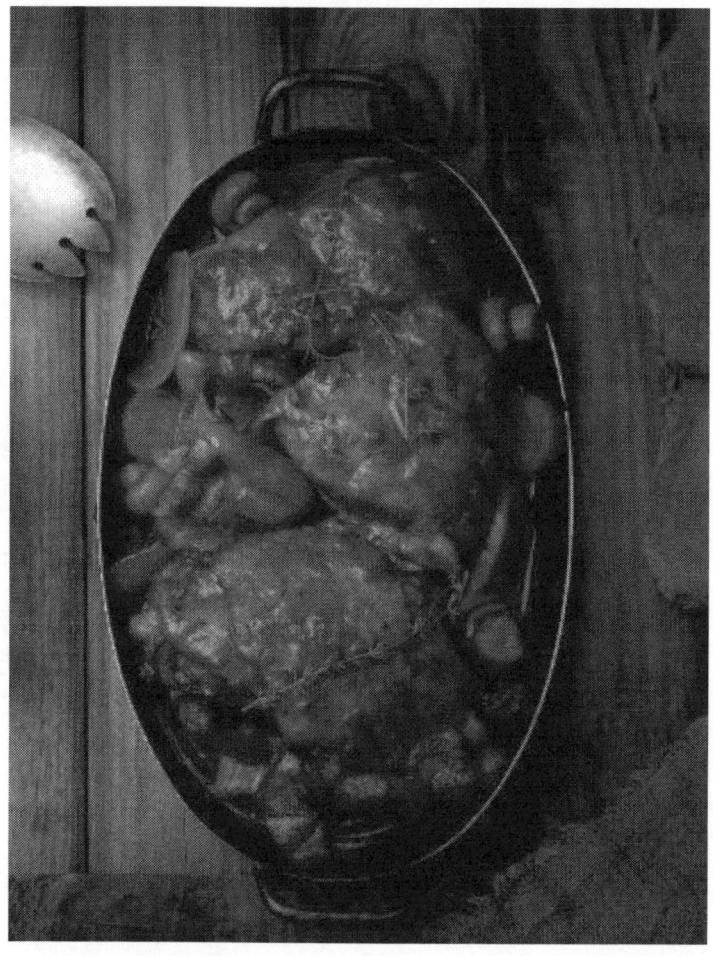

Red Peppers, Zucchini and Eggplant Casserole

Serves 8

Ingredients - Allergies: SF, GF, DF, EF, NF

- 1 chopped carrots
- 1 - 1/2 cup chopped onions
- 1 - 1/2 cup sliced red peppers
- 2 tbsp. coconut oil
- 1 cup sliced zucchini
- 1/2 tsp. salt
- 1/4 tsp. ground black pepper
- 1/2 tsp. minced garlic
- 1/2 tsp. oregano
- 2 pounds sliced eggplant

Instructions

Put all recipe ingredients in the casserole dish, cover and bake for 2 hours on 400F.

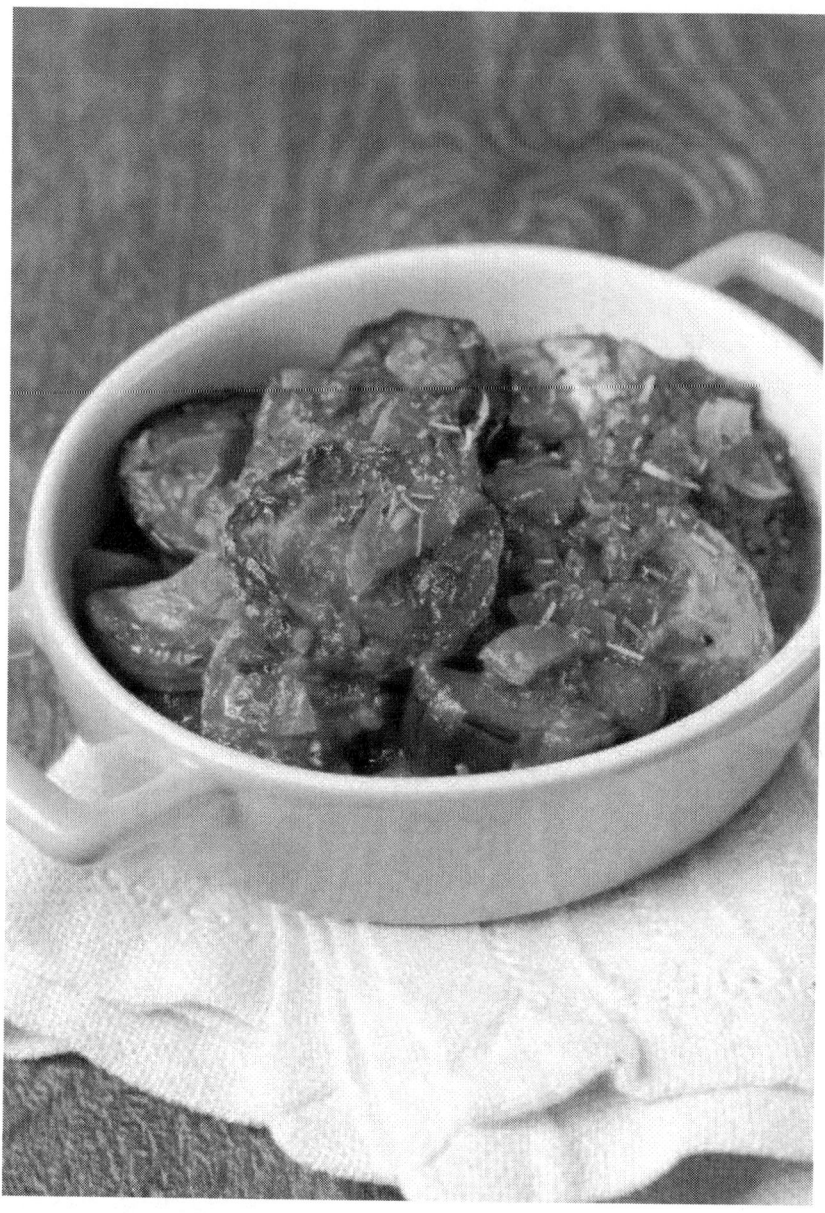

Chia, Flax & Broccoli Casserole

Serves 4

Ingredients - Allergies: SF, GF, DF, EF, NF

- 2 cups broccoli florets
- 1 cup chopped onions
- 2 tbsp. coconut oil
- 1 cup "healthy casserole sauce"
- 1/2 cup flax seeds meal
- 1/2 cup chia seeds

Instructions

Put broccoli and onion in the casserole dish, mix sauce, flax and chia seeds, pour sauce on top, cover and bake for 1 1/2 hours on 400F.

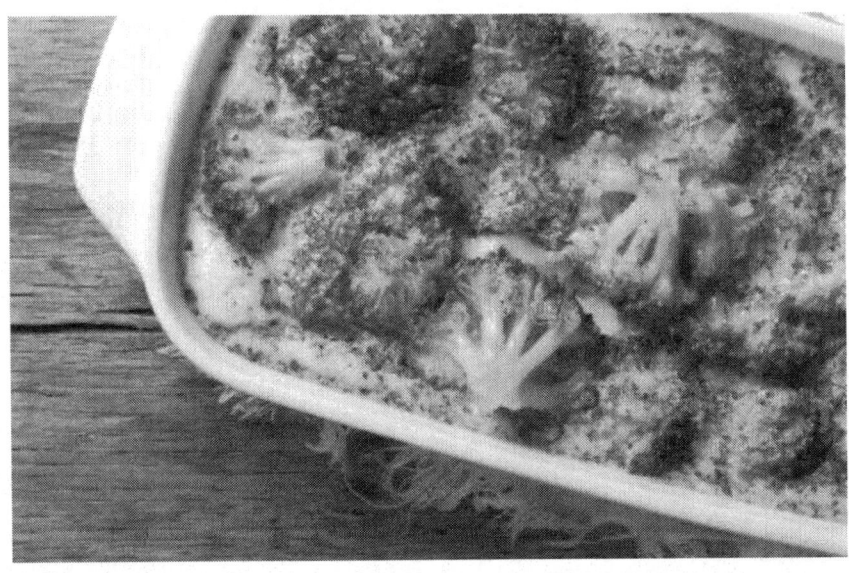

Osso Bucco Casserole

Serves 6-8

Ingredients - Allergies: SF, GF, DF, EF, NF

- 1-1/2 cups sliced mushrooms
- 1 1.2 cups chopped onions
- 2 tbsp. coconut oil
- 1 cup beef stock
- 1/2 tsp. salt
- 1/4 tsp. ground black pepper
- 1 tsp. minced garlic
- 1 tsp. chopped parsley
- 4 pounds osso bucco

Instructions

Put all recipe ingredients in the casserole dish, cover and bake for 2 hours on 400F. Onions and mushrooms should be almost melted and turned into a sauce after 2 hours. Garnish with chopped parsley.

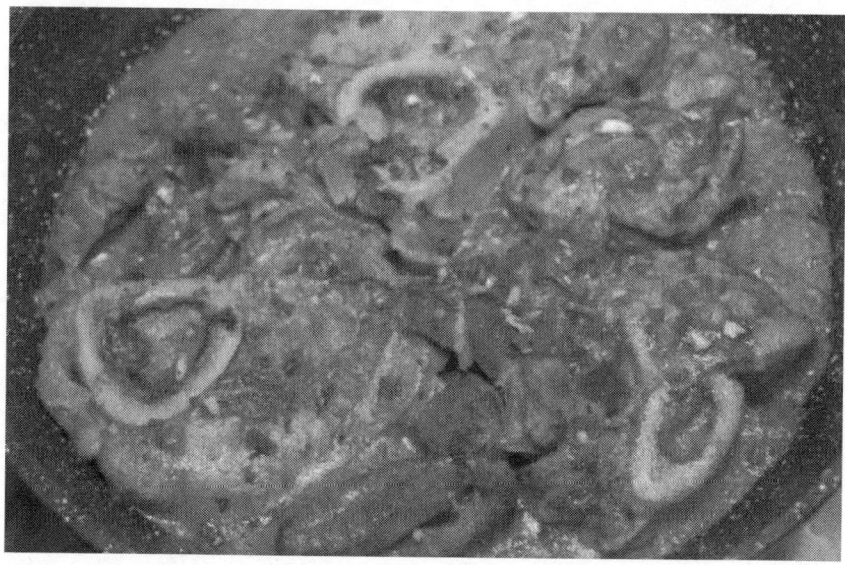

Chicken, Olives & Garlic Casserole

Serves 8

Ingredients - Allergies: SF, GF, DF, EF, NF

- 1 cup chopped onions
- 2 tbsp. coconut oil
- 1 cup Kalamata olives
- 1/4 tsp. ground black pepper
- 1 head garlic, sliced across (bake separately for 45 minutes)
- 1 Tbsp. fresh rosemary
- 4 pounds chicken pieces (dark meat) with skin on

Instructions

Put chicken, onions and olives in the casserole dish, season, cover and bake for 2 hours on 400F. Serve with baked garlic.

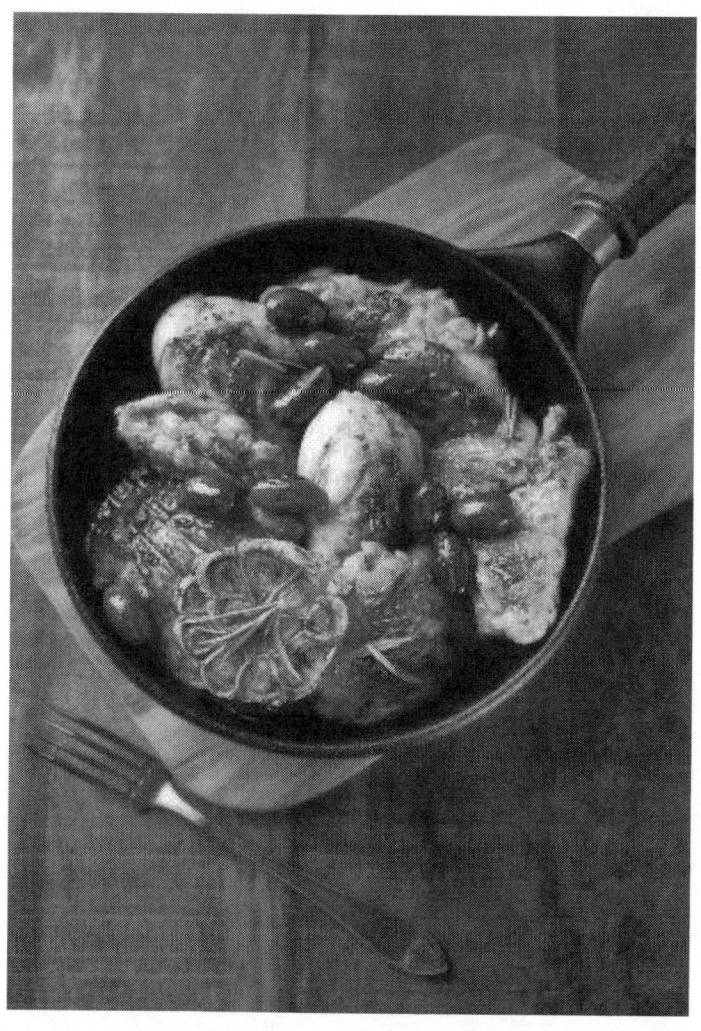

Pork, Sweet Potatoes & Tomato Casserole

Serves 8

Ingredients - Allergies: SF, GF, DF, EF, NF

- 1-1/2 cups chopped sweet potatoes
- 1 cup chopped onions
- 2 tbsp. coconut oil
- 1-1/2 cups sliced tomatoes
- 1 cup "healthy casserole sauce"
- 4 pounds cubed pork
- 1 Tbsp. chopped parsley

Instructions

Put all recipe ingredients in the casserole dish, pour sauce on top, arrange sliced tomatoes on top, cover and bake for 2 hours on 400F. Garnish with parsley.

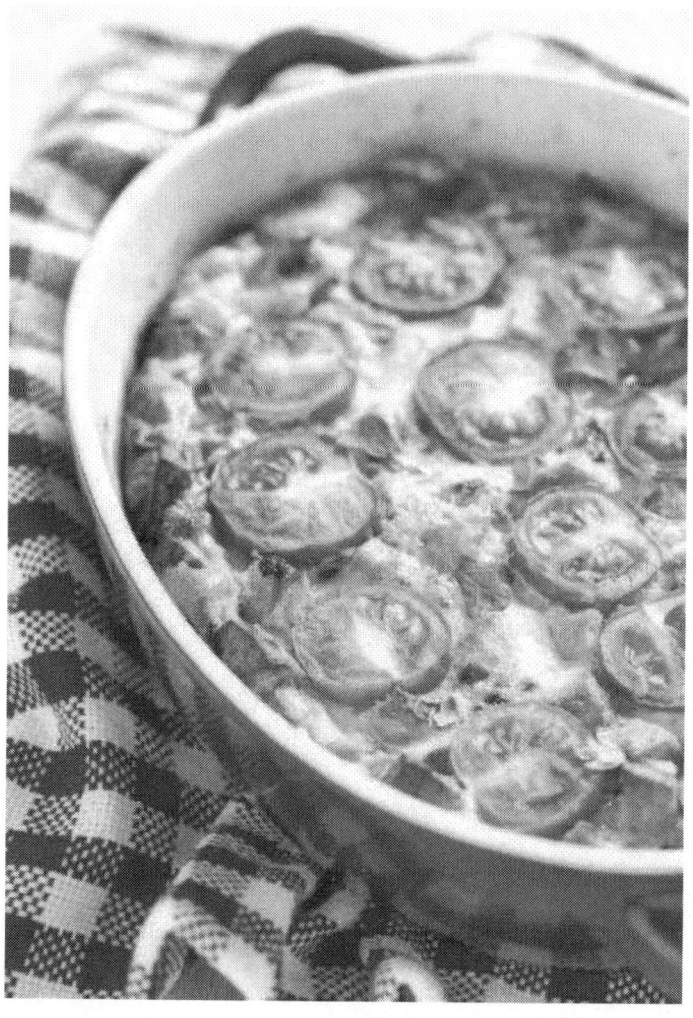

Eggplant, Zucchini and Tomato Casserole

Serves 8

Ingredients - Allergies: SF, GF, DF, EF, NF

- 1-1/2 cups sliced zucchini
- 1-1/2 cups sliced tomatoes
- 2 tbsp. coconut oil
- 1-1/2 cups sliced eggplant
- 1/2 tsp. salt
- 1/4 tsp. ground black pepper
- 1/2 tsp. minced garlic

Instructions

Arrange all ingredients in the casserole dish (see picture), cover and bake for 1 1-2 hours on 400F.

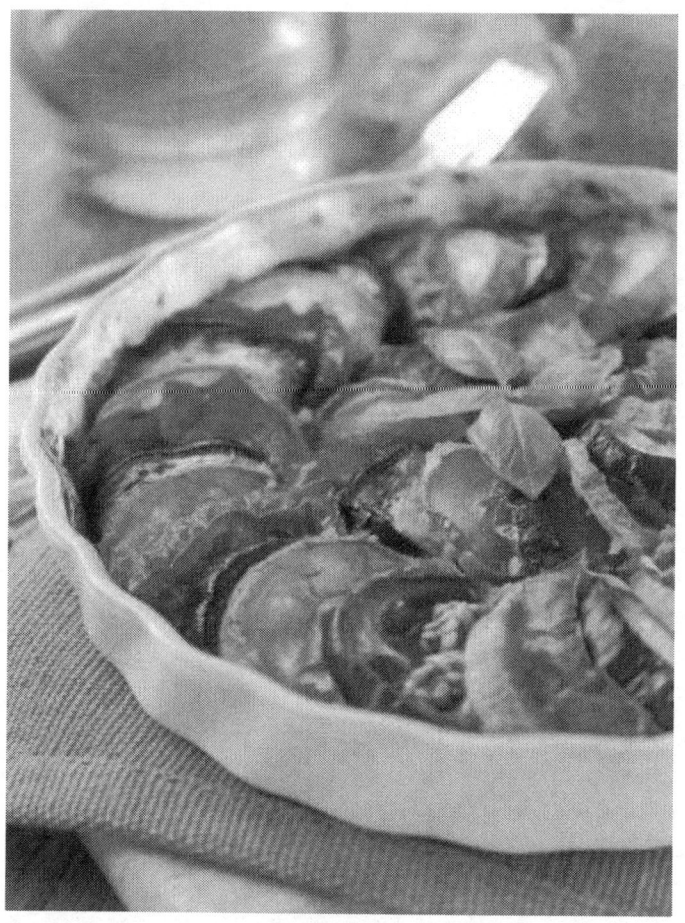

Zucchini & Chicken Casserole

Serves 8

Ingredients - Allergies: SF, GF, DF, EF, NF

- 1-1/2 cups sliced zucchini
- 1 cup chopped onions
- 2 tbsp. coconut oil
- 2 tbsp. chopped green onions
- 1 cup "healthy casserole sauce"
- 4 pounds cubed chicken

Instructions

Put ingredients in the casserole dish, pour sauce on top, cover and bake for 1 1/2 hours on 400F. Sprinkle with green onions before serving.

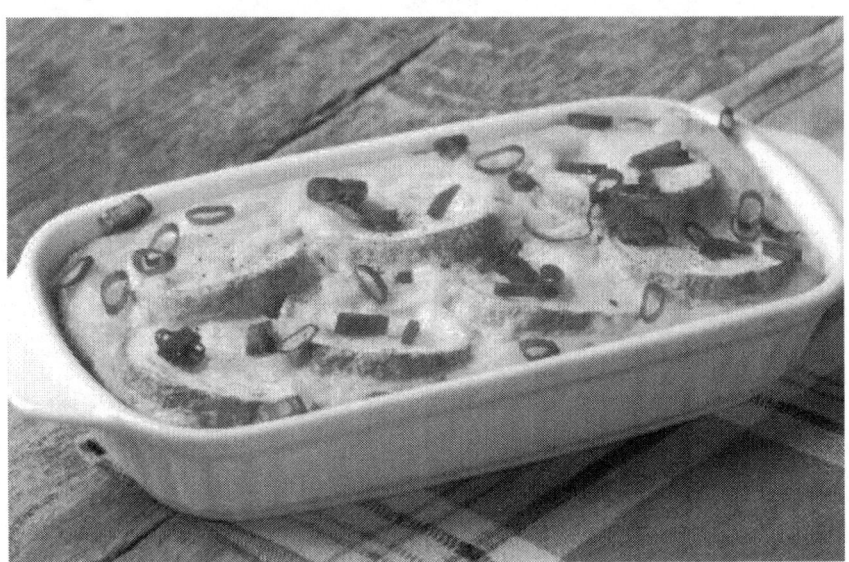

Shrimp, Tomato Paste and Red Peppers Casserole
Serves 4

Ingredients - Allergies: SF, GF, DF, EF, NF

- 1/2 cups chopped carrots
- 1 cup chopped red peppers
- 1/2 cup chopped onions
- 2 tbsp. coconut oil
- 2 cups tomato paste - see recipe at the beginning
- 1/2 tsp. salt
- 1/4 tsp. ground black pepper
- 1 tsp. minced garlic
- 2 pounds shrimp

Instructions

Put all recipe ingredients in the casserole dish, cover and bake for 2 hours on 400F.

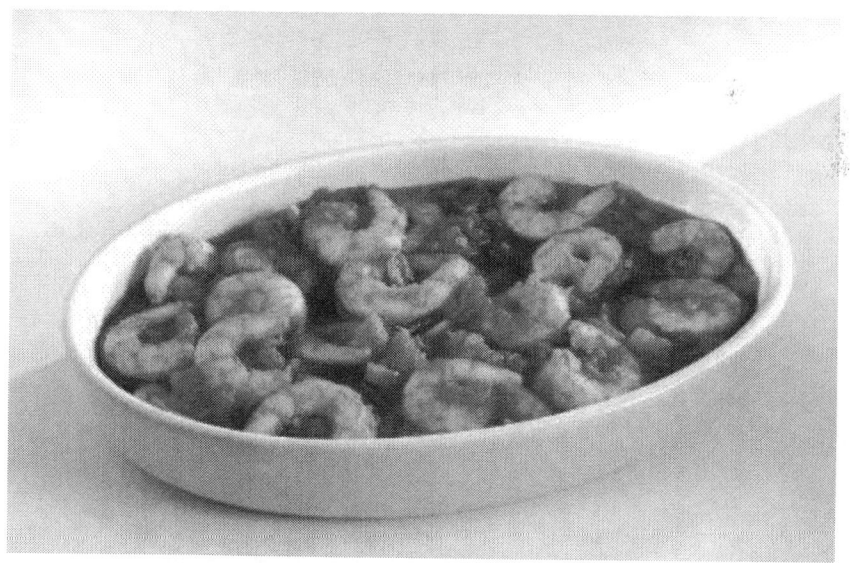

Mushrooms Casserole

Instructions – serves 4 - Allergies: SF, GF, NF

- 3 pounds sliced mushrooms (shiitake preferably)
- 1 pound sliced leeks
- Salt and ground black pepper
- 1 tbsp. chopped parsley
- 2 beaten eggs
- 1 cup of low-fat Greek yogurt
- 1/2 cup of shredded cheddar cheese, low-fat
- 1 pound cubed skinless boneless chicken (or turkey) breasts

Instructions

Heat oven to 375 degrees F. Mix beaten eggs and low-fat yogurt in a separate dish. In a casserole, place 1 layer of mushrooms, leeks and chicken cubes and season with salt, pepper, and parsley. Cover with 1/2 of a cup of eggs/yogurt mixture. Repeat process 2 more times and cover with shredded cheese. Bake until mushrooms and chicken is tender and crust is golden brown. Serve with Large Fiber Loaded salad with Italian Dressing.

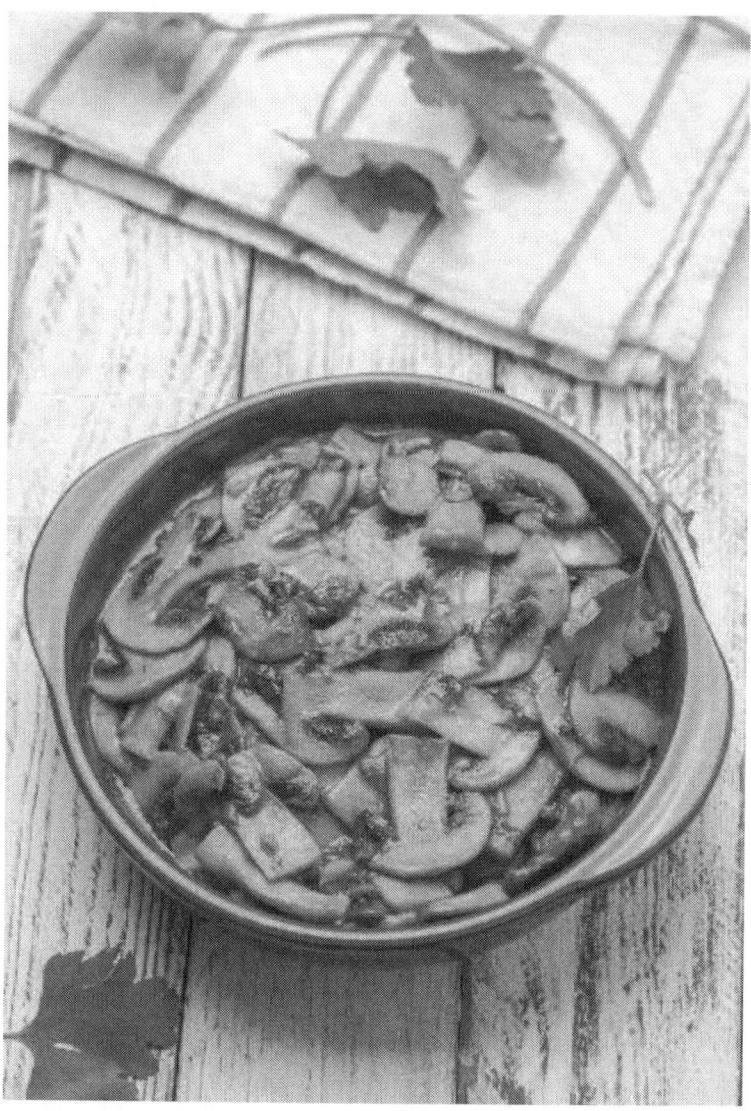

Nutrition Facts

Serving Size 647 g

Amount Per Serving

Calories 325   Calories from Fat 55

	% Daily Value*
Total Fat 6.1g	**9%**
Saturated Fat 1.7g	**9%**
Trans Fat 0.0g	
Cholesterol 143mg	**48%**
Sodium 520mg	**22%**
Potassium 1426mg	**41%**
Total Carbohydrates 30.8g	**10%**
Dietary Fiber 5.5g	**22%**
Sugars 13.5g	
Protein 44.9g	

Vitamin A 41%	•	Vitamin C 43%
Calcium 23%	•	Iron 74%

Nutrition Grade A

* Based on a 2000 calorie diet

Chicken Eggplant Casserole

Ingredients – serves 4 - Allergies: SF, GF, NF

- 3 pounds Eggplant
- Salt and ground black pepper
- 1 tbsp. chopped parsley
- 2 beaten eggs
- 1 cup of low-fat Greek yogurt
- 1/2 cup of shredded cheddar cheese, low-fat
- 1 pound cubed skinless boneless chicken (or turkey) breasts

Instructions

Preheat oven to 375 degrees F. Mix beaten eggs and low-fat yogurt in a separate dish. In a casserole, place 1 layer of eggplant and meat cubes. Sprinkle with salt, pepper, and parsley. Cover with 1/2 of a cup of eggs/yogurt mixture. Repeat process 2 more times and cover with shredded cheese. Bake until eggplant and chicken are tender and crust is golden brown, about 20 minutes. Serve with Large Fiber Loaded salad with Italian Dressing.

Nutrition Facts

Serving Size 590 g

Amount Per Serving

Calories 300	Calories from Fat 52
	% Daily Value*
Total Fat 5.8g	9%
Saturated Fat 1.7g	8%
Trans Fat 0.0g	
Cholesterol 143mg	48%
Sodium 497mg	21%
Potassium 1024mg	29%
Total Carbohydrates 31.1g	10%
Dietary Fiber 12.7g	51%
Sugars 13.3g	
Protein 36.7g	
Vitamin A 22% •	Vitamin C 36%
Calcium 20% •	Iron 37%

Nutrition Grade A

* Based on a 2000 calorie diet

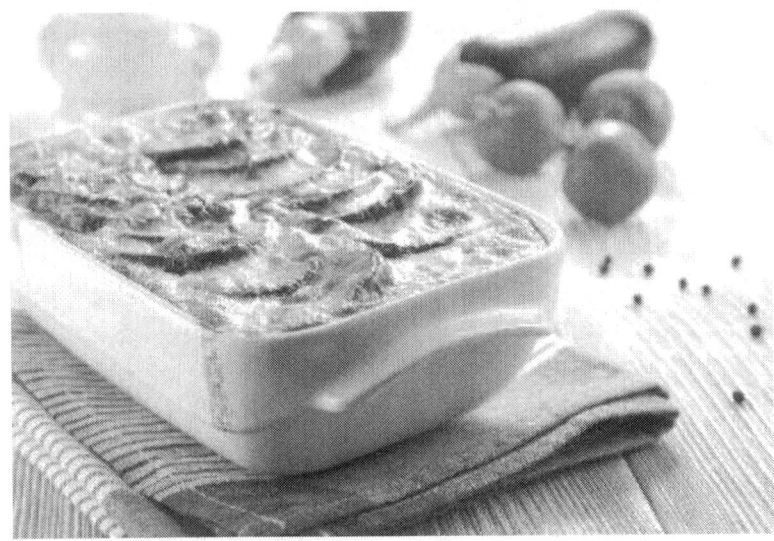

Beef Meatballs Green Beans Casserole

Serves 1

Ingredients - Allergies: SF, GF

- 1 cup green beans florets
- 5 oz. beef meatballs (see separate recipe)
- 1 tsp of almond flour
- Salt, pepper
- 1 egg - beaten

Half a cup of Yogurt Dressing

- 1/4 cup of chicken broth
- 2 tbsp. of grated low-fat cheddar cheese

Instructions

Heat oven to 400°.

Cook green beans around 5 minutes. Prepare beef meatballs as in the recipe above. Combine soup, flour, salt and pepper in a saucepan, stirring with a whisk until smooth. Bring to a boil over medium-high heat; cook 1 minute, stirring constantly. Remove from heat. Add yogurt dressing, beaten egg and then half of the cheese, stirring until well combined. Add sauce to green beans mixture; and stir gently until combined.

Put mixture in a small casserole dish oiled with some coconut oil. Sprinkle with remaining cheese. Bake at 400° for 50 minutes or until mixture bubbles at the edges and cheese begins to brown. Remove from oven and let cool for 5 minutes. Serve with large Fiber Loaded Salad with Italian Dressing.

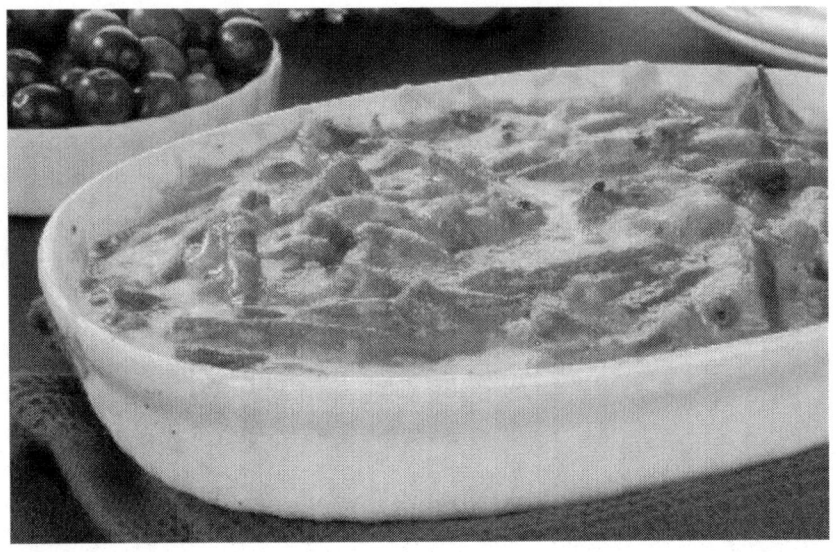

Nutrition Facts

Serving Size 368 g

Amount Per Serving	
Calories 412	Calories from Fat 146
	% Daily Value*
Total Fat 16.2g	**25%**
Saturated Fat 6.5g	**32%**
Trans Fat 0.0g	
Cholesterol 277mg	**92%**
Sodium 728mg	**30%**
Potassium 921mg	**26%**
Total Carbohydrates 12.7g	**4%**
Dietary Fiber 3.3g	**13%**
Sugars 6.2g	
Protein 51.6g	
Vitamin A 32% •	Vitamin C 28%
Calcium 30% •	Iron 130%
Nutrition Grade A-	
* Based on a 2000 calorie diet	

Chicken, Tomato Paste and Olives Casserole

Serves 4

Ingredients - Allergies: SF, GF, DF, EF, NF

- 1 cup chopped carrots
- 1/2 cup chopped red peppers
- 1/2 cup chopped onions
- 1 pound young potatoes
- 1/2 cup olives
- 2 tbsp. oil
- 2 cups tomato paste - see recipe at the beginning
- 1/2 tsp. salt
- 1/4 tsp. ground black pepper
- 1 tsp. minced garlic
- 2 pounds chicken pieces

Instructions

Put all recipe ingredients in the casserole dish, cover and bake for 2.5 hours on 400F.

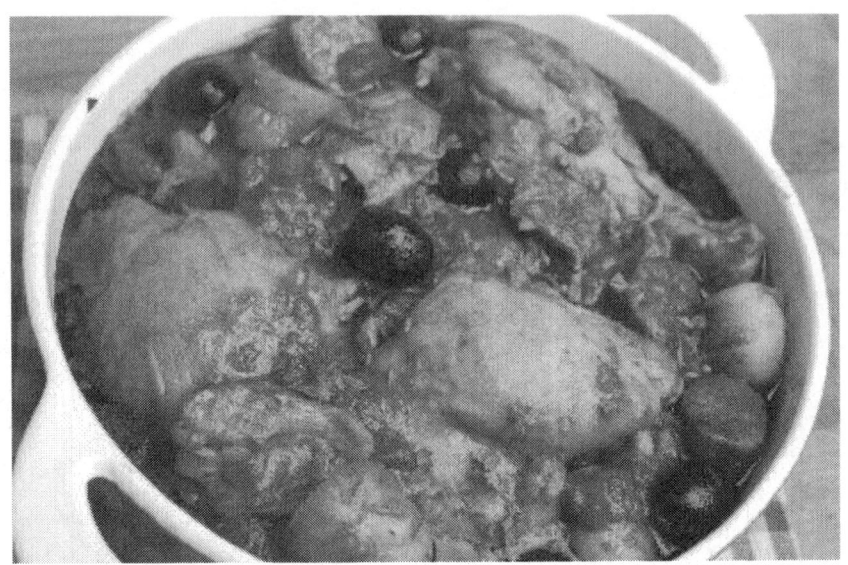

Chicken, Carrot and Mushrooms Casserole

Serves 4

Ingredients - Allergies: SF, GF, DF, EF, NF

- 2 cups chopped carrots
- 1/2 cup chopped onions
- 1 cup chicken stock
- 2 tbsp. oil
- 1/2 tsp. salt
- 1/4 tsp. ground black pepper
- 1 tsp. minced garlic
- 2 pounds chicken
- 1 Tbsp. Dill

Instructions

Put all recipe ingredients in the casserole dish, cover and bake for 2 hours on 400F.

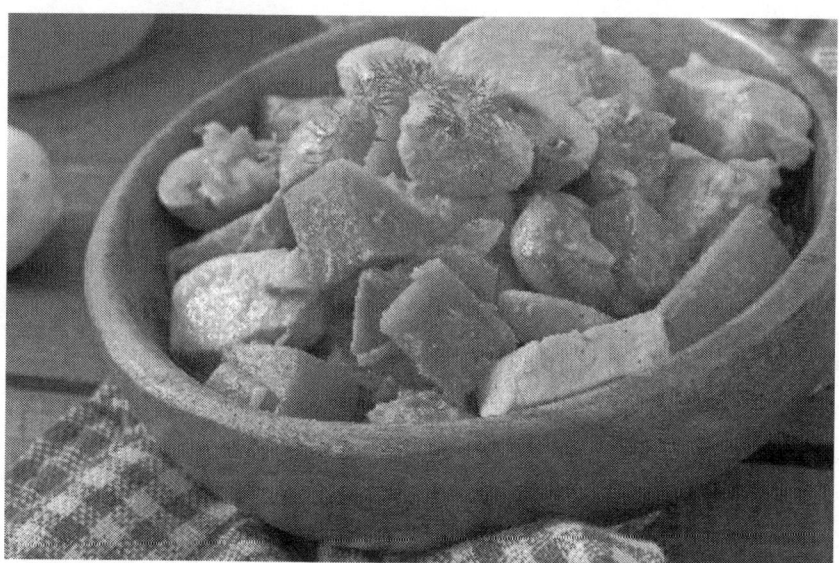

Pork Liver Casserole

Serves 4

Ingredients - Allergies: SF, GF, DF, EF, NF

- 1/2 cups chopped carrots
- 1 cup chopped red peppers
- 1 cup chopped onions
- 2 tbsp. oil
- 1 cup tomato paste - see recipe at the beginning
- 1 cup beef stock
- 1/2 tsp. salt
- 1/4 tsp. ground black pepper
- 1 tsp. minced garlic
- 2 pounds pork liver, sliced
- 1 Tsp. turmeric

Instructions

Put all recipe ingredients in the casserole dish, cover and bake for 2 hours on 400F.

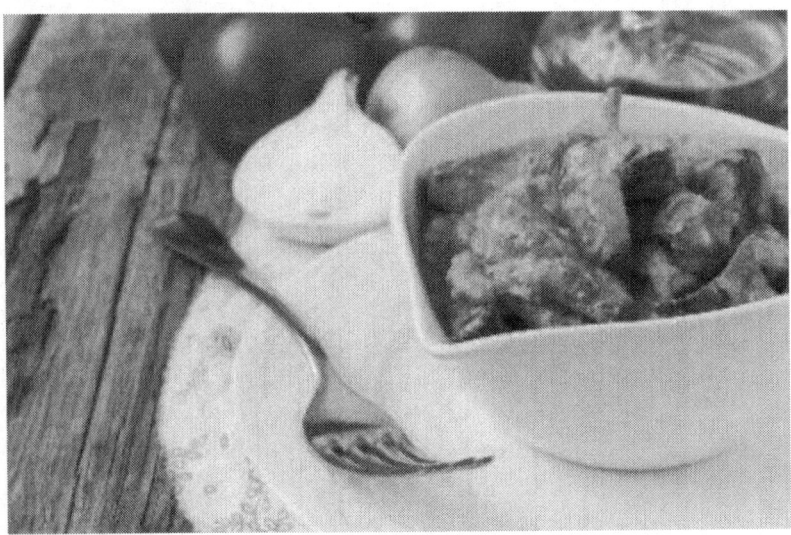

Salmon Broccoli Casserole

Serves 4

Ingredients - Allergies: SF, GF, NF

- 2 cups broccoli florets
- 1/2 cup chopped onions
- 2 tbsp. oil
- 2 cups healthy casserole sauce
- 1/2 tsp. salt
- 1/4 tsp. ground black pepper
- 1 tsp. minced garlic
- 2 pounds slamon steaks, quartered

Instructions

Put all recipe ingredients but sauce in the casserole dish, pour sauce on top, cover and bake for 2 hours on 400F.

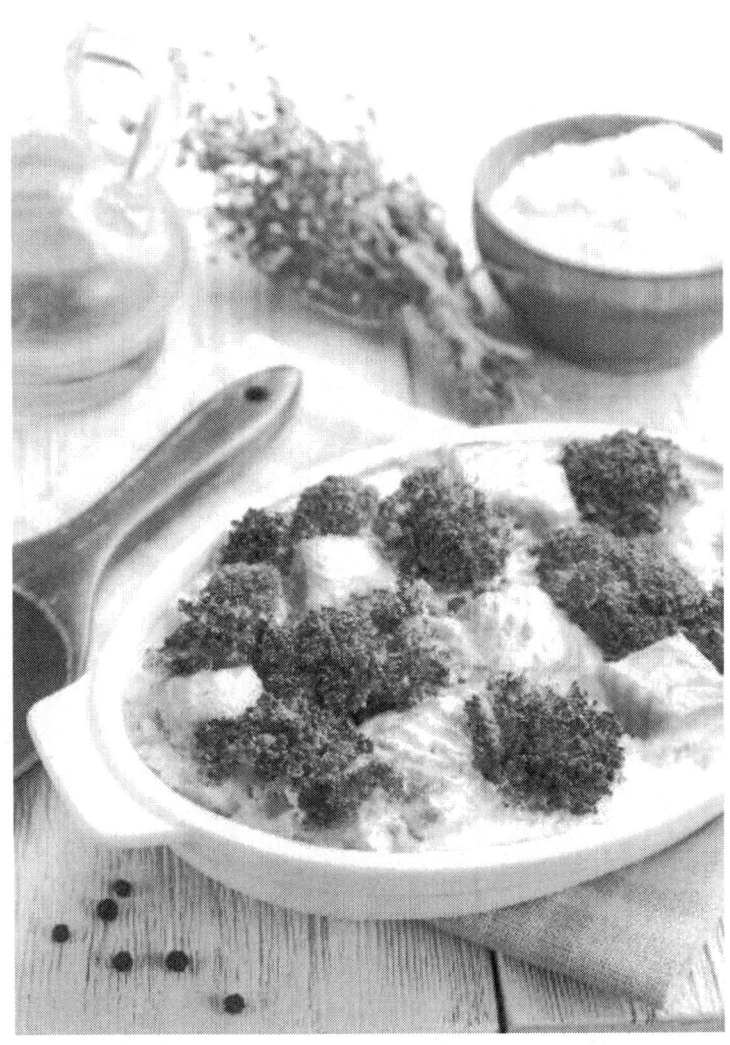

Salmon, Tomato Paste and Mushrooms Casserole

Serves 4

Ingredients - Allergies: SF, GF, DF, EF, NF

- 1/2 cups chopped carrots
- 1/2 cup chopped onions
- 2 cups chopped mushrooms
- 2 tbsp. oil
- 2 cups tomato paste - see recipe at the beginning
- 1/2 tsp. salt
- 1/4 tsp. ground black pepper
- 1 tsp. minced garlic
- 2 pounds salmon filets

Instructions

Put all recipe ingredients in the casserole dish, cover and bake for 2 hours on 400F.

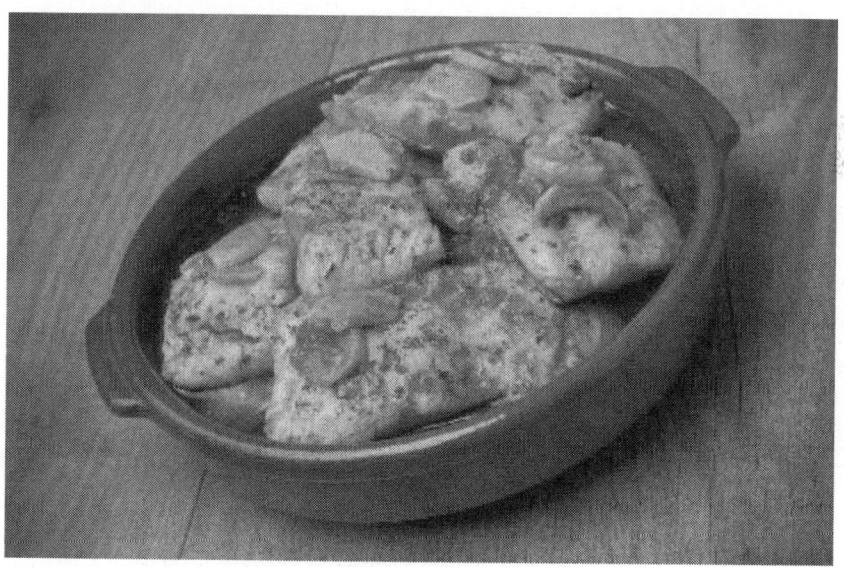

Zucchini Noodles & Slivered Almonds Casserole

Serves 4

Ingredients - Allergies: SF, GF, DF, EF, NF

- 1/2 cups chopped carrots
- 5 cups raw zucchini noodles (use spiralizer)
- 1/2 cup chopped onions
- 2 cups toasted slivered almonds
- 2 tbsp. oil
- 1/2 tsp. salt
- 1/4 tsp. ground black pepper

Instructions

Put all recipe ingredients in the casserole dish, cover and bake for 45 minutes on 400F.

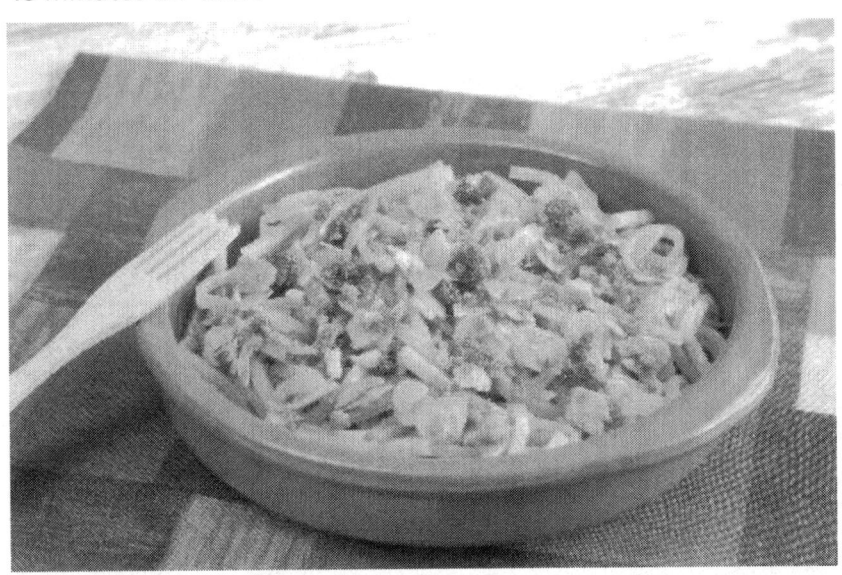

Lamb and Red Kidney Beans Casserole

Serves 4

Ingredients - Allergies: SF, GF, DF, EF, NF

- 1/2 cups chopped carrots
- 2 cups cooked red kidney beans
- 1 cup chopped onions
- 2 tbsp. oil
- 1 cups tomato paste - see recipe at the beginning
- 1/2 tsp. salt
- 1/4 tsp. ground black pepper
- 1 cup beef broth
- 1 tsp. minced garlic
- 2 pounds lamb steaks

Instructions

Put all recipe ingredients in the casserole dish, cover and bake for 2 hours on 400F.

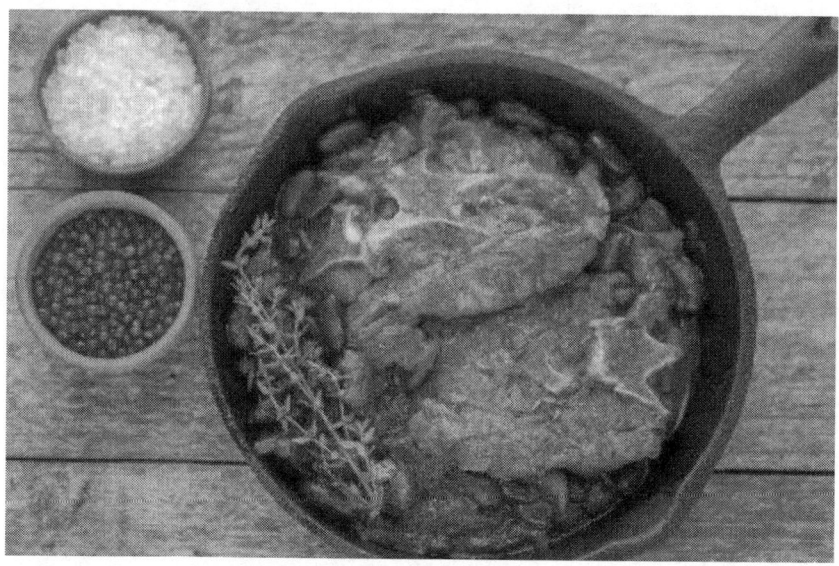

Beet & Beef Casserole

Serves 4

Ingredients - Allergies: SF, GF, DF, EF, NF

- 1 cup chopped tomatoes
- 1/2 cup chopped onions
- 2 tbsp. oil
- 2 cups chopped beets
- 1 chopped carrot
- 1 bay leaf
- 1 cup red wine - optional
- 1 Tbsp chopped rosemary
- 1/2 tsp. salt
- 1/4 tsp. ground black pepper
- 2 tsp. minced garlic
- 2 pounds beef cut into the small chunks

Instructions

Put all recipe ingredients in the casserole dish and bake for 3 hours on 400F. Garnish with dill.

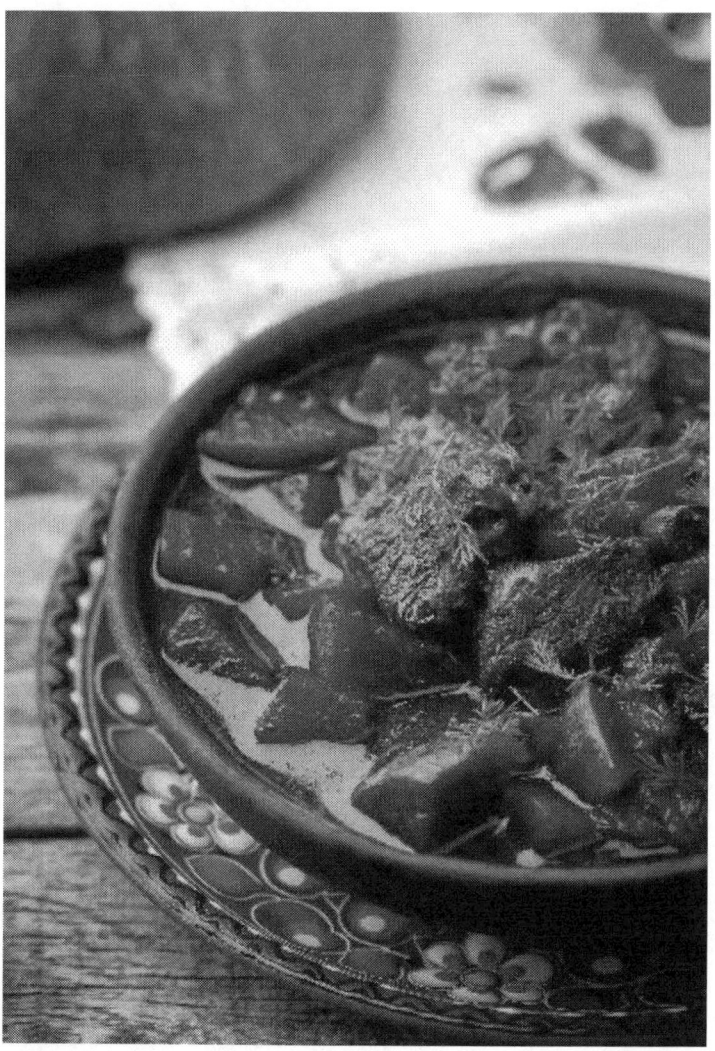

"Breaded" "fried" food
Breaded Tilapia

Ingredients - Allergies: SF, GF, DF, NF

Recipe is for 4 servings.

- 1 cup coconut meal for breading
- 1/2 tsp. pepper
- 1/2 tsp. minced garlic
- 1/2 tsp. paprika
- 1/4 tsp. salt
- 2 large egg whites (or whole eggs), beaten
- 1 pound tilapia fillets, cut into 1/2-by-3-inch strips

Instructions

Heat oven to 400°F. Set a wire rack on a baking sheet and coat with some coconut oil.

Place coconut, pepper, garlic, paprika and salt in a blender and process until finely ground. Transfer to a shallow dish.

Place egg whites in a second dish. Dip every piece of fish in the egg and then coat all sides with the coconut breading mixture. Place on the prepared rack. Sprinkle some drops of olive oil over each piece.

Bake until the fish is cooked through. Breading should be golden brown. Serve with large Fiber loaded salad.

Nutrition Facts

Serving Size 189 g

Amount Per Serving

Calories 261   Calories from Fat 130

	% Daily Value*
Total Fat 14.4g	22%
Saturated Fat 1.3g	7%
Trans Fat 0.0g	
Cholesterol 137mg	46%
Sodium 227mg	9%
Potassium 103mg	3%
Total Carbohydrates 9.6g	3%
Dietary Fiber 8.6g	34%
Sugars 0.8g	
Protein 30.3g	

Vitamin A 17%   •   Vitamin C 14%
Calcium 9%   •   Iron 18%

Nutrition Grade B-

* Based on a 2000 calorie diet

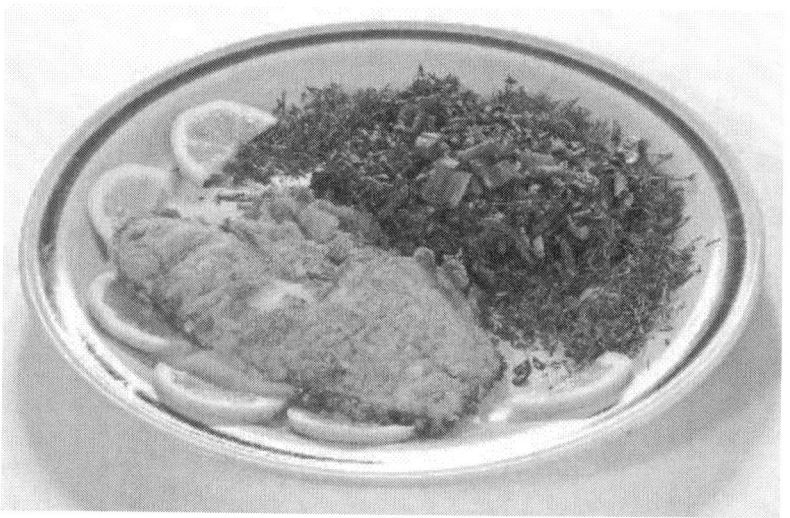

Breaded Chicken

Ingredients - Allergies: SF, GF, DF, NF

Recipe is for 4 servings.

- 1 cup flax seeds meal for breading
- 1/2 tsp. pepper
- 1/2 tsp. minced garlic
- 1/2 tsp. paprika
- 1/4 tsp. salt
- 2 large egg whites (or whole eggs), beaten
- 1 pound skinless, boneless chicken pieces

Instructions

Heat oven to 400°F. Set a wire rack on a baking sheet; coat with some coconut oil.

Place flax, pepper, garlic, paprika and salt in a food processor or blender and process until finely ground. Transfer to a shallow dish.

Place egg whites in a second dish. Dip every piece of chicken in the egg and then coat all sides with the flax breading mixture. Place on the prepared rack. Sprinkle some drops of olive oil over each piece.

Bake until the chicken is cooked through and the breading is golden brown and crisp, about 8 minutes each side. Serve with large Fiber loaded salad.

Nutrition Facts

Serving Size 189 g

Amount Per Serving

Calories 384	Calories from Fat 196
	% Daily Value*
Total Fat 21.8g	**34%**
Saturated Fat 3.2g	**16%**
Trans Fat 0.0g	
Cholesterol 183mg	**61%**
Sodium 285mg	**12%**
Potassium 378mg	**11%**
Total Carbohydrates 9.6g	**3%**
Dietary Fiber 8.6g	**34%**
Sugars 0.8g	
Protein 42.0g	
Vitamin A 18%	Vitamin C 14%
Calcium 8%	Iron 19%

Nutrition Grade B+

* Based on a 2000 calorie diet

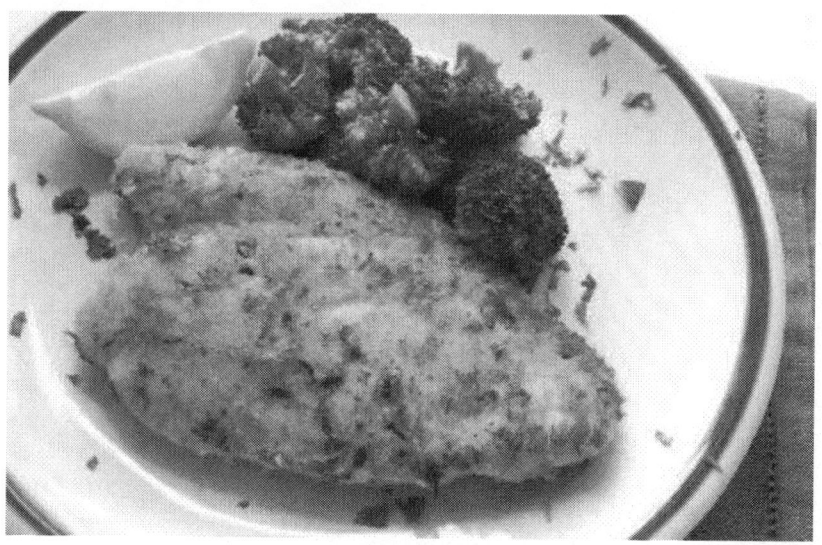

Lemon Pork with Asparagus

Serves: 3-4

Ingredients - Allergies: SF, GF, DF, EF, NF
- 1 lb. pork chops
- 1/4 cup buckwheat flour
- 1/2 tsp. salt
- 2 tbsp. coconut oil
- Pepper
- 1 cup chopped asparagus
- 2 lemons, sliced

Instructions

Place the flour and salt in a dish and gently toss each chop in the dish to coat. Melt the coconut oil in a large skillet over medium/high heat. Add the chicken and sauté until golden brown on each side. Sprinkle each side with the pepper directly in the pan.

When the chops are cooked through, transfer them to a plate. Add the lemon slices and asparagus to the pan. When the asparagus and the lemons are done, add the chops back to the pan.

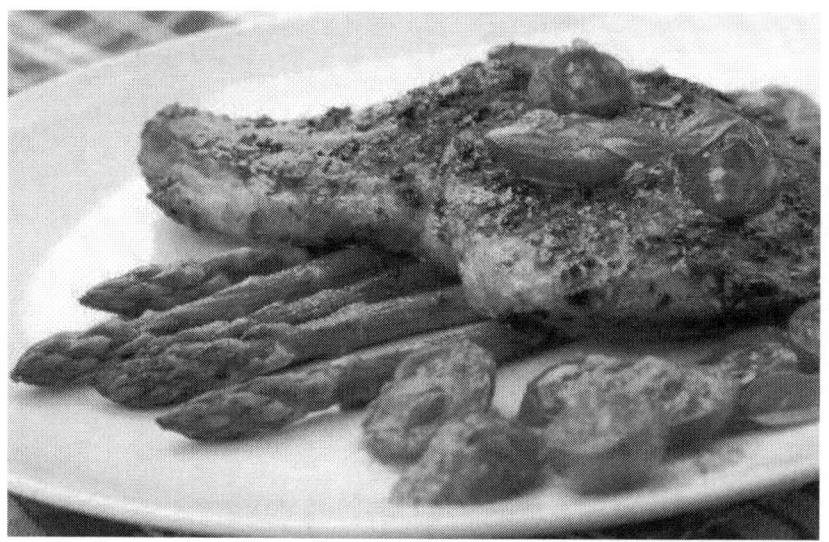

Pizza

Meat Pizza

Serves 4

Ingredients - Allergies: SF, GF, EF, NF

- 1 cup cooked and minced chicken breast
- 1 cup low-fat cheddar, shredded
- 1 tbsp. minced onion & few basil leaves
- 1 tsp garlic minced

Instructions

Preheat oven to 425 degrees Fahrenheit. Process chicken, onion and garlic together. Mixture will be a dense crumb consistency. Press chicken mixture on parchment paper on a cookie sheet. Bake for 12 minutes. Let cool for five minutes.

Top with 1/4 cup of tomato sauce, a handful of low-fat cheese, basil and mushrooms (shiitake). Bake for 6-8 minutes more, or until toppings are melted. Let cool for five minutes. Slice and serve. Alternatively, you may want to try cauliflower crust version:

Grate half of the large cauliflower and steam it for 15 minutes. Squeeze the excess water out and let cool. Mix in 2 eggs, one cup low-fat mozzarella, and salt and pepper. Pat into a 10-inch round on the prepared cookie sheet. Brush with oil and bake until golden. Add the topping as above.

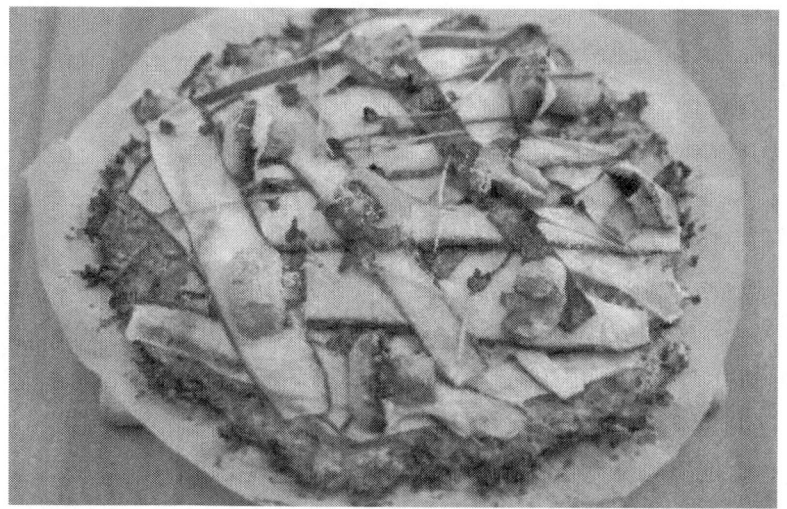

Side dishes

Roasted curried cauliflower
Serves 10

Ingredients - Allergies: SF, GF, DF, EF, NF

- 12 cups cauliflower florets
- 1 chopped large onion
- 1 tsp. coriander seeds
- 1 tsp. cumin seeds
- 3/4 cup olive oil or avocado oil
- 1/2 cup lemon juice
- 3 1/2 teaspoons curry paste
- 1 tbsp. hot paprika
- 1 3/4 teaspoons salt
- 1/4 cup chopped cilantro

Instructions

Heat oven to 450°F. Place cauliflower florets in large roasting pan. Add onions to cauliflower. Dry toast coriander and cumin seeds in a skillet over medium heat until slightly browned, about 5 minutes. Crush in mortar with pestle. Place seeds in bowl. Whisk in oil, lemon juice, curry paste, paprika, and salt. Pour dressing over vegetables and toss to coat. Spread vegetables in single layer and sprinkle with pepper.

Roast vegetables until tender, stirring occasionally, about 35 minutes.

Sprinkle cilantro and serve warm.

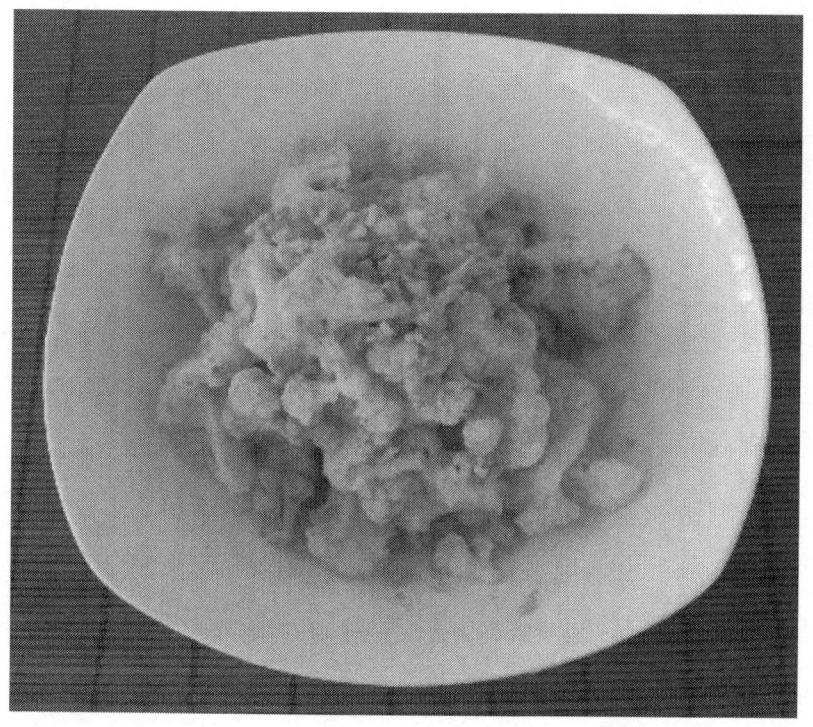

Roasted cauliflower with Tahini sauce

Serves 6

Ingredients - Allergies: SF, GF, DF, EF, V, NF

- 1/4 cup extra-virgin <u>olive</u> oil or <u>avocado</u> oil
- 4 tsp. ground cumin
- 2 heads cauliflower, cored and cut into 1 1/2" florets
- Salt and ground black pepper
- 1/2 cup tahini
- 3 cloves garlic, smashed and minced into a paste
- Juice of 1 lemon

Instructions

Roast cauliflower like in the previous recipe.
Meanwhile, combine tahini, lemon juice, garlic, and 1/2 cup water in a bowl and season with salt. Serve cauliflower hot or at room temperature with tahini sauce.

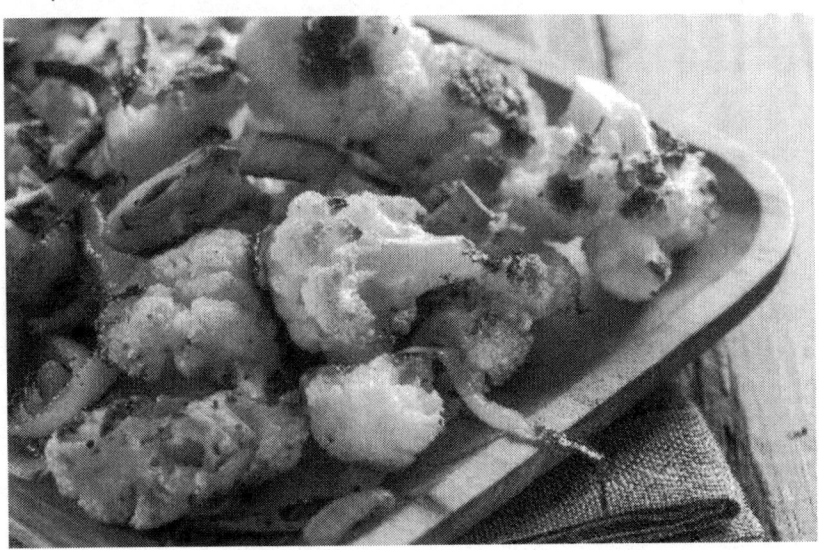

Baked Sweet Potatoes

Serves 2

Ingredients - Allergies: SF, GF, DF, EF, V, NF

- 2 medium sweet potatoes

Instructions

Heat oven to 425 degrees F. Quarter sweet potatoes and place them in a casserole with a lid. Bake until tender when pierced with a fork (40 minutes approx.).

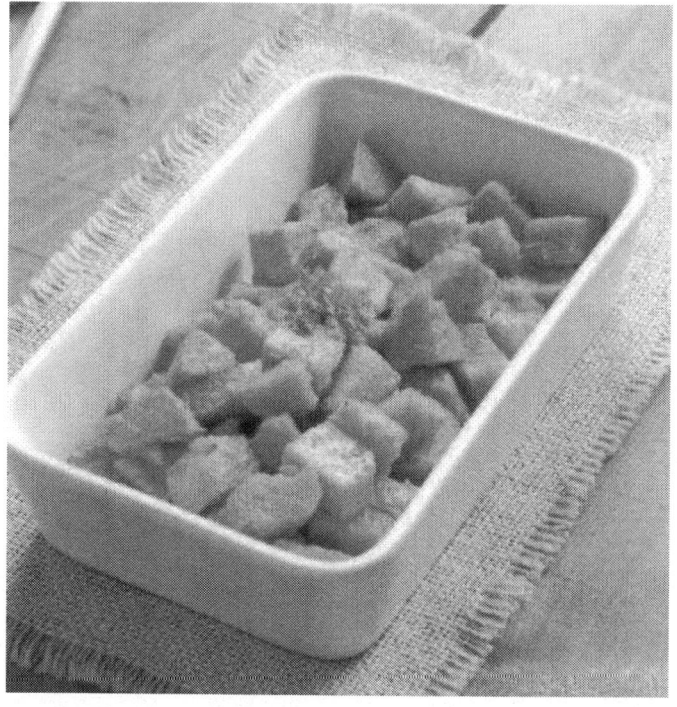

Asparagus with mushrooms and hazelnuts

Serves 4

Ingredients - Allergies: SF, GF, DF, EF, V

- 2 tbsp. lemon juice
- 1/4 tsp sea salt
- Ground black pepper, to taste
- 1 pound fresh asparagus, ends trimmed
- 2 tbsp. coconut oil
- 6 cups mushrooms
- 1/2 cup green onions, sliced
- 2 tbsp. hazelnuts, toasted and finely chopped

Instructions

Add the lemon juice, 1 tbsp. of the oil, salt, and pepper in a small bowl. Boil water in a pan and add the asparagus. Boil for few minutes. Heat the remaining 1 tbsp. oil in a pan on high heat. Add mushrooms and cook them until they are soft. Add green onions and sauté 1 more minute. Add the asparagus, and cook another 3 minutes. Remove from the heat and slowly add in the lemon juice mixture. Add the toasted hazelnuts over the top.

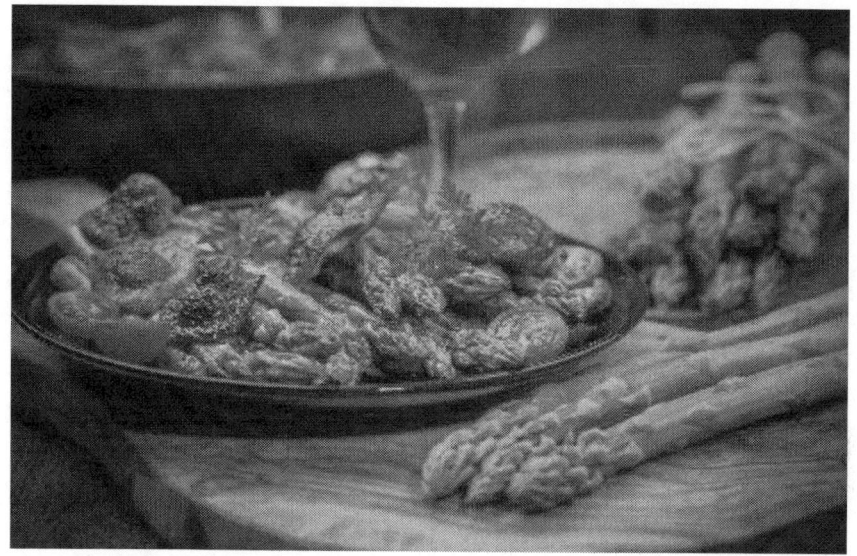

Chard and Cashew Sauté

Serves 2

Ingredients - Allergies: SF, GF, DF, EF, V, NF

- 1 bunch Swiss chard
- 1/2 cup cashews
- 1 tbsp. coconut oil
- Sea salt (optional)
- Ground black pepper

Instructions

Wash Swiss chard and remove tough stems. Heat a skillet over medium heat, and add oil when hot. Chop Swiss chard into thin strips. Add Swiss chard to the hot skillet, along with cashews. Sauté only 1 minute. Season with sea salt and ground black pepper according to taste and serve warm.

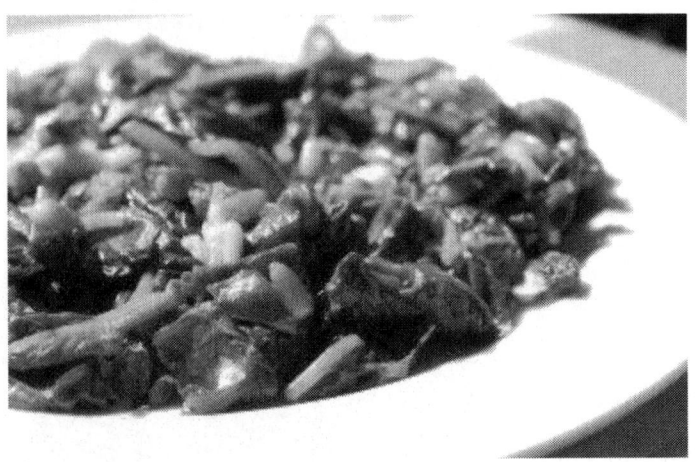

Cauliflower rice side dish

Serves 2

Ingredients - Allergies: SF, GF, DF, EF, V, NF

- 1 head cauliflower
- 2 Tbs coconut oil
- Sea salt, garlic, ginger or ground black pepper (optional seasonings)

Instructions

Place the cauliflower into a food processor and pulse it until a grainy rice-like consistency. Season with sea salt and ground black pepper. Meanwhile, heat a large pan over high heat. Add coconut oil when hot. Sauté cauliflower in a pan with oil and any additional seasonings if desired.

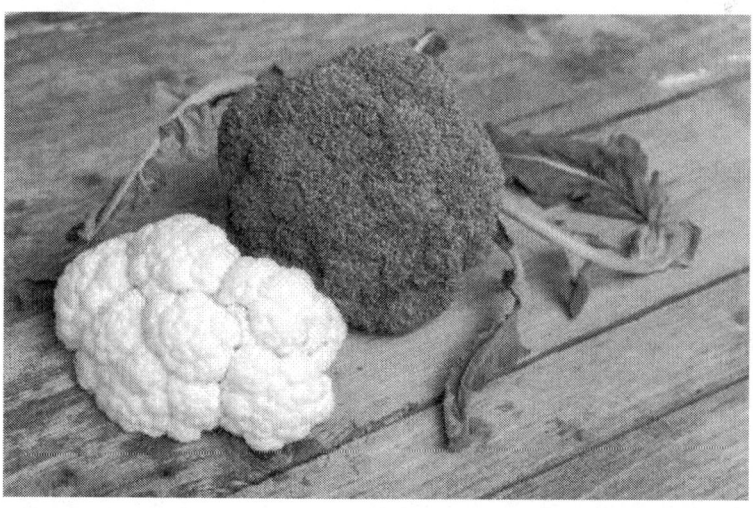

Crockpot

Slow Cooker Pepper Steak
Serves 4-6

Ingredients - Allergies: SF, GF, DF, EF, NF

- 2 pounds beef sirloin, cut into 2 inch strips
- 1 tbsp. minced garlic
- 3 tbsp. coconut oil
- 1 cup Beef Broth

- 1 tbsp. tapioca flour
- 1/2 cup chopped onion
- 2 cups carrots
- 1 cup chopped tomatoes
- 1 tsp. salt

Instructions

Sprinkle beef with minced garlic. Heat the coconut oil in a skillet and brown the seasoned beef sirloin strips. Transfer to a slow cooker.
Mix in tapioca flour in broth until dissolved. Pour broth into the slow cooker with meat. Add carrots, onion, chopped tomatoes and salt. Cover and cook on high for 3 to 4 hours, or on low for 6 to 8 hours.

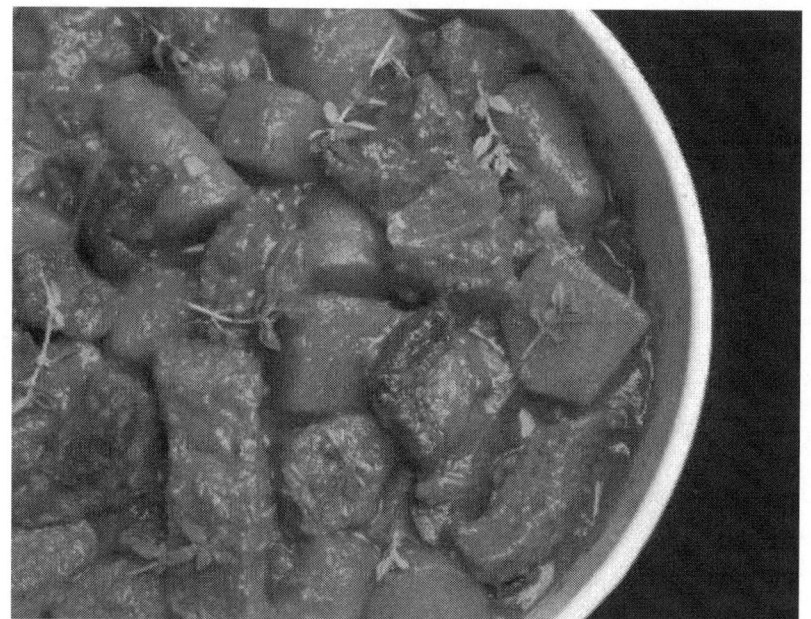

Pork Tenderloin with peppers and onions
Serves 3-4

Ingredients - Allergies: SF, GF, DF, EF, NF

- 1 tbsp. coconut oil
- 1 pound pork loin
- 1 tbsp. caraway seeds
- 1/2 tsp sea salt
- 1/4 tsp ground black pepper
- 1 red onion, thinly sliced
- 2 red bell peppers, sliced
- 4 cloves of garlic, minced
- 1/4-1/3 cup chicken broth

Instructions

Wash and chop vegetables. Slice pork loin, and season with black pepper, caraway seeds and sea salt. Heat a pan over medium/high heat. Add coconut oil when hot. Add pork loin and brown slightly. Add onions and mushrooms, and continue to sauté until onions are translucent. Add peppers, garlic and chicken broth. Simmer until vegetables are tender and pork is fully cooked.

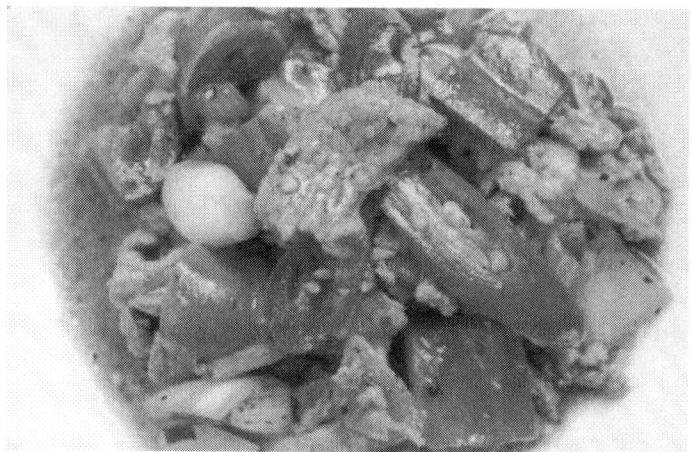

Beef Bourguinon

Serves 8-10

Ingredients - Allergies: SF, GF, DF, EF

- 4 pounds cubed lean beef
- 1 cup red wine
- 1/3 cup coconut oil
- 1 tsp. thyme
- 1 tsp. black pepper
- 2 cloves garlic, crushed
- 1 onion, diced
- 1 pound mushrooms, sliced
- 1/3 cup almond flour

Instructions

Marinate beef in wine, oil, thyme and pepper for few hours at room temperature or 6-8 hours in the fridge. Cook garlic and onion in a pan until soft. Add mushrooms. Cook until they are browned. Drain beef liquid. Place beef in slow cooker. Sprinkle flour over the beef and stir to coat. Add mushroom mixture on top. Pour reserved marinade over all. Cook on low for 7-9 hrs.

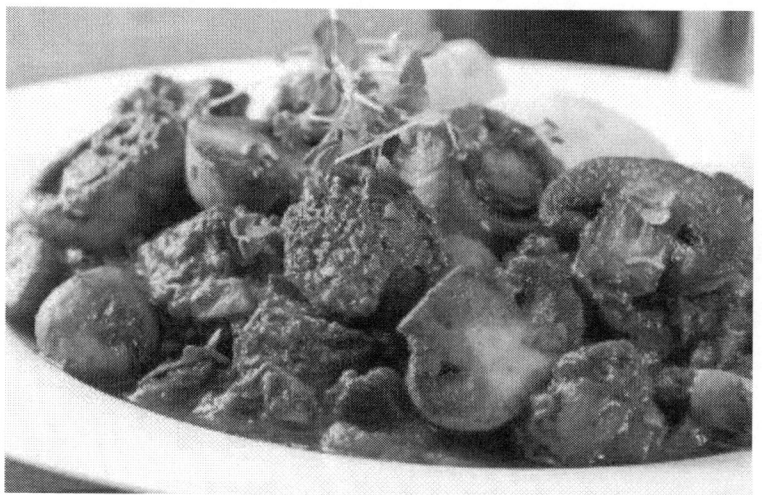

Italian Chicken

Serves 6-8

Ingredients - Allergies: SF, GF, DF, EF

- 1 skinless chicken, cut into pieces
- 1/4 cup almond flour
- 1 1/2 tsp. salt
- 1/8 tsp. pepper
- 1/2 cup chicken broth
- 1 cup sliced mushrooms
- 1/2 tsp. paprika
- 1 zucchini, sliced into medium pieces
- ground black pepper
- parsley to garnish

Instructions

Season chicken with 1 tsp. salt. Combine flour, pepper, remaining salt, and paprika. Coat chicken pieces with this mixture. Place zucchini first in a crockpot. Pour broth over zucchini. Arrange chicken on top. Cover & cook on low for 6 to 8 hours or until tender. Turn control to high, add mushrooms, cover, and cook on high for additional 10-15 minutes. Garnish with parsley and ground black pepper.

FOOD FOR DIABETICS

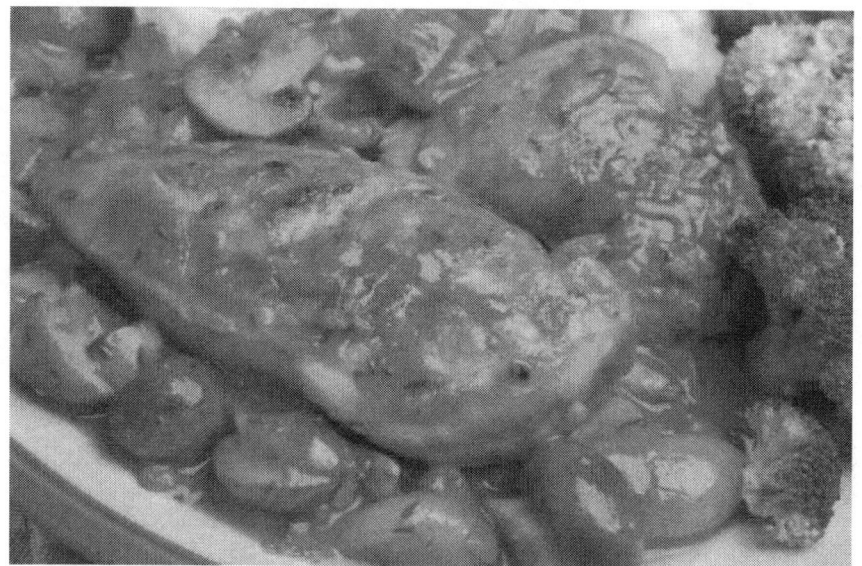

Ropa Vieja

Ingredients - Allergies: SF, GF, DF, EF, NF

6 servings

- 1 tbsp. coconut oil
- 2 pounds beef flank steak
- 1 cup beef broth
- 1 cup tomato sauce
- 1 small onion, sliced
- 1 green bell pepper sliced into strips
- 2 cloves garlic, chopped
- 1/2 cup tomato paste
- 1 tsp. ground cumin
- 1 tsp. chopped cilantro
- 1 tbsp. olive oil & 1 tbsp. lemon juice

Instructions

Heat oil in a skillet over high heat. Brown the flank steak on each side (4 minutes per side). Move the beef to a slow cooker. Add in the beef broth and tomato sauce, then add the onion, bell pepper, garlic, tomato paste, cumin, cilantro, olive oil and lemon juice. Stir until blended. Cover, and cook on high for 4 hours, or on Low for up to 8 hours. When ready to serve, shred meat and serve with brown rice or quinoa and salad.

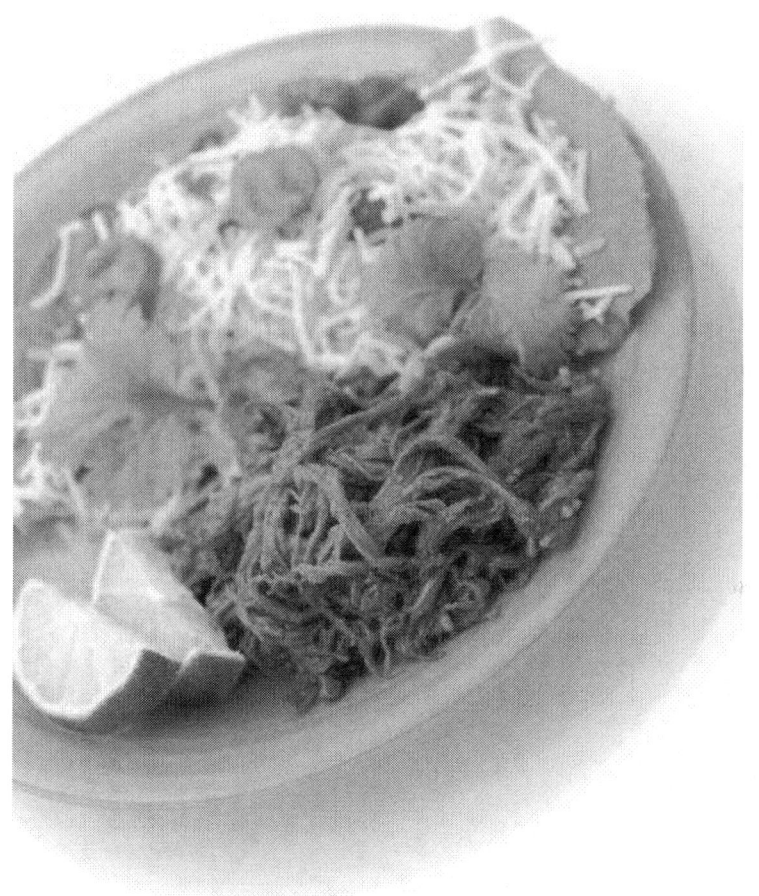

Lemon Roast Chicken

Serves 6-8

Ingredients - Allergies: SF, GF, DF, EF, NF

- 1 whole skinless chicken
- 1 dash Salt
- 1 dash Pepper
- 1 tsp. Oregano
- 2 cloves minced garlic
- 2 tbsp. coconut oil
- 1/4 cup Water
- 3 tbsp. Lemon juice

- Rosemary

Instructions

Wash chicken and season with salt and pepper. Sprinkle half of oregano and garlic inside chicken cavity. Add coconut oil to a frying pan. Brown chicken on all sides and transfer to crock pot. Sprinkle with oregano and garlic. Add water to fry pan and stir to loosen brown bits. Pour into crock pot and cover. Cook on low 7 hours. Add lemon juice when cooking is done. Transfer chicken to cutting board and carve chicken. Skim fat. Pour juice into sauce bowl. Serve with rosemary and some juice over chicken.

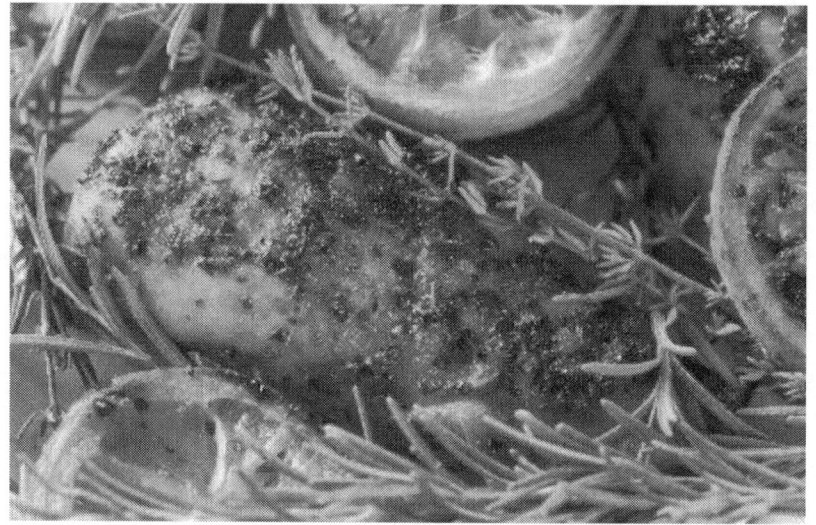

Fall Lamb and Vegetable Stew

Serves 6-8

Ingredients - Allergies: SF, GF, DF, EF, NF

- 2 pounds Lamb stew meat
- 2 chopped Tomatoes
- 1 Summer squash
- 1 Zucchini
- 1 cup Mushrooms, sliced
- 1/2 cup Bell peppers, chopped
- 1 cup Onions, chopped
- 2 teaspoons Salt
- 1 Garlic cloves, crushed
- 1/2 tsp. Thyme leaves
- 1 Bay leaves
- 2 cups chicken broth

Instructions

Cut squash and zucchini. Place vegetables and lamb in crockpot. Mix salt, garlic, thyme, and bay leaf into broth and pour over lamb and vegetables. Cover & cook on low for 7 hours. Serve over brown rice.

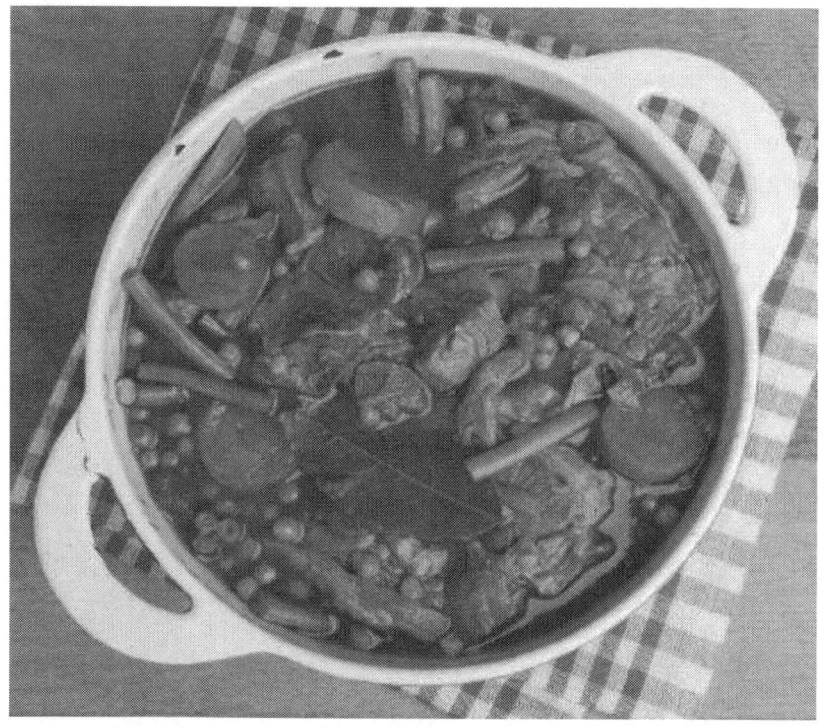

Slow cooker pork loin

Serves 4-6

Ingredients - Allergies: SF, GF, DF, EF, NF

- 1-1/2 lb pork loin
- 1 cup tomato sauce
- 2 zucchinis, sliced
- 1 head cauliflower, separated into medium florets
- 1-2 Tbs dried basil
- 1/4 tsp ground black pepper
- 1/2 tsp sea salt (optional)

Instructions

Add all of the ingredients to a crock pot.

Cook on high for 3-4 hours or low 7-8 hours.

FOOD FOR DIABETICS

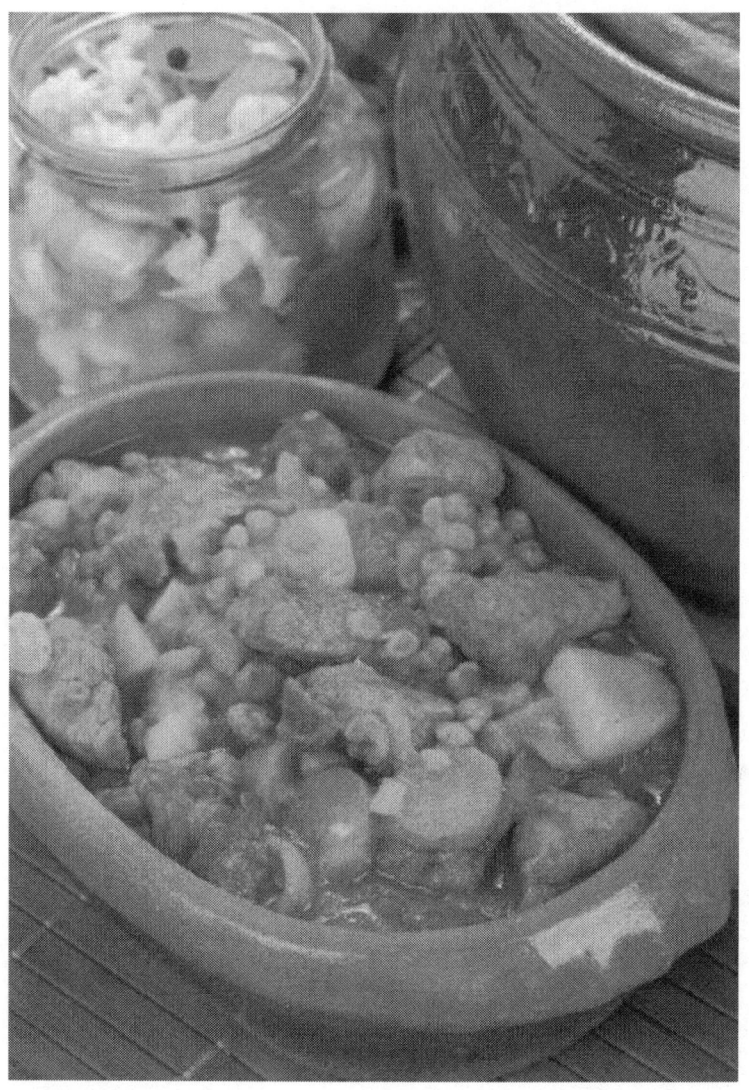

Sauerbraten

Serves 6-8

Ingredients - Allergies: SF, GF, DF, EF, NF

Marinade

- Water -- 2 cups
- Lemon juice – 1/2 cup
- Red wine -- 1 cup
- Peppercorns -- 1 tbsp.
- Juniper berries -- 8
- Whole cloves -- 4
- Bay leaves -- 2

Roast

- Beef rump or round -- 3 to 4 pounds
- Salt and pepper -- to season
- <u>coconut</u> oil -- 3 tbsp.
- Onion, thinly sliced -- 1
- Carrot, cut into thin rounds -- 2
- Celery, thinly chopped -- 1 stalk

Instructions

Place the marinade ingredients (except lemon juice) into a pot and bring to a boil. Boil for 5 minutes then remove and cool to room temperature. Add lemon juice.

Place the beef in a large glass dish and pour the marinade. Make sure that beef is covered with the marinade.

Set the roast and its marinade in the fridge and marinade for at least few hours. Turn the beef once or twice daily.

Remove the roast from the marinade and season with salt and pepper. Brown the roast well on all sides and set aside.

Add the celery, onion and carrot to the pot and sauté until the onion is cooked translucent. Put the roast to the pot and add in the marinade. Bring to a boil, then reduce heat to medium-low. Cover the pot and simmer until the roast is fork tender.

Remove the roast and set it aside. Strain the sauce and discard the solids and return the liquid to the pot. Bring to a simmer and add in the salt and pepper and simmer for few minutes more.

Variations

- **Meats**: Pork, lamb or venison.
- **Marinade Variations**: Nutmeg, ginger, thyme and coriander.

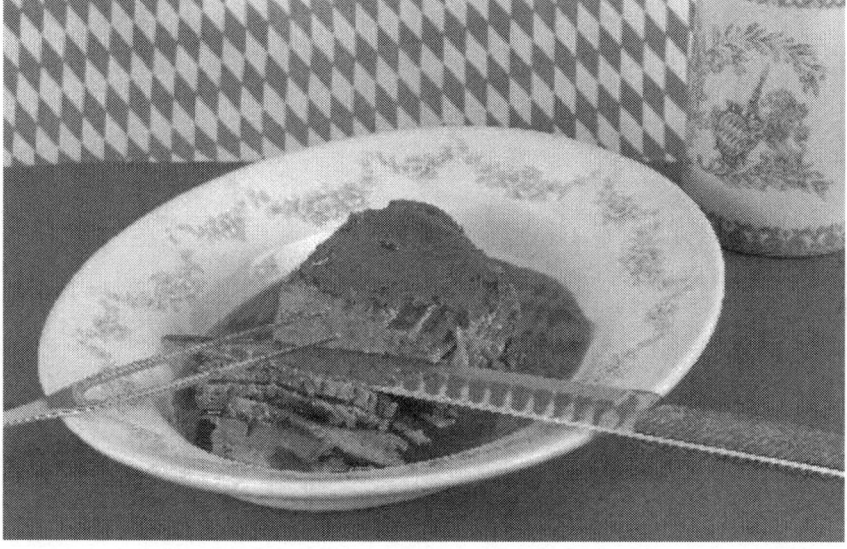

Fish

Cioppino

Serves 6

Ingredients - Allergies: SF, GF, DF, EF, NF

- 3/4 cup coconut oil
- 2 onions, chopped
- 2 cloves garlic, minced
- 1 bunch fresh parsley, chopped
- 1,5 cups stewed tomatoes
- 1,5 cups chicken broth
- 2 bay leaves
- 1 tbsp. dried basil
- 1/2 tsp. dried thyme
- 1/2 tsp. dried oregano
- 1 cup water
- 1-1/2 cups white wine
- 1-1/2 pounds peeled and deveined large shrimp
- 1-1/2 pounds bay scallops
- 18 small clams
- 18 cleaned and debearded mussels
- 1-1/2 cups crabmeat
- 1-1/2 pounds cod fillets, cubed

Instructions

Over medium heat melt coconut oil in a large stockpot and add onions, parsley and garlic. Cook slowly, stirring occasionally until onions are soft. Add tomatoes to the pot. Add chicken broth, oregano, bay leaves, basil, thyme, water and wine. Mix well.

Cover and simmer 30 minutes.

Stir in the shrimp, scallops, clams, mussels and crabmeat. Stir in fish. Bring to boil. Lower heat, cover and simmer until clams open.

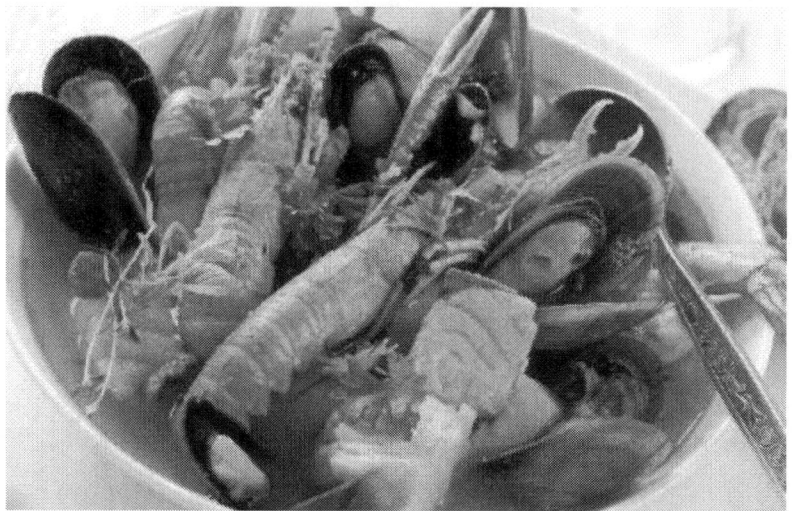

Flounder with Orange Coconut Oil
Serves 6

Ingredients - Allergies: SF, GF, DF, EF, NF

- 3 1/2 lbs. flounder
- 3 tbsp. white wine
- 3 tbsp. lemon juice
- 3 tbsp. coconut oil
- 3 tbsp. parsley
- 1 tsp. black pepper
- 2 tbsp. orange zest
- 1/2 tsp. salt
- 1/2 cup chopped scallions

Instructions

Preheat oven to 325F. Sprinkle fish with pepper and salt.
Place fish in the baking dish. Sprinkle orange zest on top of the fish. Melt remaining coconut oil and add the parsley and scallions to the coconut oil and pour over flounder. Then add in the white wine.
Place in oven and bake for 15 minutes. Serve fish with extra juice on a side.

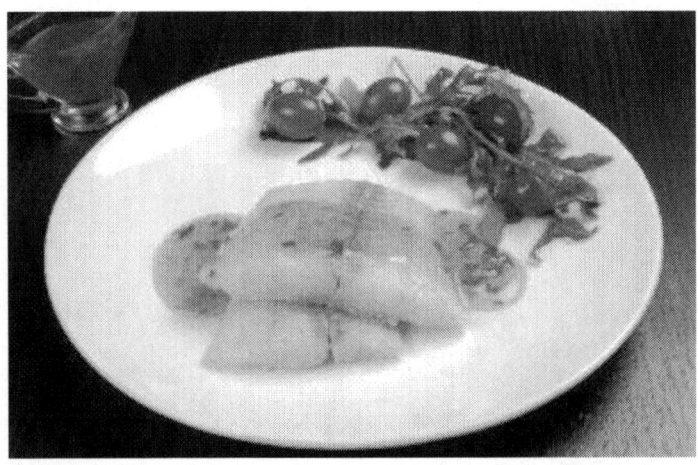

Grilled Salmon
Serves 4

Ingredients - Allergies: SF, GF, DF, EF, NF

- 4 (4 ounce) filets salmon
- 1/4 cup <u>coconut</u> oil
- 2 tbsp. fish sauce
- 2 tbsp. lemon juice
- 2 tbsp. thinly sliced green onion
- 1 clove garlic, minced & 3/4 tsp. ground ginger
- 1/2 tsp. crushed red pepper flakes
- 1/2 tsp. sesame oil
- 1/8 tsp. salt

Instructions

Whisk together coconut oil, fish sauce, garlic, ginger, red chili flakes, lemon juice, green onions, sesame oil, and salt. Put fish in a glass dish, and pour marinade over. Cover and refrigerate for 4 hours.
Preheat grill. Place salmon on grill. Grill until fish becomes tender. Turn halfway during cooking.

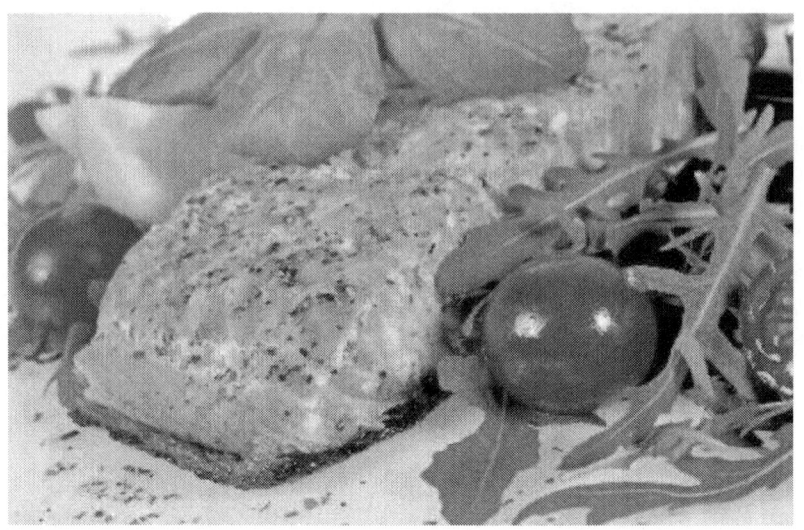

Crab Cakes
Serves 6-8

Ingredients - Allergies: SF, GF, DF, NF

- 3 lbs. crabmeat
- 3 beaten eggs
- 3 cups flax seeds meal
- 3 tbsp. mustard
- 2 tbsp. grated horseradish
- 1/2 cup coconut oil
- 1 tsp. lemon rind
- 3 tbsp. lemon juice
- 2 tbsp. parsley
- 1/2 tsp. cayenne pepper
- 2 tsp. fish sauce

Instructions

In medium bowl combine all ingredients except oil. Shape in to smallish hamburgers. In fry pan heat oil and cook patties for 3-4 minutes on each side or until golden brown. Optionally, bake them in the oven.
Serve as appetizers or as main course with large fiber salad.

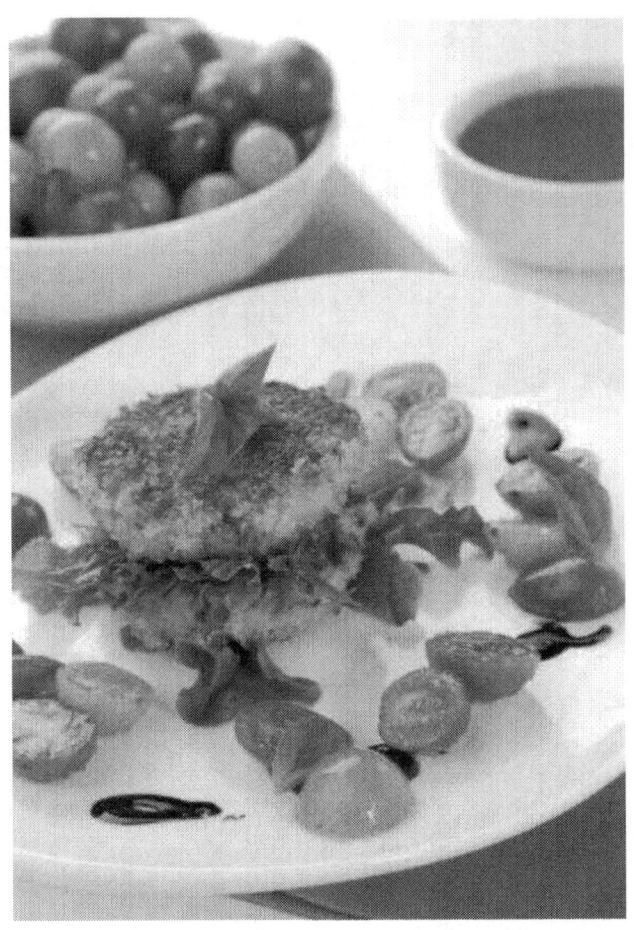

Sweets

Superfoods Dark Chocolate

Instructions - Allergies: SF, GF, DF, EF, V, NF

Mix 1/4 cup of coconut oil with 1/4 to 1/2 cup of cocoa powder (unsweetened, ideally organic and unprocessed) and some lucuma powder to taste. You really should experiment with cocoa and honey amount. Maybe start with equal amount of coconut oil, cocoa and honey, mix it and then increase amount of cocoa to your taste. Form balls or put in the ice cube tray. Put it in the fridge and 1 hour later you'll have great homemade Superfoods chocolate!

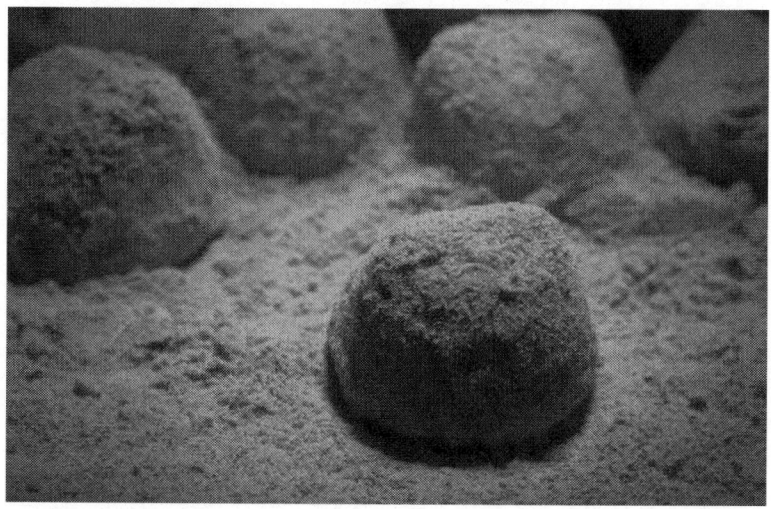

Fruits dipped in Superfoods chocolate

Ingredients - Allergies: SF, GF, DF, EF, V

- 2 apples or 2 bananas or a bowl of strawberries or any fruit that can be dipped in melted chocolate
- 1/2 cup of melted superfoods chocolate (see earlier recipe)
- 2 tbsp. chopped nuts (almond, walnut, Brazil nuts) or seeds (hemp, chia, sesame, flax seeds meal)

Instructions

Cut apple in wedges or cut banana in quarters. Melt the chocolate and chop the nuts. Dip fruit in chocolate, sprinkle with nuts or seeds and lay on tray. Transfer the tray to the fridge so the chocolate can harden; serve. If you don't want chocolate, cover fruits with almond or sunflower butter and sprinkle with chia or hemp seeds and cut it into chunks and serve.

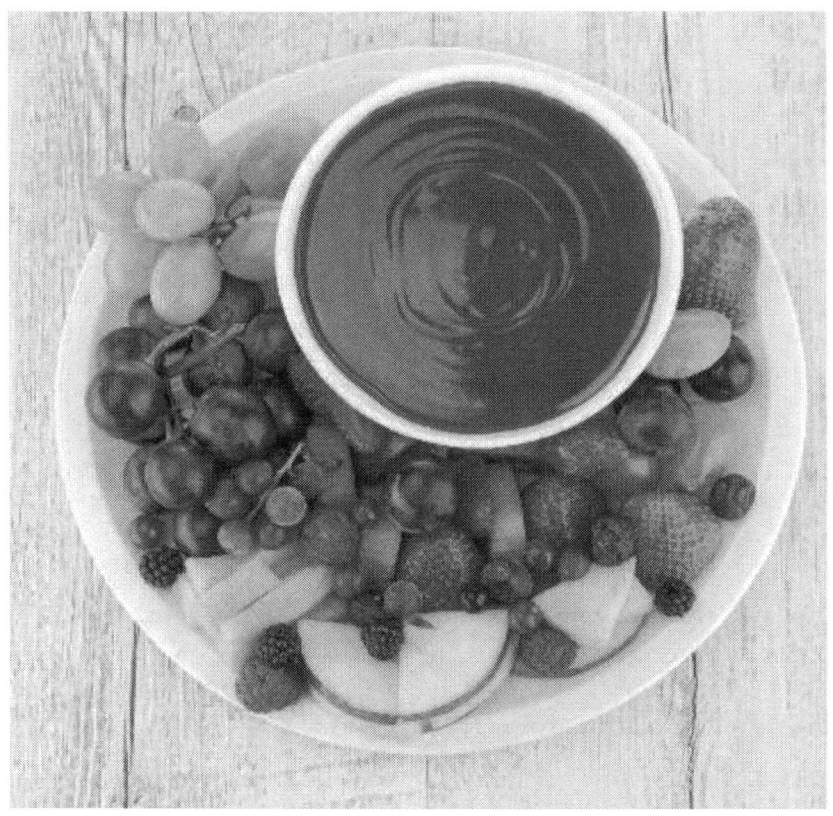

Superfoods No-Bake Cookies

Ingredients - Allergies: SF, GF, DF, EF, V

- 1/2 cup coconut milk
- 1/2 cup cocoa powder
- 1/2 cup coconut oil
- 1/2 cup lucuma powder
- 2 cups finely shredded coconut
- 1 cup large flake coconut
- 2 tsp of ground vanilla bean
- 1/2 cup chopped almonds or chia seeds (optional)
- 1/2 cup almond butter (optional)

Instructions

Combine the coconut milk, coconut oil and cacao powder in a saucepan. Cook the mixture over medium heat, stirring until it comes to a boil and then boil for around 1 minute. Remove the mixture from the heat and stir in the shredded coconut, large flake coconut, lucuma powder and the vanilla. Add additional ingredients if you want. Spoon the mixture to a parchment lined baking sheet to cool.

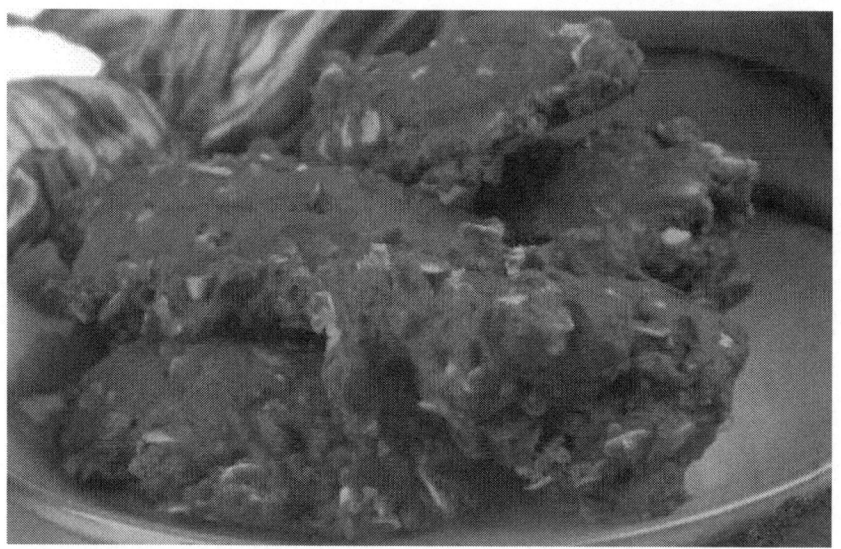

Raw Brownies

Ingredients - Allergies: SF, GF, DF, EF, V
- 1 1/2 cups walnuts
- 1/4 cup pitted dates, soaked overnight and drained
- 1/2 cup tahini
- 1 1/2 tsp. ground vanilla bean
- 1/3 cup unsweetened cocoa powder
- 1/3 cup almond butter

Instructions

Add walnuts and salt to a food processor or blender. Mix until finely ground.

Add the vanilla, dates, and cocoa powder to the blender. Mix well and optionally add a couple drops of water at a time to make the mixture stick together.

Transfer the mixture into a pan and top with almond butter.

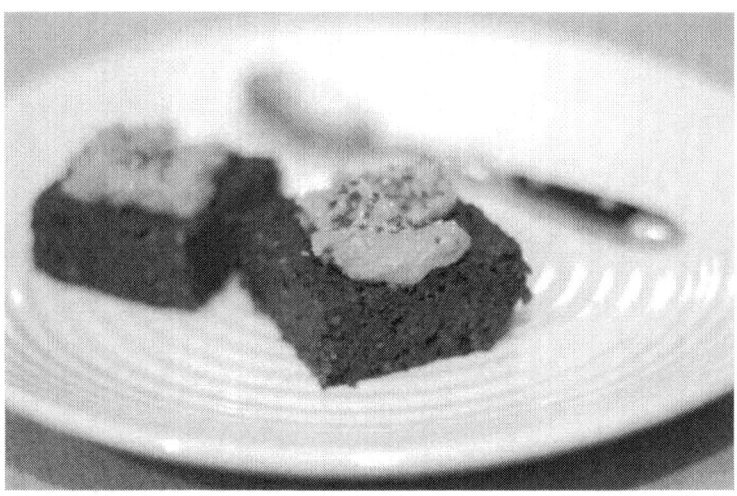

Superfoods Ice cream

Allergies: SF, GF, DF, EF, V, NF

Freeze a banana cut into chunks and process it in blender once frozen and add half a tsp. of cinnamon or 1 tsp. of cocoa or both and eat it as ice-cream.

Other option would be to add one spoon of almond butter and mix it with mashed banana, it's also a delicious ice cream.

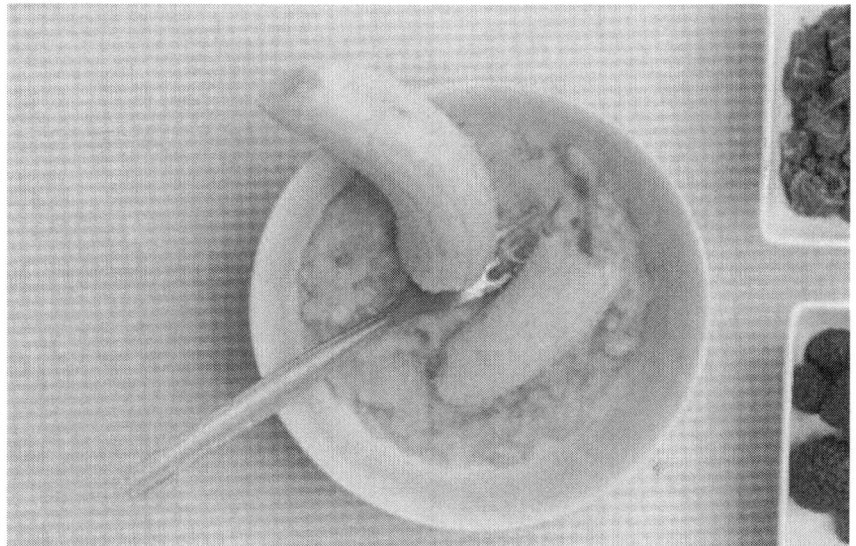

Apple Spice Cookies

Ingredients - Allergies: SF, GF, DF, EF, V

- 1 cup unsweetened almond butter
- 1/2 cup lucuma powder
- 1 egg & 1/2 tsp salt
- 1 apple, diced
- 1 tsp cinnamon
- 1/4 tsp ground cloves
- 1/8 tsp nutmeg
- 1 tsp fresh ginger, grated

Instructions

Heat oven to 350 degrees F. Combine almond butter, egg, lucuma powder and salt in a bowl. Add apple, spices, and ginger and stir. Spoon batter onto a baking sheet 1 inches apart. Bake until set. Remove cookies and allow to cool on a cooling rack.

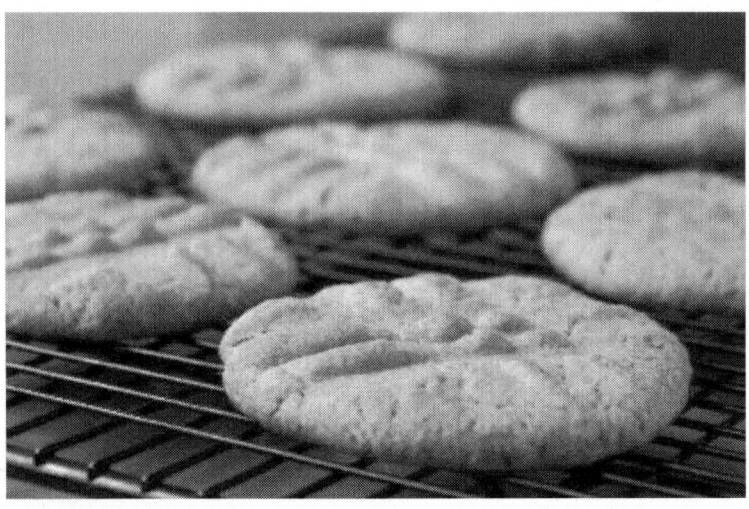

Superfoods Macaroons

Ingredients - Allergies: SF, GF, DF, NF

- 3 egg whites
- 1/2 cup lucuma powder
- 1/4 tsp. salt
- 1 cup unsweetened flaked coconut
- 1/2 cup soft dried apricots, coarsely chopped (3 ounces)

Heat the oven to 325 degrees. Whisk together egg whites, sugar, and salt in a bowl until frothy. Add apricots and coconut and mix to combine.

Shape mixture into mounds with hands and place one inch apart on baking sheet.

Bake until lightly golden, 35 to 40 minutes. Rotate sheet halfway through. You can cover them with Superfoods Dark Chocolate.

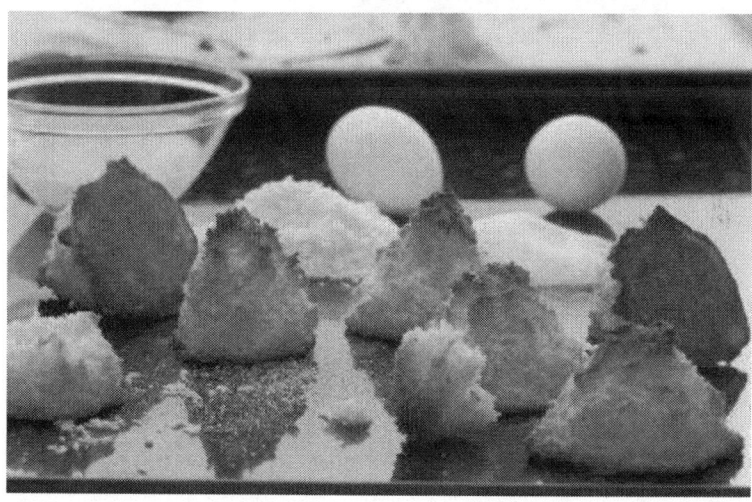

Superfoods Stuffed Apples

Allergies: SF, GF, DF, EF, V

Core 10 apples, fill them with Superfoods No Bake Balls mix and bake them in the oven for 25-30 minutes.

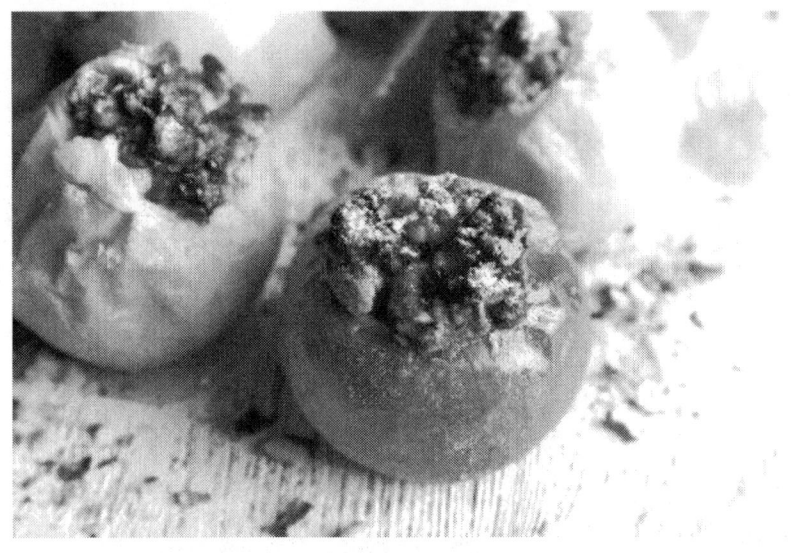

Whipped Coconut cream

Ingredients - Allergies: SF, GF, DF, EF, V, NF

- 4 cups of any fresh berries
- 2 lemons
- 1 can full fat coconut milk (14 oz.), refrigerated overnight
- 1 tsp of ground vanilla bean
- 2 Tbsp. lucuma powder
- Dash of cardamom, nutmeg and clove (optional)

Instructions

Separate coconut cream from the milk by putting it overnight in the fridge. Don't shake it before opening.
Open the can of coconut milk and scrape out the cream into a bowl. Use the saved milk for smoothies or other recipes.
Add cardamom, lucuma powder and vanilla. Whip the cream with a hand mixer until fluffy. Put in the fridge.
Wash berries and place in serving bowls or glasses. Squeeze the lemon over the berries. Place a big scoop of cream on top of the berries and serve.

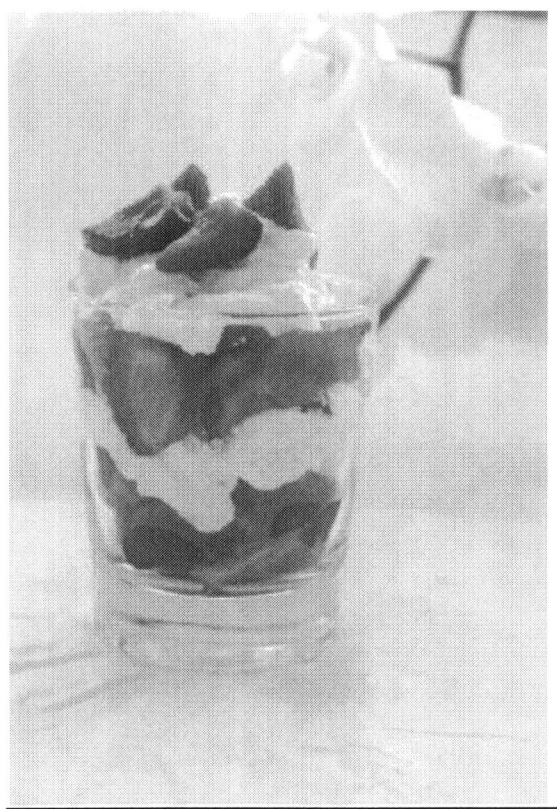

Granola Mix

Ingredients - Allergies: SF, GF, DF, EF, V

- 10 Cup Rolled Oats
- 1/2 Pound Shredded Coconut
- 2 Cup Raw Sunflower Seeds
- 1 Cup Sesame Seeds or chia seeds
- 3 Cup Chopped Nuts
- 1-1/2 Cup -Water
- 1-1/2 Cup coconut oil
- 1 Cup lucuma powder
- 1-1/2 Tsp. Salt
- 2 Tsp. Cinnamon
- 1 tbsp. of ground vanilla bean
- Dried cranberries

Instructions

Turn the oven on and heat oven to 300F. Combine oats, coconut, sunflower seeds, sesame seed, cranberries and nuts (can include almonds, pecans, walnuts, or a combination of all of them). Blend well.
Combine water, oil, lucuma powder, salt, cinnamon and vanilla in a large pan. Heat until lucuma powder is dissolved, but don't boil. Pour the honey over the dry ingredients and stir well. Spread onto cookie sheets. Bake 25 to 30 minutes, and stir occasionally. Let it cool. Store in a cool dry place.

FOOD FOR DIABETICS

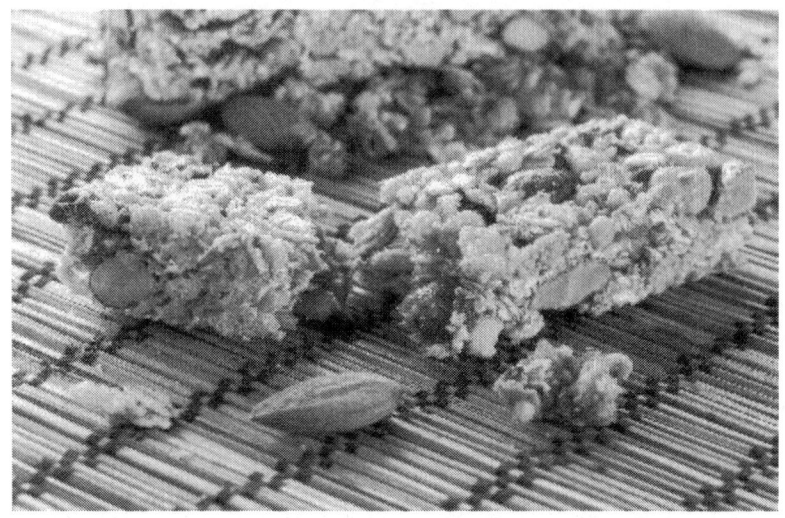

Upside down Apple Cake

Ingredients - Allergies: SF, GF, DF

Bottom Fruit Layer:

- 2 tbsp. coconut oil, melted
- 1 apple, sliced, or 1/4 cup blueberries, plums, banana etc.
- 2 tbsp. walnut chunks
- 2 tbsp. lucuma powder
- 1 tsp ground cinnamon.

Top Cake Layer:

- 2 eggs, beaten.
- 1/3 cup lucuma powder
- 1/4 cup unsweetened coconut milk, or unsweetened almond milk.
- 1 tsp ground vanilla bean
- 1 tsp lemon juice.
- 1 banana, mashed, or 1/4 cup blueberries
- 1/3 cup coconut flour

Instructions

Heat the oven (350 F), and grease a 9 inch cake pan.

Place 2 tbsps. coconut oil into cake pan, and put pan into preheating oven for a couple minutes to melt oil. Make sure oil is evenly distributed all over the bottom of the pan.

Sprinkle 2 tbsps. lucuma powder all over the oil.

Sprinkle 1 tsp cinnamon on top of sweetened layer.

Layer apple slices or blueberries on top of sweetened layer. Add optional walnut pieces to fruit layer. Set aside.

Combine all the "top cake layer" ingredients in a large mixing bowl except for the coconut flour. Mix and add the coconut flour and mix well.

Spoon batter on top of fruit layer and spread evenly.

Bake until center is set.

Remove from oven and let cool.

Slide a butter knife between cake and edge of pan to loosen cake. Turn the pan upside down onto a serving platter. Cake should fall onto plate. If not, use spatula to take the cake out.

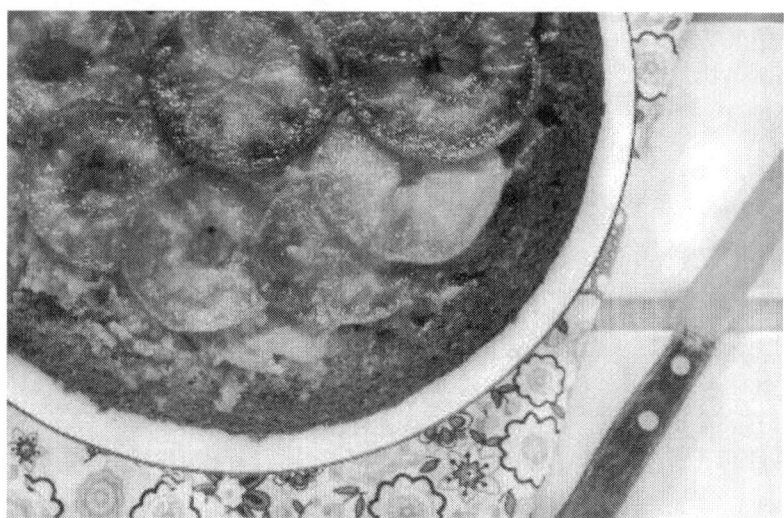

Raw Vegan Reese's Cups

"Peanut" Butter Filling
- 1/2 cup sunflower seeds butter
- 1/2 cup almond butter
- 1 Tbsp. lucuma powder
- 2 Tbsp. melted coconut oil

Superfoods Chocolate Part:
- 1/2 cup cacao powder
- 2 Tbsp. lucuma powder
- 1/3 cup coconut oil (melted)

Instructions

Mix the "Peanut" butter filling ingredients. Put a spoonful of the mixture into each muffin cup.

Refrigerate. Mix Superfoods chocolate ingredients. Put a spoonful of the Superfoods chocolate mixture over the "peanut" butter mixture. Freeze!

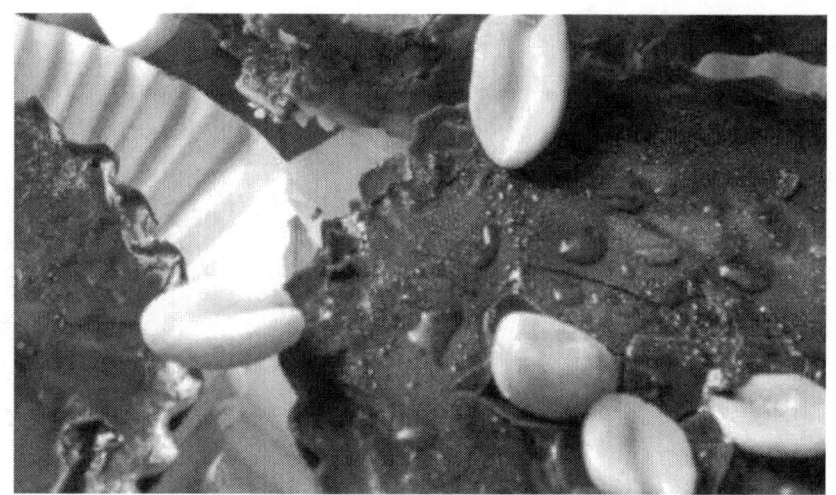

Raw Vegan Coffee Cashew Cream Cake

Coffee Cashew Cream
- 2 cups raw cashews
- 1 tsp. of ground vanilla bean
- 3 tablespoons melted coconut oil
- 1/4 cup lucuma powder
- 1/3 cup very strong coffee or triple espresso shot

Crust
See recipe for Raw Walnuts Pie Crust

Instructions
Blend all ingredients for the cream, pour it onto the crust and refrigerate. Garnish with coffee beans.

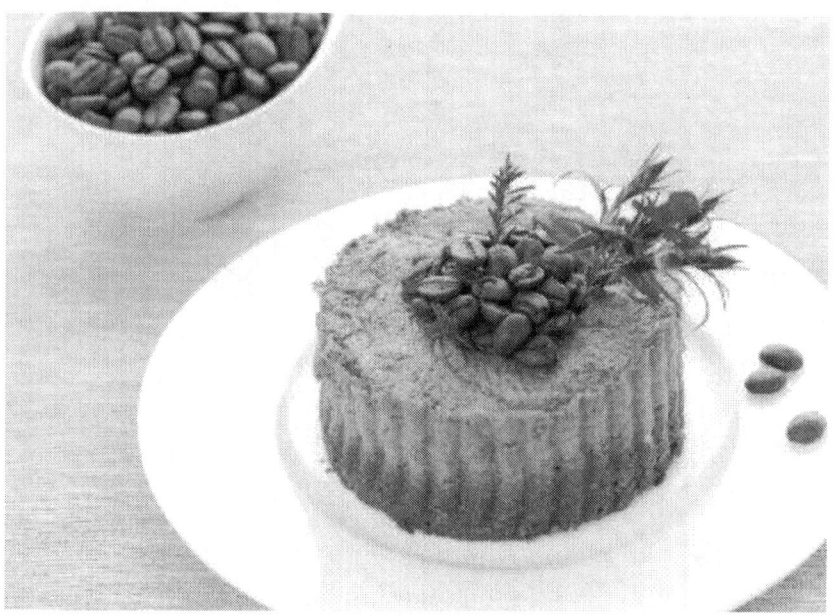

Raw Vegan Chocolate Cashew Truffles

Ingredients

- 1 cup ground cashews
- 1 tsp. of ground vanilla bean
- 1/2 cup coconut oil
- 1/4 cup lucuma powder
- 2 tbsp. flax seeds meal
- 2 tbsp. hemp hearts
- 2 tbsp. cacao powder

Instructions

Mix all ingredients and make truffles. Sprinkle coconut flakes on top.

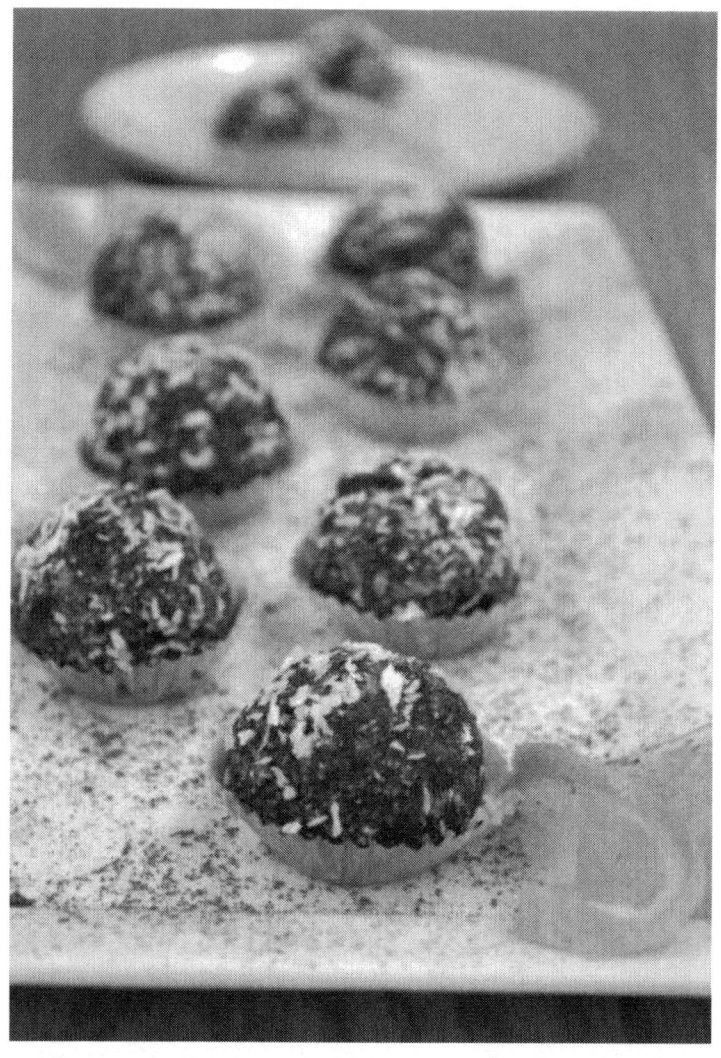

Raw Vegan Double Almond Raw Chocolate Tart

Ingredients

- 1½ cups raw almonds
- ¼ cup coconut oil, melted
- 1 tablespoon lucuma powder or royal jelly
- 8 ounces dark chocolate, chopped
- 1 cup coconut milk
- 1/2 cup unsweetened shredded coconut

Instructions

Crust

Ground almonds and add melted coconut oil, lucuma powder and combine. Using a spatula, spread this mixture into the tart or pie pan.

Filling

Put chopped chocolate in a bowl, heat coconut milk and pour over chocolate and whisk together. Pour filling into tart shell. Refrigerate. Toast almond slivers chips and sprinkle over tart.

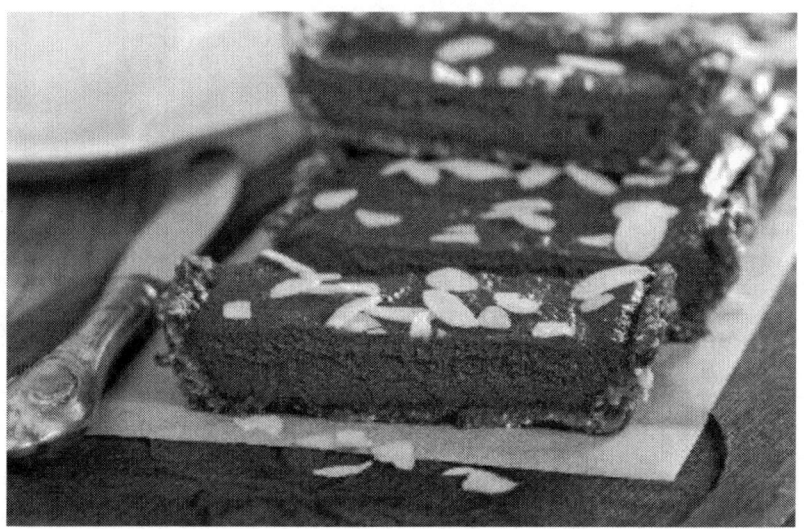

Raw Vegan Bounty Bars

"Peanut" Butter Filling

- 2 cups desiccated coconut
- 3 Tbsp. coconut oil - melted
- 1 cup coconut cream - full fat
- 4 Tbsp. of lucuma powder
- 1 Tsp. ground vanilla bean
- pinch of sea salt

Superfoods Chocolate Part:

- 1/2 cup cacao powder
- 2 Tbsp. lucuma powder
- 1/3 cup coconut oil (melted)

Instructions

Mix coconut oil, coconut cream, honey, vanilla and salt. Pour over desiccated coconut and mix well. Mold coconut mixture into balls, small bars similar to bounty and freeze. Or pour whole mixture into a tray, freeze and cut into small bars.

Make Superfoods Chocolate mixture, warm it up and dip frozen coconut into chocolate and put on a tray and freeze again.

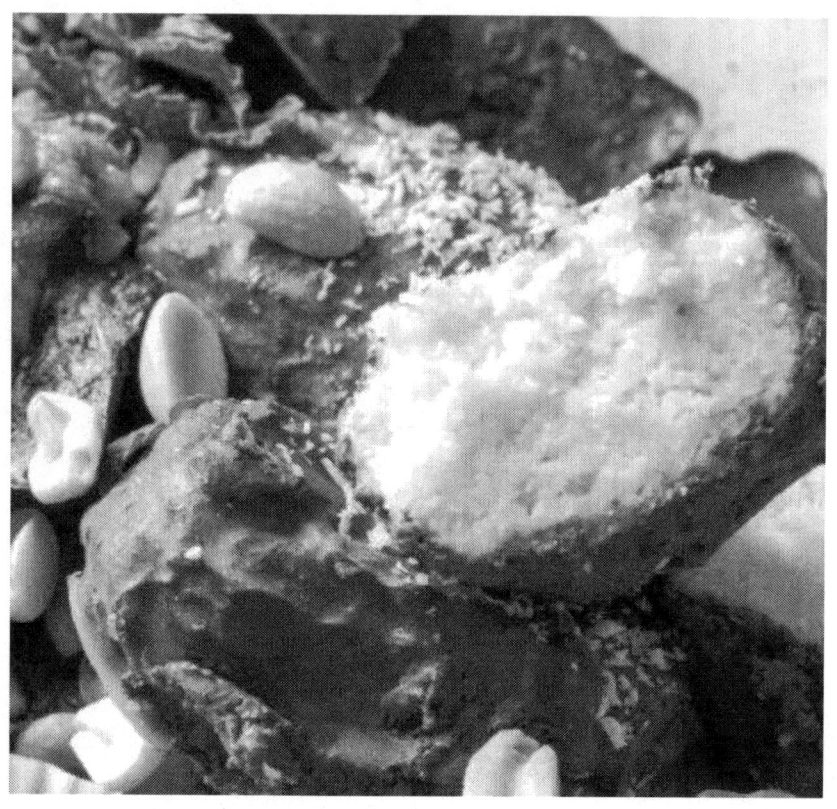

Raw Vegan Tartlets with Coconut Cream

Crust:

See recipe for Raw Walnuts Pie Crust. Make tartlets.

Pudding:

- 1 avocado
- 2 tablespoons coconut oil
- 2 tablespoons lucuma powder
- 2 tablespoons cacao powder
- 1 teaspoon ground vanilla bean
- Pinch of salt
- 1/4 cup Almond milk, as needed

Coconut cream:

See recipe for "Whipped Coconut Cream". Add 1/2 tsp. cinnamon and whip again.

To make the pudding: blend all the ingredients in the food processor until smooth and thick. Spread evenly into tartlet crusts. Optionally, put some goji berries on top of the pudding layer.

Make the coconut cream, spread it on top of the pudding layer, and put back in the fridge overnight. Serve with one blueberry on top of each tartlet.

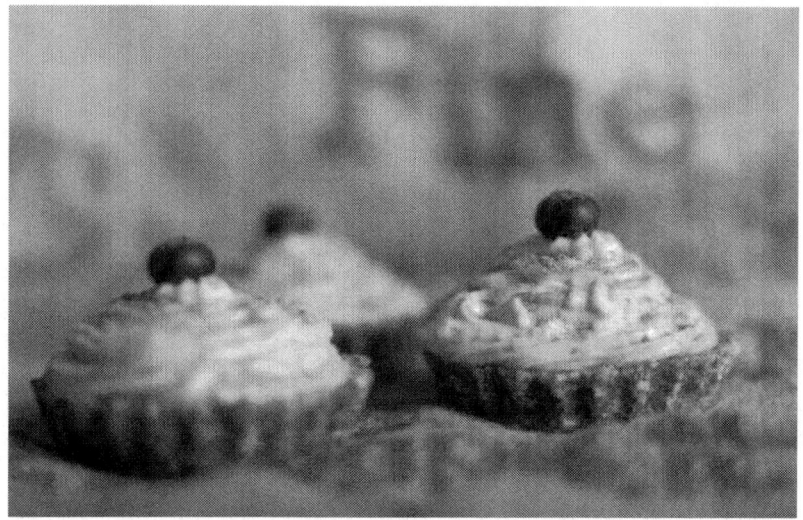

Raw Vegan "Peanut" Butter Truffles

Ingredients

- 5 tbsp. sunflower seed butter
- 1 tbsp. coconut oil
- 1 tbsp. lucuma powder
- 1 teaspoons ground vanilla bean
- 3/4 cup almond flour
- 1 tbsp. flax seeds meal
- pinch of salt
- 1 tbsp. cacao butter
- hemp hearts (optional)
- 1/4 cup Superfoods Chocolate

Instructions

Add sunflower seed butter, coconut oil, lucuma powder, vanilla, almond flour, flaxseed meal and salt to a large bowl.

Mix until all ingredients are incorporated.

Roll the dough into 1-inch balls, place them on parchment paper and refrigerate for half an hour (yield about 14 truffles)

Dip each truffle in the melted Superfoods Chocolate, one at the time, and place them back on the pan with parchment paper or coat them in cocoa powder or coconut flakes.

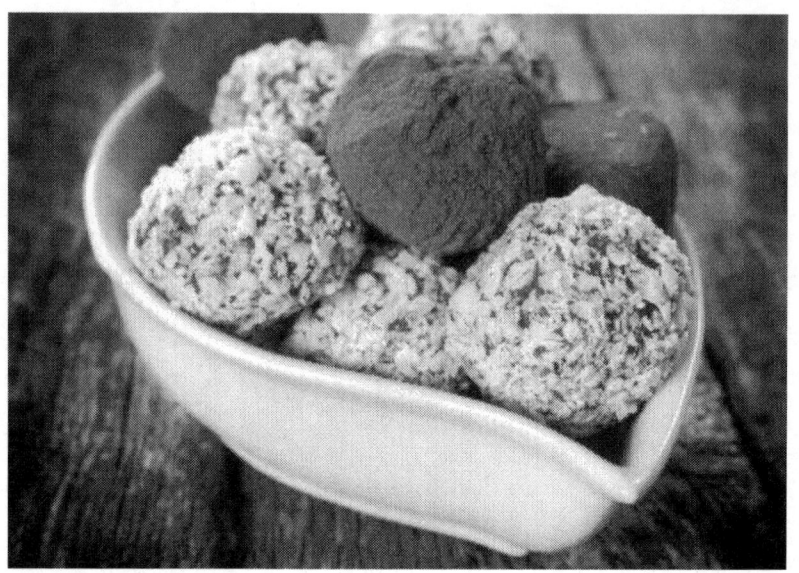

Raw Vegan Chocolate Pie

Crust

- 2 cups almonds, soaked overnight and drained
- 1 cup pitted dates, soaked overnight and drained
- 1 cup chopped dried apricots
- 1 1/2 tsp. ground vanilla bean
- 2 tsp. chia seeds
- 1 banana

Filling

- 4 Tbsp. raw cacao powder
- 3 Tbsp. lucuma powder
- 2 ripe avocados
- 2 Tbsp. organic coconut oil
- 2 Tbsp. almond milk (if needed, check for consistency first)

Instructions

Add almonds and banana to a food processor or blender. Mix until it forms a thick ball. Add the vanilla, dates, and apricot chunks to the blender. Mix well and optionally add a couple drops of water at a time to make the mixture stick together.

Spread in a 10 inch dis.

Mix filling ingredients in a blender and add almond milk if necessary. Add filling to the crust and refrigerate.

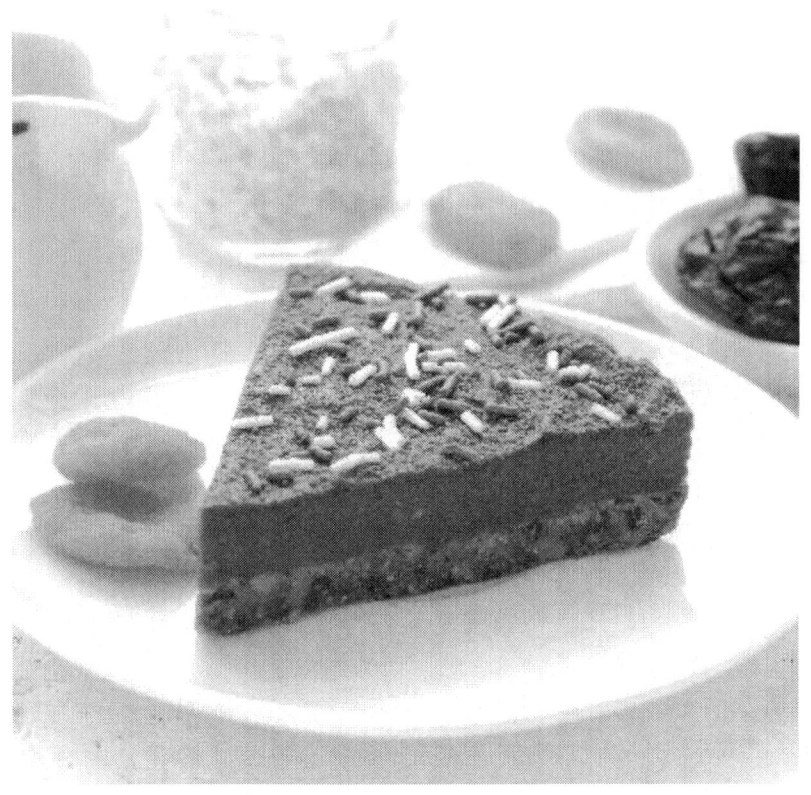

Raw Vegan Chocolate Walnut Truffles

Ingredients
- 1 cup ground walnuts
- 1 tsp. cinnamon
- 1/2 cup coconut oil
- 1/4 cup lucuma powder
- 2 tbsp. chia seeds
- 2 tbsp. cacao powder

Instructions

Mix all ingredients and make truffles. Coat with cinnamon, coconut flakes or chopped almonds.

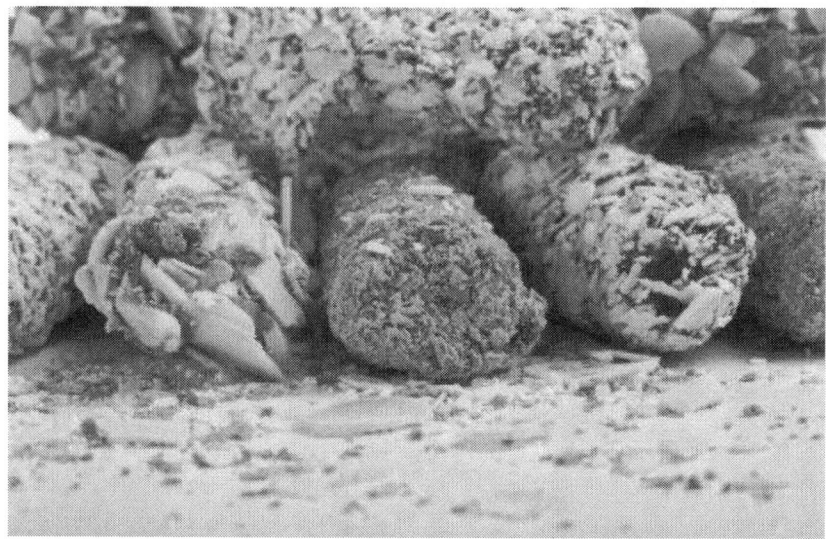

Your Free Gift

As a way of saying thanks for your purchase, I'm offering you my FREE eBook that is exclusive to my book and blog readers.

Superfoods Cookbook Book Two has over 70 Superfoods recipes and complements Superfoods Cookbook Book One and it contains Superfoods Salads, Superfoods Smoothies and Superfoods Deserts with ultra-healthy non-refined ingredients. All ingredients are 100% Superfoods.

It also contains Superfoods Reference book which is organized by Superfoods (more than 60 of them, with the list of their benefits), Superfoods spices, all vitamins, minerals and antioxidants. Superfoods Reference Book lists Superfoods that can help with 12 diseases and 9 types of cancer.

http://www.SuperfoodsToday.com/FREE

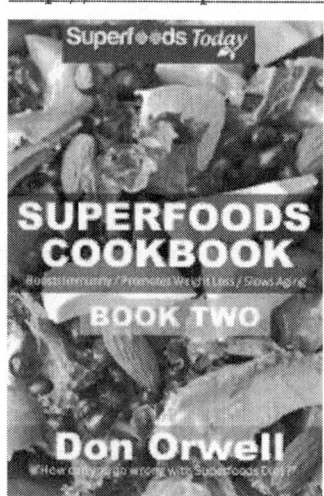

Other Books from this Author

Superfoods Today Diet is a Kindle Superfoods Diet book that gives you 4 week Superfoods Diet meal plan as well as 2 weeks maintenance meal plan and recipes for weight loss success. It is an extension of Detox book and it's written for people who want to switch to Superfoods lifestyle.

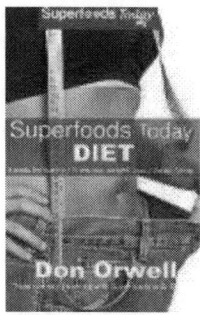

Superfoods Today Body Care is a Kindle book with over 50 Natural Recipes for beautiful skin and hair. It has body scrubs, facial masks and hair care recipes made with the best Superfoods like avocado honey, coconut, olive oil, oatmeal, yogurt, banana and Superfoods herbs like lavender, rosemary, mint, sage, hibiscus, rose.

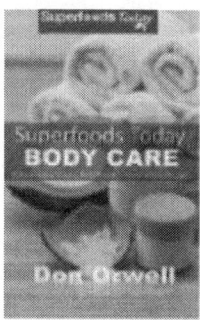

Superfoods Today Cookbook is a Kindle book that contains over 160 Superfoods recipes created with 100% Superfoods ingredients. Most of the meals can be prepared in under 30 minutes and some are really quick ones that can be done in 10 minutes only. Each recipe combines Superfoods ingredients that deliver astonishing amounts of antioxidants, essential fatty acids (like omega-3), minerals, vitamins, and more.

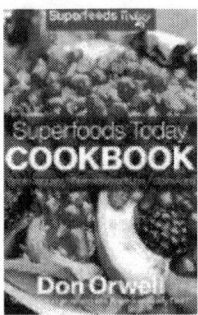

Superfoods Today Smoothies is a Kindle Superfoods Smoothies book with over 70+ 100% Superfoods smoothies. Featured are Red, Purple, Green and Yellow Smoothies

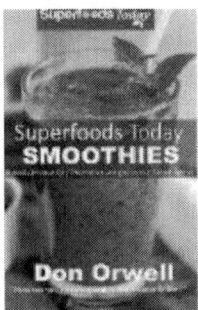

Low Carb Recipes for Diabetics is a Kindle Superfoods book with Low Carb Recipes for Diabetics.

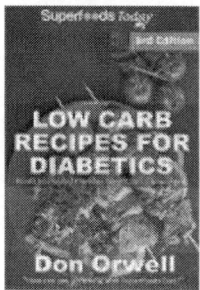

Diabetes Recipes is a Kindle Superfoods book with Superfoods Diabetes Recipes suitable for Diabetes Type-2.

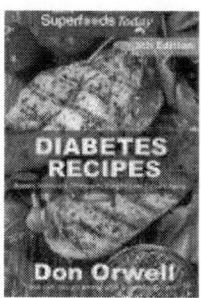

Diabetic Cookbook for One is a Kindle Superfoods book with Diabetes Recipes for One suitable for Diabetes Type-2

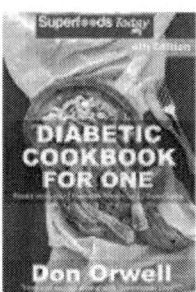

Diabetic Meal Plans is a Kindle book with Superfoods Diabetes Meal Plans suitable for Diabetes Type-2

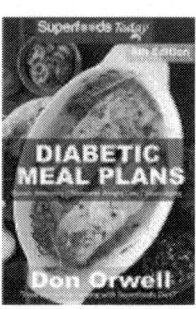

One Pot Cookbook is a Kindle Superfoods book with Superfoods One Pot Recipes.

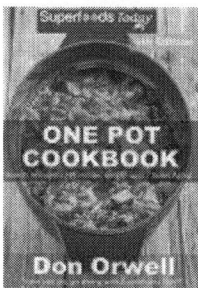

Low Carb Dump Meals is a Kindle book with Low Carb Dump Meals Superfoods Recipes.

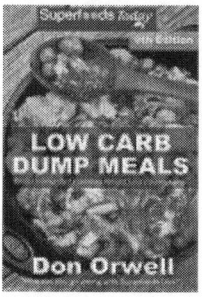

Superfoods Today Salads is a Kindle book that contains over 60 Superfoods Salads recipes created with 100% Superfoods ingredients. Most of the salads can be prepared in 10 minutes and most are measured for two. Each recipe combines Superfoods ingredients that deliver astonishing amounts of antioxidants, essential fatty acids (like omega-3), minerals, vitamins, and more.

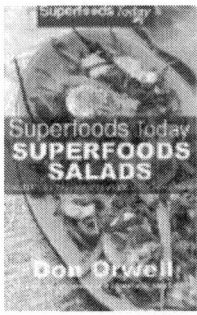

Superfoods Today Kettlebells is a Kindle Kettlebells beginner's book aimed at 30+ office workers who want to improve their health and build stronger body without fat.

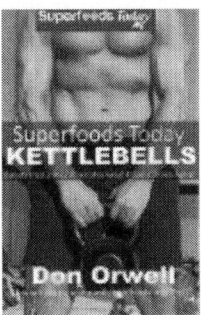

Superfoods Today Red Smoothies is a Kindle Superfoods Smoothies book with more than 40 Red Smoothies.

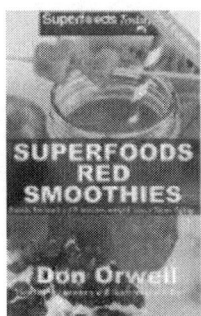

Superfoods Today 14 Days Detox is a Kindle Superfoods Detox book that gives you 2 week Superfoods Detox meal plan and recipes for Detox success.

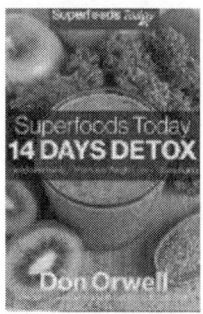

Superfoods Today Yellow Smoothies is a Kindle Superfoods Smoothies book with more than 40 Yellow Smoothies.

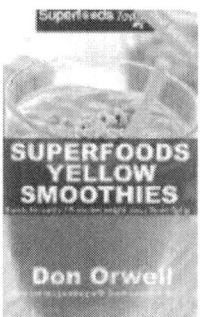

Superfoods Today Green Smoothies is a Kindle Superfoods Smoothies book with more than 35 Green Smoothies.

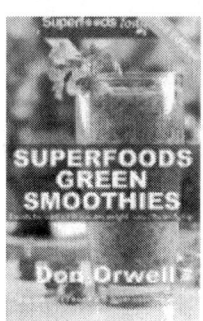

Superfoods Today Purple Smoothies is a Kindle Superfoods Smoothies book with more than 40 Purple Smoothies.

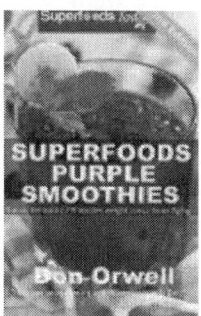

Superfoods Cooking For Two is a Kindle book that contains over 150 Superfoods recipes for two created with 100% Superfoods ingredients.

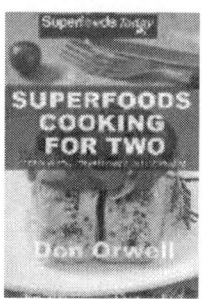

Nighttime Eater is a Kindle book that deals with Nighttime Eating Syndrome (NES). Don Orwell is a life-long Nighttime Eater that has lost his weight with Superfoods and engineered a solution around Nighttime Eating problem. Don still eats at night☺. Don't fight your nature, you can continue to eat at night, be binge free and maintain low weight.

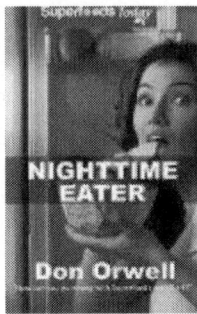

Superfoods Today Smart Carbs 20 Days Detox is a Kindle Superfoods book that will teach you how to detox your body and start losing weight with Smart Carbs. The book has over 470+ pages with over 160+ 100% Superfoods recipes.

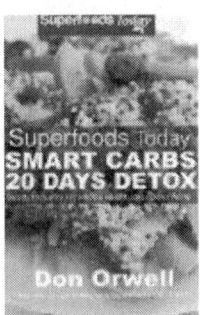

Superfoods Today Vegetarian Salads is a Kindle book that contains over 40 Superfoods Vegetarian Salads recipes created with 100% Superfoods ingredients. Most of the salads can be prepared in 10 minutes and most are measured for two.

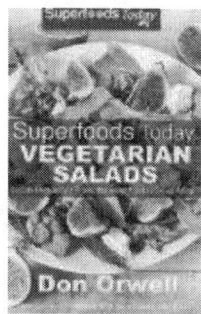

Superfoods Today Vegan Salads is a Kindle book that contains over 30 Superfoods Vegan Salads recipes created with 100% Superfoods ingredients. Most of the salads can be prepared in 10 minutes and most are measured for two.

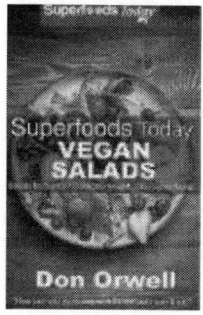

Superfoods Today Soups & Stews is a Kindle book that contains over 70 Superfoods Soups and Stews recipes created with 100% Superfoods ingredients.

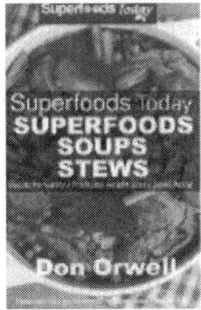

Superfoods Desserts is a Kindle Superfoods Desserts book with more than 60 Superfoods Recipes.

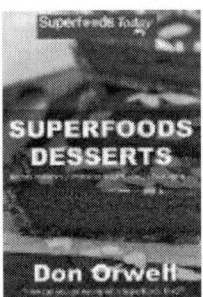

Smoothies for Diabetics is a Kindle book that contains over 70 Superfoods Smoothies adjusted for diabetics.

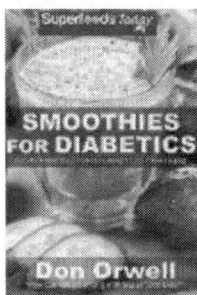

50 Shades of Superfoods for Two is a Kindle book that contains over 150 Superfoods recipes for two created with 100% Superfoods ingredients.

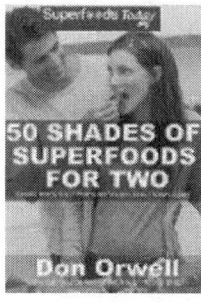

50 Shades of Smoothies is a Kindle book that contains over 70 Superfoods Smoothies.

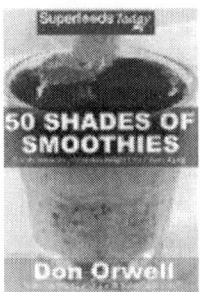

50 Shades of Superfoods Salads is a Kindle book that contains over 60 Superfoods Salads recipes created with 100% Superfoods ingredients. Most of the salads can be prepared in 10 minutes and most are measured for two. Each recipe combines Superfoods ingredients that deliver astonishing amounts of antioxidants, essential fatty acids (like omega-3), minerals, vitamins, and more.

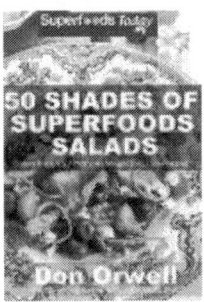

Superfoods Vegan Desserts is a Kindle Vegan Dessert book with 100% Vegan Superfoods Recipes.

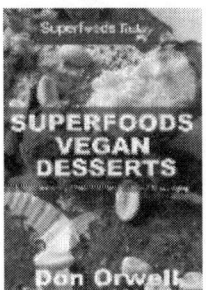

Desserts for Two is a Kindle Superfoods Desserts book with more than 40 Superfoods Desserts Recipes for two.

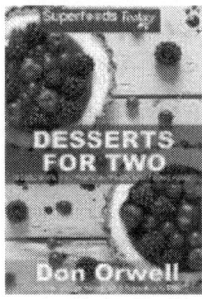

Superfoods Paleo Cookbook is a Kindle Paleo book with more than 150 100% Superfoods Paleo Recipes.

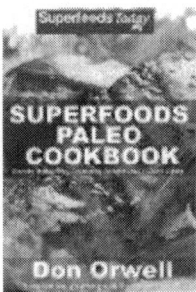

Superfoods Breakfasts is a Kindle Superfoods book with more than 40 100% Superfoods Breakfasts Recipes.

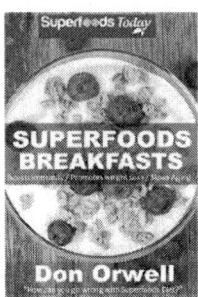

Superfoods Dump Dinners is a Kindle Superfoods book with Superfoods Dump Dinners Recipes.

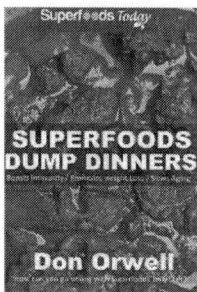

Healthy Desserts is a Kindle Desserts book with more than 50 100% Superfoods Healthy Desserts Recipes.

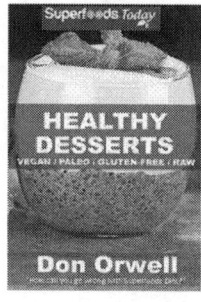

Superfoods Salads in a Jar is a Kindle Salads in a Jar book with more than 35 100% Superfoods Salads Recipes.

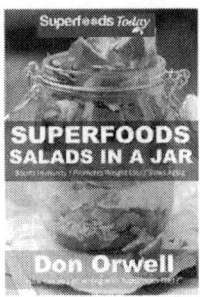

Smoothies for Kids is a Kindle Smoothies book with more than 80 100% Superfoods Smoothies for Kids Recipes.

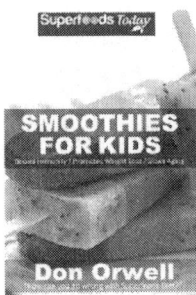

Vegan Cookbook for Beginners is a Kindle Vegan book with more than 75 100% Superfoods Vegan Recipes.

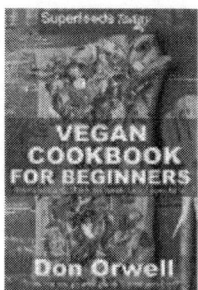

Vegetarian Cooking for Beginners is a Kindle Vegetarian book with more than 150 100% Superfoods Paleo Recipes.

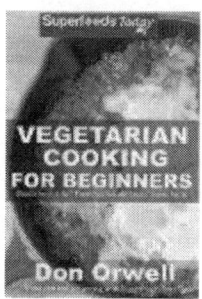

Foods for Diabetics is a Kindle book with more than 170 100% Superfoods Diabetics Recipes.

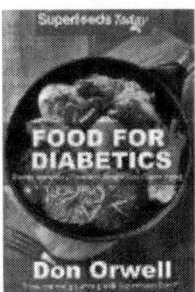

Healthy Kids Cookbook is a Kindle book with Superfoods Kids friendly Recipes.

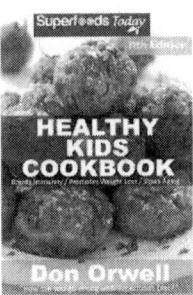

Superfoods Beans Recipes is a Kindle book with Superfoods Beans Recipes.

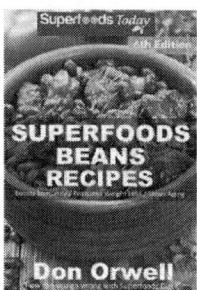

Diabetic Slow Cooker Recipes is a Kindle book with Superfoods Slow Cooker Diabetic Recipes.

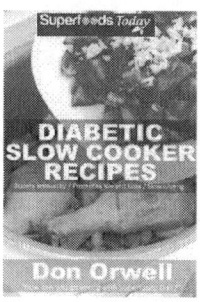

Ketogenic Crockpot Recipes is a Kindle book with Superfoods Ketogenic Crockpot Recipes.

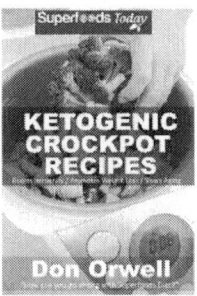

Stir Fry Cooking is a Kindle book with Stir Fry Superfoods Recipes.

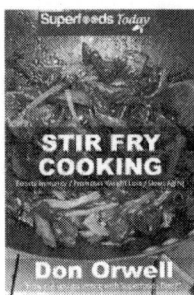

Sirt Food Diet Cookbook is a Kindle book with Superfoods Sirt Food Recipes.

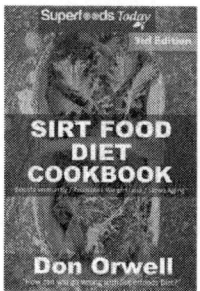

Made in the USA
Lexington, KY
07 March 2018